Baillière's
CLINICAL
RHEUMATOLOGY
INTERNATIONAL PRACTICE AND RESEARCH

Baillière's

CLINICAL RHEUMATOLOGY

INTERNATIONAL PRACTICE AND RESEARCH

Volume 4/Number 2
August 1990

Controversies in the Management of Rheumatic Diseases

N. BELLAMY MD, MSc, FRCP(Glas), FRCP(Edin), FRCP(C), FACP
Guest Editor

Baillière Tindall
London Philadelphia Sydney Tokyo Toronto

This book is printed on acid-free paper.

Baillière Tindall   24–28 Oval Road
W.B. Saunders   London NW1 7DX, UK

The Curtis Center, Independence Square West
Philadelphia, PA 19106–3399, USA

55 Horner Avenue
Toronto, Ontario M8Z 4X6, Canada

Harcourt Brace Jovanovich Group (Australia) Pty Ltd
30–52 Smidmore Street, Marrickville, NSW 2204, Australia

Harcourt Brace Jovanovich Japan, Inc
Ichibancho Central Building, 22–1 Ichibancho
Chiyoda-ku, Tokyo 102, Japan

ISSN 0950–3579

ISBN 0–7020–1480–X (single copy)

Baillière's Clinical Rheumatology is published three times each year by Baillière Tindall. Annual subscription prices are:

TERRITORY	ANNUAL SUBSCRIPTION	SINGLE ISSUE
1. UK	£41.00 post free	£22.50 post free
2. Europe	£47.00 post free	£22.50 post free
3. All other countries	Consult your local Harcourt Brace Jovanovich office for dollar price	

The editor of this publication is Katharine Hinton, Baillière Tindall, 24–28 Oval Road, London NW1 7DX, UK.

Baillière's Clinical Rheumatology was published from 1975 to 1986 as *Clinics in Rheumatic Diseases*.

Typeset by Phoenix Photosetting, Chatham.
Printed and bound in Great Britain by Mackays of Chatham PLC, Chatham, Kent.

Contributors to this issue

NICHOLAS BELLAMY MD, MSc, FRCP(Glas), FRCP(Edin), FRCP(C), FACP, Associate Professor of Medicine and Epidemiology, University of Western Ontario, London, Ontario, N6A 4G5, Canada.

PETER BROOKS MD, BS, FRACP, FACRM, Florance and Cope Professor of Rheumatology, University of Sydney at The Royal North Shore Hospital, Sydney, Australia.

W. WATSON BUCHANAN MD, FRCP(Glas, Edin & C), FACP, Room 2F10, Rheumatic Diseases Unit, McMaster University, Faculty of Health Sciences, 1200 Main Street West, Hamilton, Ontario, L8N 3Z5, Canada.

CYRUS COOPER MA, MB BS, DM, MRCP, Senior Registrar, Rheumatology Unit, Bristol Royal Infirmary, Bristol, BS2 8HW; Honorary Lecturer, University of Bristol, UK.

ADEL G. FAM MD, FRCP(C), FACP, MRCP(UK), Head, Division of Rheumatology, Professor of Medicine, Department of Medicine, Sunnybrook Health Science Centre, University of Toronto, 2075 Bayview Avenue, Toronto, Ontario, M4N 3M5, Canada.

PETER GHOSH BSc, PhD, ARIC, FRACI, Associate Professor, Dept of Surgery, University of Sydney, Director Raymond Purves Research Laboratories, Royal North Shore Hospital, St Leonards 2065, Australia.

D. M. GRENNAN MD, PhD, FRCP, Reader in Rheumatology, University of Manchester and Honorary Consultant Physician, Hope Hospital, Salford, UK.

JOHN HOWARD MD, FRCPC, Assistant Professor, University of Western Ontario, Attending Physician, Victoria Hospital, 375 South Street, London, Ontario, Canada N6A 4G5.

RICHARD H. HUNT FRCP, FRCPC, FRCP(Edin), FACG, Professor, Dept of Medicine; Head, Division of Gastroenterology, McMaster University Health Sciences Centre, Hamilton, Ontario, L8N 3Z5, Canada.

WALTER F. KEAN MB ChB, FRCP(C), FACP, MD(Glas), Associate Clinical Professor of Medicine, McMaster University; Associate, Department of Chemistry, McMaster University Health Sciences Center, Hamilton, Ontario, L8N 3Z5, Canada.

JOHN R. KIRWAN BSc, MB BS, MD, MRCP(UK), Consultant Senior Lecturer in Rheumatology, Rheumatology Unit, University Department of Medicine, Bristol Royal Infirmary, Bristol BS8 2UR, UK.

RODGER LAURENT MD, FRACP, Staff Specialist in Rheumatology, Department of Rheumatology, Royal North Shore Hospital, St. Leonards, Sydney, NSW 2065, Australia.

PETER LEE MB ChB, MD, FRCPC, FRACP, Associate Professor of Medicine, University of Toronto, Staff Rheumatologist, The Wellesley Hospital, 160 Wellesley Street East, Toronto, Ontario, M4Y 1J3, Canada.

NICOLE G. H. LE RICHE MD FRCPC, Assistant Professor, University of Western Ontario, London, Ontario, Canada N6A 5C1; Attending Physician, St Joseph's Health Centre, 268 Grosvenor Street, London, Ontario, Canada, N6A 4V2, Canada.

ALFONSE T. MASI MD DrPH, Professor of Medicine, Department of Medicine, University of Illinois College of Medicine at Peoria, One Illini Drive, Box 1649, Peoria, IL 61656, USA.

K. D. RAINSFORD PhD, MRCPath, FRSC, Professor of Rheumatology and Pathology, Director, Pharmacology of Rheumatic Diseases, McMaster University Faculty of Health Sciences, Hamilton, Ontario, Canada.

PATRICK J. ROONEY MD(Hons), FRCP(Glasg), FRCPE, FACP, Associate Professor of Medicine, McMaster University, Room 70, Holbrook Building, Chedoke McMaster Hospitals, Hamilton, Ontario, L8N 3Z5, Canada.

PAUL A. SANDERS MBChB, MRCP(UK), MD, Senior Registrar Rheumatology, Rheumatic Diseases Centre, Hope Hospital, Eccles Old Road, Salford, M6 8HD, UK.

M. B. UROWITZ MD, FRCP(C), Professor of Medicine, University of Toronto; Physician-in-Chief, Wellesley Hospital, 160 Wellesley Street East, StE 649, Toronto, Ontario, M4Y 1J3, Canada.

MUHAMMAD B. YUNUS MD, MRCP, FACP, Associate Professor of Medicine, Department of Medicine, University of Illinois College of Medicine at Peoria, One Illini Drive, Box 1649, Peoria, IL 61656, USA.

Table of contents

PREVIOUS ISSUES

August 1987
The Foot in Arthritis
M. I. V. JAYSON & L. A. SMIDT

December 1987
Epidemiological, Sociological and Environmental Aspects of Rheumatology
J. A. D. ANDERSON

April 1988
Biochemical Aspects of Rheumatic Diseases
J. DIXON & H. BIRD

August 1988
Anti-rheumatic Drugs
P. M. BROOKS

December 1988
Genetics of Rheumatic Diseases
D. M. GRENNAN

April 1989
Occupational Rheumatic Diseases
G. P. BÁLINT & W. W. BUCHANAN

August 1989
The Gut and Rheumatic Disease
P. J. ROONEY

December 1989
The Shoulder Joint
B. L. HAZLEMAN & P. A. DIEPPE

April 1990
Pregnancy and the Rheumatic Diseases
A. L. PARKE

FORTHCOMING ISSUES

December 1990
Slow-acting Antirheumatic Drugs and Immunosuppressives
P. M. BROOKS

April 1991
Drug Induced Rheumatic Diseases
M.-F. KAHN

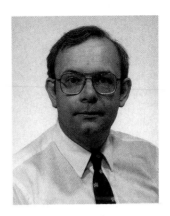

Foreword

This issue of *Baillière's Clinical Rheumatology* is concerned with those areas of therapeutic rheumatology in which the decision to treat is attended by a lack of clear consensus regarding risks and/or benefits. If clinicians are to make rational decisions regarding drug prescribing, and patients to give their informed consent, then either such controversy requires resolution or at least the nature of the controversy requires adequate understanding by both provider and recipient. In some cases controversies are recent and have arisen as the result of new developments in basic science. In other instances they are long-standing and remain unresolved.

In this book an international panel of contributors has addressed many important issues, combining their own experience with critical but constructive appraisals of the medical literature. In the first chapter Dr Fam discusses key issues relevant to the management of hyperuricaemia providing guidance as to who should be treated, when treatment should be initiated, which agent should be used, and what precautions should be followed. In the next chapter Drs Urowitz and Lee review the risks to specific organs from each of three slow-acting anti-rheumatic drugs. All of these drugs have been shown to be efficacious in specific conditions and yet some patients continue to refuse them for fear of their side-effects; a fear that is often exaggerated, particularly when viewed in the context of potential benefits and the risks of other life events. In recent years there has been concern regarding the safety of anti-rheumatic drugs, particularly those of the non-steroidal anti-inflammatory (NSAID) class. Indeed patients have become alarmed by adverse reporting in the media and yet many are dependent on such drugs for the successful management of their arthritis. Consequently, four chapters have been dedicated to NSAID therapy. These chapters examine the risk of upper gastrointestinal haemorrhage (Drs Rooney and Hunt), compare ASA and non-acetylated salicylates (Drs Rainsford and Buchanan), review the effects of NSAIDs on cartilage (Professor Brooks), and compare the effects of NSAIDs with those obtainable from simple analgesic management (Drs Sanders and Grennan). In recent years the emergence of several different classes of agents with which to prevent and/or treat NSAID gastropathy has created diversity in practice styles. Doctors Howard and Le Riche provide a rational approach to this confusing area of therapeutic rheumatology. The emergence of oral gold, as an alternative, to the more traditional intramuscular formulation, has required that rheumatologists choose the preferred agent based on risks, benefits, costs and convenience. The decision which formulation to use is not simple but Dr Kean has provided a critical appraisal of the relevant characteristics of each agent. It seems that patients are frequently confused regarding the differential effects of local versus systemic corticosteroid drugs. While such agents are not new the review by Drs Cooper and Kirwan of the risks and potential benefits of this potent class of anti-rheumatic drugs contains much useful information for both clinicians and patients. There has been an almost explosive interest in the condition currently termed fibromyalgia. Despite the availability of several different treatment modalities, therapists remain perplexed as to which is the best approach for individual patients. The review by Drs Masi and Yunus puts our current knowledge into perspective and provides direction in the management of this ubiquitous condition. Finally, while we still struggle to comprehend the definition of disease modification in rheumatoid arthritis, Dr Laurent has reviewed the evidence that similar drugs may also modify the progress of ankylosing spondylitis.

Much of the literature which contributors have reviewed is not easy to interpret and is at times conflicting. However, the therapeutic needs of musculoskeletal patients demand to be met now, at a time when the aforementioned controversies have not been resolved. This book, therefore, should be of considerable assistance to individuals actively involved in the management of patients with musculoskeletal disease, as well as those training in general internal medicine and rheumatology.

NICHOLAS BELLAMY

1

Strategies and controversies in the treatment of
gout and hyperuricaemia

ADEL G. FAM

Gout is one of the better understood of the rheumatic diseases, and certainly one of the most satisfactory to treat. It is characterized by chronic hyperuricaemia, recurrent attacks of acute arthritis provoked by the release of monosodium urate crystals into synovial cavities, and development in some patients of gross urate deposits (tophi). It chiefly affects middle-aged and elderly men, and occurs in three overlapping stages: a long phase of asymptomatic hyperuricaemia, a period of recurrent acute gouty attacks separated by asymptomatic intervals (intercritical gout), followed in about 10% of patients by chronic tophaceous gouty arthritis (Becker, 1988).

When gout is diagnosed, the patient is usually committed to some form of long-term therapy. It is important, therefore, to establish a firm diagnosis at the outset. This can be secured by the demonstration of intracellular or extracellular urate crystals in joint effusions, or aspirates from tophaceous deposits (Fam, 1986). However, this may not be possible in all patients because of factors such as the absence of a detectable joint effusion or visible tophi, inaccessible joints, small number of crystals, lack of experience with joint aspiration or evaluation of effusions for crystals, and excessive delay in the examination of synovial fluid following aspiration (Wade and Liang, 1988; Kerolus et al, 1989). Under these circumstances, the diagnosis of gout can be made on the basis of a typical clinical history (middle-aged or elderly male, self-limited attacks of acute monoarticular or oligoarticular arthritis in lower extremities, especially the big toes, with severe local pain, tenderness, swelling and redness, followed by a return to normal joint function), in association with documented hyperuricaemia.

Hyperuricaemia—elevated serum urate over 450 μmol/l (7.0 mg/dl) in men and 350 μmol/l ((6.0 mg/dl) in women—is the biochemical hallmark of gout. However, it is improper to equate the finding of hyperuricaemia with gout; many people who have lifelong hyperuricaemia do not develop gouty arthritis (asymptomatic hyperuricaemia), and serum urate levels may initially be normal in some patients with gout (Becker, 1988; Wade and Liang, 1988).

Gouty arthritis nearly always occurs in the setting of chronic hyperuricaemia. The management of a patient with gout, therefore, requires that two objectives be considered independently: immediate control of the acute

Baillière's Clinical Rheumatology—
Vol. 4, No. 2, August 1990
ISBN 0–7020–1480–X

gouty episode, and treatment of the chronic hyperuricaemia, in order to prevent subsequent attacks and long-term complications such as chronic tophaceous gouty arthritis, tophi, uric acid urolithiasis and urate nephropathy (Ross and Seegmiller, 1979; Rodnan, 1982; Fam, 1988; Wallace and Singer, 1988a). The therapeutic approaches to these goals are entirely different. Anti-inflammatory drugs used to control acute gouty arthritis do not affect hyperuricaemia or prevent gouty complications, and drugs used to treat hyperuricaemia (such as allopurinol or uricosurics) are not effective in the control of acute gouty paroxysms.

MANAGING ACUTE GOUTY ARTHRITIS

Successful treatment of an acute gouty attack depends upon the administration of an effective, well-tolerated anti-inflammatory drug in full dosage. The earlier such therapy is initiated after the onset of an acute episode, the more effective it will be. Although acute gouty episodes run a self-limited course, complete resolution of a severe attack over a period of seven days is unlikely without the use of an effective anti-inflammatory medication (Ahern et al, 1987; Bellamy et al, 1987; Agudelo, 1989).

Three types of drugs are used in the treatment of acute gout: non-steroidal anti-inflammatory drugs (NSAIDs), colchicine and corticosteroids including corticotrophin (ACTH) (Table 1). Urate-lowering drugs should be continued as usual if the patient is already being so treated, but they must not be started for the first time during an acute attack. A major change in serum urate concentration induced by stopping or initiating one of these drugs may prolong an attack already in progress (Bellamy et al, 1988; Fam, 1988; Wallace and Singer, 1988a).

Once considered the mainstay in the treatment of acute gout, colchicine has now fallen into relative disuse because of its frequent adverse reactions and unpredictable effects (Rodnan, 1982; Bellamy et al, 1988; Fam, 1988; Wallace and Singer, 1988a). Abdominal cramps, diarrhoea and nausea occur in about 80% of patients treated with oral colchicine, making it unsuitable for routine clinical use. NSAIDs are generally better tolerated

Table 1. Drugs in the treatment of acute gouty arthritis.

Non-steroidal anti-inflammatory drugs (NSAIDs)	
indomethacin: 50 mg four times daily ⎫	
naproxen: 500 mg twice daily ⎬ for 5–8 days	
ketoprofen: 50 mg four times daily ⎭	
Colchicine	
oral:	0.6 mg every 1–2 hours to a maximum of 4–5 mg
intravenous:	1–2 mg, then 1 mg IV every 6–12 hours to a maximum of 4 mg
Corticosteroids and corticotrophin (ACTH)	
prednisone:	20–40 mg once daily for 1–3 days, then gradual tapering
ACTH:	single i.m. injection of 40 i.u. ACTH
intra-articular	
dexamethasone phosphate:	1–6 mg into one to three affected joints

and more predictable in their effect than colchicine. Aspirin has no place in the treatment of acute gout; low doses do not relieve symptoms and increase serum urate, and high doses (more than 3 g daily) produce uricosuria but do not ease symptoms. Phenylbutazone and its congener oxyphenbutazone are no longer used because of their rare but serious myelotoxicity.

Non-steroidal anti-inflammatory drugs

NSAIDs are now preferred by most clinicians as the drugs of first choice for the treatment of acute gouty arthritis. Indomethacin, in doses of 50 mg three or four times daily by mouth (or by suppository 100 mg twice daily) for five to eight days, is effective therapy in the majority of patients. The newer NSAIDs, such as naproxen (500 mg twice daily), ibuprofen (600 mg four times daily), ketoprofen (50 mg four times daily), sulindac (200 mg twice daily), tolmetin sodium (600 mg four times daily), diclofenac sodium (50 mg three times daily) and piroxicam (20 mg once daily), have all been shown to be equally efficacious, but extensive clinical experience with their use in acute gout is limited (Wilkens and Case, 1973; Altman et al, 1988). Whatever drug is used, it should be started as early as possible during the acute attack, in maximum initial doses. It is useful, therefore, to supply the patient with the appropriate medication (preferably to be kept in a convenient pocket, for all too often gout strikes when the patient is far from home), and instructions on how to self-treat the acute attack. The patient is instructed to start the drug at the first 'twinge' of a gouty episode. With this approach it is often possible to terminate an attack within three days using less than the full therapeutic course of the drug. Self-treatment with indomethacin or other NSAID has proved effective and safe under these circumstances.

The rate of resolution of the acute attack is strikingly modified by NSAID therapy. More than 90% of patients experience pain relief within one day and complete resolution of the attack within five to eight days (Altman et al, 1988; Agudelo, 1989). Although adverse reactions (e.g. dyspepsia, nausea and diarrhoea) may occur, the duration of NSAID therapy is short, and serious toxicity leading to drug withdrawal (e.g. gastrointestinal bleeding) is rare, occurring in fewer than 10% of patients (Altman et al, 1988).

Colchicine

Colchicine, an anti-inflammatory antimitotic drug, is one of the oldest remedies for gout. It is an alkaloid derived from the roots of the autumn crocus (*Colchicum autumnale*). The drug acts by two mechanisms in acute gout: suppression of the production of a urate crystal-induced chemotactic factor from polymorphonuclear leucocytes (PMN), and dissolution of PMN microtubules, hence interfering with PMN migration, chemotaxis and phagocytic activity (Ahern et al, 1987; Wallace and Singer, 1988a). Because of its effects on leucocyte function and chemotaxis, colchicine is more effective when used within 24 hours of onset of an acute gouty episode (Wallace and Singer, 1988a).

Colchicine is metabolized in the liver, and the greater part of the drug and its metabolites are excreted in the bile. About 20% of the drug is excreted unchanged in the urine. It is administered orally in a dose of one 0.6 mg tablet every one to two hours until acute joint pain is relieved, the patient develops gastrointestinal toxicity or the patient has received a maximum of 4–6 mg per day. In a recent placebo-controlled study, oral colchicine was shown to be efficacious in two-thirds of patients presenting with acute gout (Ahern et al, 1987). However, most patients given colchicine experienced gastrointestinal upset (nausea, diarrhoea and abdominal pain) before full clinical improvement, and all developed diarrhoea after a median time of 24 hours and a mean dose of 6.7 mg colchicine (Ahern et al, 1987). The narrow benefit-to-toxicity ratio of colchicine has led many clinicians to limit its use to patients in whom effective and less toxic NSAIDs are poorly tolerated or are contraindicated (Ahern et al, 1987; Roberts et al, 1987; Bellamy et al, 1988; Fam, 1988).

Intravenous administration of colchicine in acute gout produces a more prompt response (within 6–12 hours in most patients) with fewer gastro-intestinal side-effects. It is given in an initial dose of 1–2 mg diluted in 20 ml normal saline, followed if necessary by an additional 1 mg every 6–12 hours to a maximum total cumulative dose of 4 mg (Roberts et al, 1987; Wallace and Singer, 1988b). The drug should be administered cautiously and slowly to minimize the risk of local extravasation (Roberts et al, 1987; Wallace and Singer, 1988b), which can lead to thrombophlebitis, painful tissue necrosis and sloughing, median nerve neuritis and arteriovenous fistula formation. The relative absence of warning gastrointestinal symptoms after intravenous administration makes this route more risky than oral administration (Roberts et al, 1987; Wallace and Singer, 1988b). Serious toxic reactions, including bone marrow suppression, disseminated intravascular coagulation, vomiting, diarrhoea, oliguric renal failure, liver cell injury, alopecia, seizures and death have been reported (Roberts et al, 1987; Wallace and Singer, 1988b). The dose should be lowered in elderly patients and in those with hepatic or renal dysfunction. Intravenous colchicine is not recommended in patients with combined renal and hepatic disease, those with a creatinine clearance less than 10 ml/min, and in the presence of extrahepatic biliary obstruction.

Although systemic toxicity can be largely prevented by strict adherence to dose guidelines, the clinical usefulness of intravenous colchicine is limited by its small benefit-to-risk ratio. Many physicians now restrict its use to patients who have difficulty taking oral medications, when safer alternate treatments are unavailable or contraindicated (Roberts et al, 1987).

Corticosteroids including corticotrophin

Since NSAIDs have become widely available, systemic corticosteroids and corticotrophin (adrenocorticotrophic hormone, ACTH) are infrequently used in the treatment of acute gout. Exceptions include severe polyarticular gouty arthritis refractory to conventional therapy, and intolerance or contraindication to both NSAIDs and colchicine. In such circumstances, prednisone 20–40 mg daily, or intramuscular ACTH 40–80 units every 6–12 hours for one to three days, followed by gradual tapering, can be used. However, rebound attacks after discontinuation of therapy may occur (Rodnan, 1982; Wallace and Singer, 1988a).

Treatment with a single intramuscular injection of 40 iu of ACTH compared favourably with indomethacin 50 mg four times daily in a recent unblinded study of 76 patients with acute gout. Patients treated with ACTH had more rapid pain relief (3 ± 1 hours) compared with patients treated with indomethacin (24 ± 10 hours). No toxicity or rebound attacks were noted in the ACTH-treated group (Axelrod and Preston, 1988). Since oral NSAIDs may require from 24 to 72 hours to relieve pain, single-dose intramuscular ACTH may provide a more rapid alternative therapy, particularly in patients with resistant gouty attacks, and in those with altered renal function (Axelrod and Preston, 1988). However, controlled double-blinded studies are needed to confirm the efficacy and lack of toxicity of single-dose intramuscular ACTH.

An intra-articular injection of a corticosteroid into one to three affected joints often provides prompt and lasting relief. A soluble, short-acting preparation, such as dexamethasone phosphate 1–6 mg intra-articularly, is preferred because of its rapid onset of action and absence of paradoxical exacerbation of inflammation that might occur following intra-articular injection of an insoluble corticosteroid (post-injection flare) (Fam, 1988).

Intra-articular corticosteroids are particularly indicated in patients with one to three involved joints who are unable to take oral medications (e.g. because of coincidental upper gastrointestinal bleeding, vomiting or gastrointestinal suction, or in the postoperative period), in those with significant renal or liver disease, and in patients who are intolerant to both NSAIDs and colchicine.

In summary, non-salicylate NSAIDs are the drugs of first choice in the management of acute gouty arthritis. Alternative therapies in patients who cannot take oral medications include intra-articular dexamethasone phosphate, single-dose intramuscular ACTH, parenteral corticosteroids, indomethacin, naproxen or other NSAID by suppository, and intravenous colchicine (Fam, 1988).

PROPHYLAXIS OF GOUTY ARTHRITIS

It is important to identify and correct any secondary causes of hyperuricaemia, including drugs (e.g. thiazide diuretics, aspirin, nicotinic acid, and laxative abuse), and excessive alcohol ingestion (Becker, 1988). Consideration should be given to restriction of purine-rich foods, and weight reduction for obese patients. These measures constitute sufficient therapy for many patients with gout, particularly those with infrequent attacks (not more than three per year) and without significant hyperuricaemia (Table 2).

While the ultimate prevention of gouty paroxysms in patients with established gout depends on the restoration of normal serum urate concentrations, the frequency and severity of attacks can be reduced by prophylactic colchicine 0.6 mg once or twice daily. However, prolonged colchicine

Table 2. Treatment of hyperuricaemia.

Correction of predisposing factors
  Elimination of drugs causing hyperuricaemia, e.g. thiazides, aspirin
  Control of alcohol intake
  Gradual weight reduction for obese patients

Urate-lowering drugs
  Allopurinol 200–800 mg/day (single dose)
  Uricosuric drugs
    probenecid 1–3 g/day (divided doses)
    sulphinpyrazone 100–800 mg/day (divided doses)
  Others
    polyethylene glycol-modified uricase
    oxypurinol

Dietary restriction of purine-rich foods   Liver, kidney, brain, meat extractives, meats, sweetbreads, sardines, other fish, beans, lentils and peas
Surgical excision of bulky tophi

therapy does not reverse the hyperuricaemia, and can lead to a number of toxic reactions including proximal myopathy, neuropathy, myelotoxicity with leucopenia or thrombocytopenia, alopecia, malabsorption syndrome, hepatic cell injury and seizures (Neuss et al, 1986; Kuncl et al, 1987). Additionally, most patients who experience frequent attacks also have significant hyperuricaemia and require treatment with urate-lowering agents.

TREATMENT OF HYPERURICAEMIA AND TOPHACEOUS GOUT

The ultimate treatment of gout and its complications requires long-term control of hyperuricaemia. Two types of urate-lowering drugs are available (Tables 2, 3): allopurinol, a xanthine oxidase inhibitor which decreases uric acid synthesis; and uricosuric agents, including probenecid, sulphinpyrazone, and benzbromarone, which act by competitive inhibition of post-secretory renal tubular reabsorption of urate, thus increasing urate excretion and lowering serum urate.

  Laboratory evaluation of a patient with gout includes determination of serum urate and creatinine, creatinine clearance and (in those with normal renal function) 24-hour urinary uric acid excretion (Becker, 1988). These measurements are best made on two consecutive days, five days after initiation of an isocaloric purine-free diet. A purine-free diet excludes liver, brain, kidneys, sweetbreads, sardines, anchovies, mussels and meat extracts such as broth, soups, and gravies, with moderate reductions in meats, other fish, beans, lentils and peas. Under these conditions, uric acid excretion provides an estimate of purine and uric acid production. Excretion of uric acid in excess of 3.8 mmol (600 mg) per 24 hours indicates uric acid over-production. If dietary purine restriction proves impractical, determining a 24-hour uric acid excretion on a regular diet will suffice. Daily uric acid excretion greater than 4.5–5.5 mmol (800–1000 mg) is regarded as excessive. A knowledge of the patient's urinary uric acid excretion, and hence uric acid

Table 3. Choice of therapy.

Indications for urate-lowering agents
Frequent gouty attacks (more than 4 attacks/year)
Tophi
Chronic tophaceous gouty arthritis
Urate nephropathy
Uric acid urolithiasis
Hyperuricosuria > 4.5–5.5 mmol (800–1000 mg) per day on a regular diet
Prevention and treatment of hyperuricaemia in patients with myeloproliferative disorders, leukaemia or lymphoma treated with cytotoxic drugs and/or radiotherapy
Calcium oxalate urinary calculi associated with hyperuricosuria

Indications for allopurinol therapy
Major uric acid overproduction (uric acid urinary excretion > 900 mg/day on a regular diet), including patients with partial or complete HGPRTase deficiency and PRPP synthetase overactivity
Chronic tophaceous gouty arthritis
Gout complicated by urate nephropathy, uric acid nephrolithiasis and/or renal impairment
Secondary hyperuricaemia associated with leukaemia, myeloproliferative disorders or lymphoma treated with cytotoxics and/or radiotherapy
Failure of uricosuric therapy due to intolerance, lack of efficacy, renal insufficiency or poor patient compliance
Recurrent calcium oxalate urinary calculi associated with hyperuricosuria

Indications for uricosuric therapy
Patients who are allergic or intolerant to allopurinol
Combined allopurinol–uricosuric treatment in patients with massive tophaceous deposits
Possibly as first choice in patients with gout who are under 50 years old and who have normal renal function and urinary uric acid excretion and no history of renal calculi

production, will assist in the selection of a urate-lowering drug, whether allopurinol or a uricosuric.

Other studies such as enzyme assays and determination of rates of uric acid synthesis by *in vivo* isotope labelling methods are indicated in selected patients; for example those suspected to have an inherited enzyme defect (Becker, 1988).

Not every patient with gout will require treatment with urate-lowering drugs (Table 3). Although there are data to indicate that synovial microtophi are commonly present in joints of patients with gout, there is no convincing evidence that these microtophi invariably lead to joint damage, and that antihyperuricaemic treatment should be given to all patients (Wallace and Singer, 1988a; Agudelo, 1989).

When the decision is made to use an antihyperuricaemic drug, it is important to discuss the objectives of treatment with the patient (Fam, 1988). The following aspects are set out to educate the patient in understanding the rationale behind the use of urate-lowering drugs.

1. The administration of drugs to normalize serum urate is usually a lifelong commitment to regular therapy. The patient must be convinced of the necessity of undertaking such long-term treatment, and must realize that withdrawal of treatment or irregular intake of the medication can cause return of hyperuricaemia which in turn is likely to be followed by a recurrence of gouty attacks.

2. The patient should be advised about possible toxic reactions associated with antihyperuricaemic drugs and the risks that might occur without such treatment: recurrent gouty attacks, chronic gouty arthritis, uric acid renal stones and urate nephropathy.
3. The patient should be warned that gouty episodes may still occur during the first six months or so after initiation of antihyperuricaemic therapy, and that temporary use of an NSAID may be needed to control these attacks.

Frequent measurements of serum urate concentrations are important in monitoring patient compliance and effectiveness of urate-lowering treatment. The goal of therapy is to reduce and maintain serum urate below 250–350 µmol/l (4–6 mg/dl)—well below the concentration at which serum urate saturates the extracellular fluid (400 µmol/l or 6.4 mg/dl) (Fam, 1988; Wallace and Singer, 1988a). This will prevent subsequent attacks, promote resorption of tophaceous deposits and reduce further damage to the joints.

The sharp reduction in serum urate level that takes place early in the course of urate-lowering treatment may be associated with recurrence of gouty episodes. Some physicians advocate the additional administration of colchicine 0.6 mg once or twice daily (or indomethacin 25 mg twice daily in patients intolerant to colchicine) as prophylaxis against acute gouty attacks during the first six months or so after initiation of antihyperuricaemic therapy (Wallace and Singer, 1988a; Bellamy et al, 1988). However, this practice of introducing urate-lowering agents under cover of an anti-inflammatory drug cannot be routinely recommended, given the potential toxicity of prolonged use of colchicine or indomethacin, and the fact that only a minority (10–24%) of patients develop more frequent gouty episodes after initiation of allopurinol or uricosuric treatment (Fam, 1988). Instead, many clinicians advocate the use of supplemental indomethacin or other NSAID for gouty paroxysms that may occur during the first few months after initiation of urate-lowering therapy.

Allopurinol

Allopurinol is a potent antihyperuricaemic agent which is structurally similar to hypoxanthine (Rastegar and Thier, 1972; Ross and Seegmiller, 1979). As a xanthine oxidase inhibitor, allopurinol prevents the conversion of hypoxanthine to xanthine and of xanthine to uric acid. As a result, hypoxanthine and xanthine accumulate in the blood and are subsequently excreted in the urine. Administration of allopurinol is, therefore, associated with a reduction in serum and urinary urate concentrations and a con-comitant increase in serum and urinary oxypurines (hypoxanthine and xanthine). The renal clearance of oxypurines is much greater than that of uric acid and the solubility of hypoxanthine and xanthine exceeds that of uric acid. Thus, despite the presence of large amounts of oxypurines in the urine of patients receiving allopurinol, xanthine stone formation is extremely rare (Rastegar and Thier, 1972).

Allopurinol also reduces *de novo* purine synthesis by three mechanisms.

First, the conversion of excess hypoxanthine into inosinic acid leads to negative feedback inhibition of the enzyme amidophosphoribosyl transferase, the rate-limiting enzyme of *de novo* purine synthesis. Second, allopurinol depletes intracellular concentration of phosphoribosyl pyrophosphate (PRPP), the main substrate for the enzyme amidophosphoribosyl transferase. This results from the enzymatic conversion of allopurinol to allopurinol ribonucleotide, a process that consumes PRPP. Third, allopurinol ribonucleotide acts as a pseudo-feedback inhibitor of the enzyme amidophosphoribosyl transferase (Rastegar and Thier, 1972; Ross and Seegmiller, 1979).

Allopurinol is rapidly oxidized in the body to its metabolite oxypurinol (alloxanthine), which is also a potent inhibitor of xanthine oxidase. The half-life of allopurinol is only 1–3 hours, while that of oxypurinol is 16–20 hours in subjects with normal renal function. Thus, allopurinol need not be given in divided doses and can be taken as a single daily dose (Rodnan et al, 1975). Oxypurinol is less well absorbed from the gastrointestinal tract than allopurinol. It is cleared from the body through the kidneys, and accordingly the dosage of allopurinol should be reduced in patients with renal impairment.

Allopurinol is an extremely effective drug in the treatment of gout and other hyperuricaemic states. It is administered orally in a single daily dose of 200–800 mg (average 300 mg daily; formulations 100-mg, 200-mg and 300-mg tablets). It is important to titrate the dose against the serum urate level. Reduction of serum urate concentration is noted within 2 days of starting treatment. The level usually falls to normal within 7–14 days, although it may take much longer in patients with extensive tophaceous deposits. Gouty attacks often cease within 3–6 months of continuous therapy, while dissolution of the tophi may take 6–24 months. Discontinuation of allopurinol is followed by a rapid rise of serum urate concentration to pre-treatment levels, although recurrence of acute gouty attacks may not occur for long periods (Loebl and Scott, 1974).

Allopurinol is well tolerated by the majority of patients and adverse reactions are rare (about 3.5%). Precipitation of acute gouty arthritis and allergic dermatitis are the most common adverse reactions. Cautious reintroduction of allopurinol after cutaneous reactions may be possible using a schedule of gradually increasing doses (Fam et al, 1980). Another strategy in patients allergic to allopurinol is a trial administration of the active metabolite oxypurinol at a dose of 50–100 mg orally (Lockard et al, 1976; Earll and Saavedra, 1983). However, this should be carefully monitored since some of these patients may exhibit cross-reactivity to both allopurinol and oxypurinol (Lockard et al, 1976; Earll and Saavedra, 1983). More recently, intramuscular polyethylene glycol-modified *Arthrobacter protoformiae* uricase has been used successfully to treat hyperuricaemia in a patient with non-Hodgkin's lymphoma, renal insufficiency and allergy to allopurinol (Chua et al, 1988).

The syndrome of hypersensitivity vasculitis is the most serious complication of allopurinol therapy (Hande et al, 1984; Singer and Wallace, 1986). This rare, life-threatening toxic reaction is characterized by some or all of the following: fever, severe dermatitis (usually toxic epidermal necrolysis), hepatitis, progressive renal failure, eosinophilia and leucocytosis. It occurs most frequently in elderly patients with hypertension and renal impairment who are receiving thiazide diuretics (Hande et al, 1984; Singer and Wallace, 1986). Elevated plasma concentrations of the active metabolite oxypurinol in patients with renal insufficiency, in whom the dose of allopurinol has not been reduced appropriately, appear to correlate with the development of this severe hypersensitivity syndrome (Hande et al, 1984). A T-cell mediated immune response to oxypurinol has been postulated (Hande et al, 1984; Emmerson et al, 1988). Oxypurinol renal excretion is directly proportional to that of creatinine, and as renal function decreases, serum oxypurinol half-life and concentration increase (Hande et al, 1984; Emmerson et al, 1987; Day et al, 1988). It is important, therefore, to adjust the dose of allopurinol according to the creatinine clearance in patients with renal insufficiency (Hande et al, 1984). Thiazide diuretics interfere with renal excretion of oxypurinol, leading to further elevation of its plasma levels.

Direct measurements of plasma oxypurinol concentrations have recently become available, and have been used to monitor allopurinol therapy in patients with gout including those with renal impairment (Emmerson et al, 1987; Day et al, 1988). Preliminary studies indicate that plasma oxypurinol concentrations in the range of 30–100 μmol/l may be optimal for effective control of hyperuricaemia (Emmerson et al, 1987).

Measurements of plasma concentrations of oxypurinol and xanthine may also be useful in patients with gout who are still hyperuricaemic despite seemingly adequate allopurinol therapy (Emmerson et al, 1987). If oxypurinol concentrations are in the therapeutic range (30–100 μmol/l) and if plasma xanthine concentrations have increased to 6–9 μmol/l (indicating effective xanthine oxidase inhibition), further increases in allopurinol doses in these patients are less likely to control the hyperuricaemia, and may in fact lead to toxic reactions (Emmerson et al, 1987). Under these circumstances, additional or alternate therapies—such as a uricosuric drug or strict dietary control—should be considered.

Several drug interactions with allopurinol have been described (Rodnan, 1982; Wallace and Singer, 1988a). Allopurinol potentiates the effects of 6-mercaptopurine and azathioprine, which are normally inactivated by xanthine oxidase. The dose of these drugs must therefore be reduced if allopurinol is also administered. An increased incidence of bone marrow suppression occurs when allopurinol is given to a patient taking cyclophosphamide. A threefold increase in the frequency of ampicillin-induced rash has been noted in patients receiving allopurinol. Allopurinol potentiates the effects of dicoumarol. There is also evidence that allergic skin reactions are common in patients treated with both allopurinol and the anticancer drug 2-deoxycoformycin (Steinmetz et al, 1989).

Uricosuric drugs

Uricosuric drugs increase the renal excretion of urate and thereby reduce serum concentration (Thompson et al, 1962; Ross and Seegmiller, 1979;

Rodnan, 1982; Wallace and Singer, 1988a). To minimize the risk of renal calculi associated with the initial transient increase in urate excretion, and to prevent the precipitation of acute gouty attacks associated with rapid decline in serum urate concentration, uricosuric drugs should be started at low doses and gradually increased over one to three weeks. Maintenance of a large urine volume (over 2 l/day) and/or alkalization of urine with sodium bicarbonate (2–6 g/day) or acetazolamide (500 mg once daily) further reduce the risk of uric acid stones. This is particularly desirable in the first few weeks of therapy when the uricosuria is greatest. Once serum urate normalizes, the intense uricosuria subsides and renal excretion of urate approaches pre-treatment levels.

Because of its relatively short biologic half-life, probenecid is given in divided doses: 250 mg twice daily, gradually increasing until the desired serum urate concentration is achieved to a maximum dose of 3000 mg/day. Sulphinpyrazone is administered in an initial dose of 50–100 mg twice daily, gradually increasing until the optimal serum urate concentration is attained, to a maximum dose of 800 mg/day.

Anorexia, nausea, vomiting and abdominal pain are the most frequent side-effects of uricosuric drugs. Other toxic reactions include allergic rash, precipitation of gouty attacks, urinary uric acid stone formation and, rarely, aplastic anaemia (both probenecid and sulphinpyrazone), nephrotic syndrome (probenecid) and hepatic cell necrosis (probenecid) (Thompson et al, 1962; Rodnan, 1982).

Both probenecid and sulphinpyrazone have proved effective in the long-term management of hyperuricaemia and gout (Thompson et al, 1962). It is estimated that 75% of patients will respond to such therapy with restoration of normal serum urate concentration, reduction in the frequency of gouty attacks and dissolution of tophaceous deposits. Most failures, in the remaining 25% of patients, are due to intolerable side-effects, particularly gastrointestinal upset (in about 5% of patients); concomitant intake of salicylates (which nullify the uricosuric action); or the presence of renal impairment (Thompson et al, 1962; Rodnan, 1982; Wallace and Singer, 1988a). Uricosurics are generally ineffective at a creatinine clearance of less than 30–50 ml/min.

SELECTION OF ANTIHYPERURICAEMIC THERAPY

In recent years, allopurinol has increasingly become the drug of choice in the treatment of gout and hyperuricaemia (Rodnan, 1982; Bellamy et al, 1988; Fam, 1988). The drug is particularly indicated in patients who are gross 'overproducers' and 'overexcretors' of uric acid, with urinary urate excretion greater than 4.5–5.5 mmol (800–1000 mg) per day on a regular diet (Table 3). This includes gross secondary hyperuricaemia associated with myeloproliferative and lymphoproliferative disorders, treated with cytotoxic drugs or radiotherapy, rare individuals with partial or complete hypoxanthine guanine phosphoribosyl transferase deficiency and those with

PRPP synthetase overactivity. Other clear-cut indications for allopurinol include patients with extensive tophaceous gout, gout complicated by uric acid urolithiasis, urate nephropathy or renal impairment, patients who fail to respond or are intolerant to uricosuric therapy, and in those with recurrent calcium oxalate urinary calculi associated with hyperuricosuria.

The therapeutic usefulness of uricosuric drugs in the treatment of hyperuricaemia is limited by a number of factors: presence of renal impairment, concomitant ingestion of salicylate, poor patient compliance and drug intolerance (Rodnan, 1982; Fam, 1988). Specific indications for the use of uricosurics include patients who are allergic or intolerant to allopurinol, and those with massive tophaceous deposits who may require treatment with both allopurinol to block uric acid synthesis and a uricosuric to increase uric acid excretion (Table 3). It must be recalled, however, that probenecid used concurrently with allopurinol may block tubular reabsorption of oxypurinol, thus increasing its excretion which in turn will reduce effective inhibition of uric acid synthesis leading to a paradoxical rise of serum urate (Rastegar and Thier, 1972; Rodnan, 1982). Therefore, when a uricosuric drug is added to a regimen including allopurinol, the serum urate should be closely monitored.

In the absence of clear-cut indications for treatment with allopurinol, some rheumatologists recommend that uricosuric drugs be tried first, since these agents are not known to influence purine or pyrimidine metabolism as allopurinol does, and they have been shown to be relatively safe after more than thirty years of clinical experience (Wallace and Singer, 1988a; Kelley et al, 1989). The candidate for uricosuric therapy is the patient with gout who is under 50 years old, with normal renal function and 24-hour urinary uric acid values and no gross tophi or history of urinary calculi. There is very little to choose between probenecid and sulphinpyrazone, but the latter drug is preferred by some physicians because of its added antiplatelet effects.

DIET

Long-term dietary restriction of purines is generally impractical, and has now been superseded by more effective urate-lowering therapy (Rastegar and Thier, 1972; Rodnan, 1982; Wallace and Singer, 1988a). The only consideration currently given to diet is avoidance of purine-rich food such as liver, kidney, sardines, anchovies, sweetbreads and gravies, particularly in patients with massive tophaceous deposits. Excessive alcohol ingestion and severe dietary restriction for control of obesity should be avoided.

There is some experimental evidence to indicate that diets enriched in gamma-linolenic acid (in plant seed oil) and eicosapentaenoic acid (in fish oil) can significantly suppress urate crystal-induced inflammation in the rat subcutaneous air pouch model (Tate et al, 1988). The significance of these findings and the effects of dietary manipulation, including combined diets enriched with fish oil and plant (primrose) seed oil, on the course of clinical gout have not been studied.

SURGERY

Since the introduction of effective urate-lowering agents, surgery is less often required in the management of gout. Surgery may be indicated for the debridement and excision of large tophi eroding into the skin, and the removal of bulky tophi located in areas subjected to excessive pressure or mechanically interfering with joint movements (Larmon, 1970). Other surgical procedures include arthroplasty for severely damaged joints, and tenoplasty for tendons damaged by tophaceous deposits.

TREATMENT OF EXTENSIVE TOPHACEOUS GOUT

Every so often, a patient presents with widespread, massive tophaceous deposits. In such patients effective lowering of serum urate levels may not be achieved by a single drug, whether allopurinol or a uricosuric agent. Combined therapy, with allopurinol and probenecid or sulphinpyrazone, is usually required (Wallace and Singer, 1988a). Serum urate concentration should be kept consistently below 250–350 μmol/l (4–6 mg/dl) to ensure complete resolution of the tophaceous deposits. These patients may also require surgical excision of massive tophi, and dietary restriction of purine-rich foods. Liberal use of alcoholic beverages should be discouraged.

TREATMENT OF ASYMPTOMATIC HYPERURICAEMIA

Controversy exists regarding the optimal management of subjects with asymptomatic hyperuricaemia (Rodnan, 1982; Bellamy et al, 1988; Fam, 1988; Wallace and Singer, 1988a). The vast majority of these individuals do not develop clinical manifestations of gout (Campion et al, 1987; Liang and Fries, 1978; Wallace and Singer, 1988a). Hyperuricaemia *per se* does not seem to affect renal function or lead to progressive renal damage (Liang and Fries, 1978; Fessell, 1979; Campion et al, 1987). The development of renal impairment in patients with gout is largely the consequence of aging, hypertension, diabetes mellitus and renovascular disease (Liang and Fries, 1978; Fessell, 1979; Campion et al, 1987; Wallace and Singer, 1988a).

In general, therefore, there seems to be no rationale for treating individuals with asymptomatic hyperuricaemia with urate-lowering drugs. Heightened awareness of the costs and potential hazards of unnecessary treatment has resulted in increased conservatism in the use of long-term antihyperuricaemic therapy in these individuals (Liang and Fries, 1978; Fessel, 1979; Campion et al, 1987; Bellamy et al, 1988; Wallace and Singer, 1988a). Corrective measures that may constitute sufficient treatment for many of these subjects include weight reduction, control of alcohol intake, elimination of drugs such as thiazides or aspirin, avoidance of purine-rich foods and periodic re-evaluation (Fessel, 1979; Auböck and Fritsch, 1985; Campion et al, 1987).

However, the likelihood of clinical gout developing increases with rising serum urate concentration (Campion et al, 1987). Individuals with sustained, significant hyperuricaemia—over 500–650 μmol/l (9–11 mg/dl)—should have their 24-hour urinary uric acid excretion measured. Those with gross uric acid overproduction—more than 4.5–5.5 mmol (800–1000 mg) per day on a regular diet—who do not respond to simple corrective measures are at a higher risk for developing uric acid calculi, and should perhaps be treated with long-term allopurinol to reduce both serum and urinary urate levels (Becker, 1988; Fam, 1988; Wallace and Singer, 1988a; Kelley et al, 1989).

CONCLUSION

Hyperuricaemia is the biochemical hallmark of gout. Non-salicylate, non-steroidal anti-inflammatory drugs such as indomethacin and naproxen are the drugs of choice in the treatment of acute gouty arthritis. Alternative therapies include colchicine, intra-articular corticosteroids and single-dose intramuscular corticotrophin. Allopurinol is the preferred urate-lowering drug for patients with frequent gouty attacks, uric acid overproduction (hyperuricosuria greater than 4.5–5.5 mmol per day), tophi, uric acid urolithiasis or urate nephropathy. Uricosuric drugs, including probenecid and sulphinpyrazone, are mainly used in patients who are allergic to allopurinol, and in combination with allopurinol in those with massive tophaceous deposits. Asymptomatic hyperuricaemia requires no treatment with urate-lowering drugs except in patients with significant persistent hyperuricaemia (greater than 500–650 μmol/l) and hyperuricosuria (greater than 4.5–5.5 mmol per day).

REFERENCES

Agudelo CA (1989) Gout and hyperuricemia. *Current Opinions in Rheumatology* **1:** 286–293.
Ahern MJ, Reid C, Gordon TP, McCredie M, Brooks PM & Jones M (1987) Does colchicine work? The results of the first controlled study in acute gout. *Australia and New Zealand Journal of Medicine* **17:** 301–304.
Altman RD, Honig S, Levin JM & Lightfoot RW (1988) Ketoprofen versus indomethacin in patients with acute gouty arthritis: a multicenter, double blind comparative study. *Journal of Rheumatology* **15:** 1422–1426.
Auböck A & Fritsch P (1985) Asymptomatic hyperuricemia and allopurinol induced toxic epidermal necrolysis. *British Medical Journal* **290:** 1969–1970.
Axelrod D & Preston S (1988) Comparison of parenteral adrenocorticotropic hormone with oral indomethacin in the treatment of acute gout. *Arthritis and Rheumatism* **31:** 803–805.
Becker MA (1988) Clinical aspects of monosodium urate monohydrate crystal deposition disease (gout). *Rheumatic Disease Clinics of North America* **14:** 377–394.
Bellamy N, Downie WW & Buchanan WW (1987) Observations on spontaneous improvement in patients with podagra: implications for therapeutic trials of non-steroidal anti-inflammatory drugs. *British Journal of Clinical Pharmacology* **24:** 33–36.
Bellamy N, Gilbert JR, Brooks PM, Emmerson BT & Campbell J (1988) A survey of current prescribing practices of antiinflammatory and urate lowering drugs in gouty arthritis in the Province of Ontario. *Journal of Rheumatology* **15:** 1841–1847.
Campion EW, Glynn RJ & DeLarbry LO (1987) Asymptomatic hyperuricemia. Risks and consequences in the normative aging study. *American Journal of Medicine* **82:** 421–426.

Chua CC, Greenberg ML, Viau AT, Nucci M, Brenckman WD & Hershfield MS (1988) Use of polyethylene glycol-modified uricase (PEG-uricase) to treat hyperuricemia in a patient with non-Hodgkin lymphoma. *Annals of Internal Medicine* **109:** 114–117.

Day RO, Minero JO, Birkett DJ et al (1988) Allopurinol dosage selection: relationship between dose and plasma oxypurinol and urate concentrations and urinary urate excretion. *British Journal of Clinical Pharmacology* **26:** 423–428.

Earll JM & Saavedra M (1983) Oxypurinol therapy in allopurinol allergic patients. *American Family Physician* **28:** 147–148.

Emmerson BT, Gordon RB, Cross M & Thomson DB (1987) Plasma oxypurinol concentrations during allopurinol therapy. *British Journal of Rheumatology* **26:** 445–449.

Emmerson BT, Hazelton RA & Frazer IH (1988) Some adverse reactions to allopurinol may be mediated by lymphocyte reactivity to oxypurinol. *Arthritis and Rheumatism* **31:** 436–440.

Fam AG (1986) Acute monoarthritis: uncovering the cause. *Diagnosis* **3:** 29–41.

Fam AG (1988) Strategies for treating gout and hyperuricemia. *Journal of Musculoskeletal Medicine* **5:** 83–98.

Fam AG, Paton TW & Chaiton A (1980) Reinstitution of allopurinol therapy for gouty arthritis after cutaneous reactions. *Canadian Medical Association Journal* **123:** 128–129.

Fessel WJ (1979) Renal outcomes of gout and hyperuricemia. *American Journal of Medicine* **67:** 74–82.

Hande KR, Noone RM & Stone WJ (1984) Severe allopurinol toxicity. Description and guidelines for prevention in patients with renal insufficiency. *American Journal of Medicine* **76:** 47–56.

Kelley WN, Fox IH & Palella TD (1989) Gout and related disorders of purine metabolism. In Kelley WN, Harris ED, Ruddy S & Sledge CG (eds) *Textbook of Rheumatology*, 3rd edn, pp 1395–1448. Philadelphia: WB Saunders.

Kerolus G, Clayburne G & Schumacher HR (1989) Is it mandatory to examine synovial fluids promptly after arthrocentesis? *Arthritis and Rheumatism* **32:** 271–278.

Kuncl RW, Duncan G, Watson D, Alderson K, Rogawski MA & Peper M (1987) Colchicine myopathy and neuropathy. *New England Journal of Medicine* **316:** 1562–1568.

Larmon WA (1970) Surgical management of tophaceous gout. *Clinical Orthopaedics* **71:** 56–59.

Liang MH & Fries JF (1978) Asymptomatic hyperuricemia: the case for conservative management. *Annals of Internal Medicine* **88:** 666–670.

Lockard O, Harmon C, Nolph K & Irvin W (1976) Allergic reaction to allopurinol with cross reactivity to oxypurinol. *Annals of Internal Medicine* **85:** 333–335.

Loebl WY, Scott JT (1974) Withdrawal of allopurinol in patients with gout. *Annals of the Rheumatic Diseases* **33:** 304–307.

Neuss MN, McCallum RM, Brenckman WD & Silberman HR (1986) Long-term colchicine administration leading to colchicine toxicity and death. *Arthritis and Rheumatism* **29:** 448–449.

Rastegar A & Thier SO (1972) The physiologic approach to hyperuricemia. *New England Journal of Medicine* **286:** 470–476.

Roberts WN, Liang MH & Stern SH (1987) Colchicine in acute gout. Reassessment of risks and benefits. *Journal of the American Medical Association* **257:** 1920–1922.

Rodnan GP (1982) Treatment of gout and other forms of crystal-induced arthritis. *Bulletin on the Rheumatic Diseases* **32:** 43–53.

Rodnan GP, Robin JA, Tolchin SF & Elion GB (1975) Allopurinol and gouty hyperuricemia. Efficacy of a single daily dose. *Journal of the American Medical Association* **231:** 1143–1147.

Ross GA & Seegmiller JE (1979) Hyperuricemia and gout: classification, complications and management. *New England Journal of Medicine* **300:** 1459–1468.

Singer JZ & Wallace SL (1986) The allopurinol hypersensitivity syndrome, unnecessary morbidity and mortality. *Arthritis and Rheumatism* **29:** 82–87.

Steinmetz JC, De Conti R & Ginsberg R (1989) Hypersensitivity vasculitis associated with 2-deoxycoformycin and allopurinol therapy. *American Journal of Medicine* **86:** 499–500.

Tate GA, Mandell BF, Karmali RA et al (1988) Suppression of monosodium urate crystal-induced acute inflammation by diets enriched with gamma-linolenic acid and eicosapentaenoic acid. *Arthritis and Rheumatism* **31:** 1543–1551.

Thompson GR, Duff IF, Robinson WD, Mikkelsen WM & Galindez H (1962) Long term uricosuric therapy in gout. *Arthritis and Rheumatism* **5:** 384–396.

Wade JP & Liang MH (1988) Avoiding common pitfalls in the diagnosis of gout. *Journal of Musculoskeletal Medicine* **5:** 16–27.

Wallace SL & Singer JZ (1988a) Therapy in gout. *Rheumatic Disease Clinics of North America* **14:** 441–457.

Wallace SL & Singer JZ (1988b) Review: systemic toxicity associated with the intravenous administration of colchicine—guidelines for use. *Journal of Rheumatology* **15:** 495–499.

Wilkens RE & Case JB (1973) Treatment of acute gout with naproxen. *Scandinavian Journal of Rheumatology* **2 (supplement):** 69–71.

2

The risks of antimalarial retinopathy, azathioprine lymphoma and methotrexate hepatotoxicity during the treatment of rheumatoid arthritis

MURRAY B. UROWITZ
PETER LEE

THE RISKS OF ANTIMALARIAL RETINOPATHY

The antimalarial drugs chloroquine and hydroxychloroquine became widely used in the treatment of rheumatoid arthritis and discoid and systemic lupus erythematosus, following their introduction in the early 1950s. However, the initial enthusiasm for these drugs was dampened considerably following the discovery of their potentially serious ocular side-effects (Cambioggi, 1957; Hobbs and Calnan, 1958; Fuld, 1959; Henkind and Rothfield, 1963). However, more recent data indicate the drugs to be less hazardous to the eyes than was originally thought. While corneal deposits are the most frequently observed ocular manifestation associated with chloroquine therapy (Easterbrook, 1988), it is the retinopathy that is of greatest concern.

Incidence

The reported incidence of retinopathy associated with the antimalarial drugs varies from less than 1% to more than 45% (Okun et al, 1963; Nozik et al, 1964; Percival and Behrman, 1969). Such wide differences are due to variations in the definition of retinopathy and methods employed for its detection, in addition to important dose-related factors.

Current definitions of definite chloroquine retinopathy require the demonstration of permanent functional loss, for example the presence of bilateral paracentral field defects confirmed by static perimetry (Mackenzie and Scherbel, 1980; Easterbrook, 1987). With such criteria, the incidence of antimalarial-related retinopathy is much lower. Bernstein (1983) estimated the risk to be 10% for patients treated with chloroquine and 3–4% with hydroxychloroquine. Even these figures are likely to be overestimates for present-day practice with proper dose adjustment and careful monitoring.

Baillière's Clinical Rheumatology—
Vol. 4, No. 2, August 1990
ISBN 0–7020–1480–X

Mechanism of retinal damage

Chloroquine has an affinity for melanin and the retinopathy associated with the antimalarials is thought to occur through the selective deposition of these drugs in the retinal pigment epithelium (Okun et al, 1963). The normal function of the retinal pigment epithelium is to phagocytose and digest discarded outer segments of aged photoreceptor cells as they are shed (Elner et al, 1981). The accumulation of chloroquine at this site interferes with essential cell function through the inhibition of membrane transport enzymes (Fedorko, 1967; Rubin, 1968) and eventually results in secondary damage to the cones and rods and nerve fibre layer (Bernstein and Ginsberg, 1964; Francois and Maudgal, 1967). Since the outer segments of the photoreceptor cells are shed diurnally under the influence of light, excess light (exposure) may potentiate chloroquine-induced retinal damage (Rubin and Slonicki, 1966; Mackenzie and Szilagyi, 1968). It has been recommended that patients on antimalarial drugs wear dark glasses if prolonged exposure to sunlight is anticipated.

The earliest clinical findings are an increased granularity and oedema of the retina. The changes are bilateral, generalized and symmetrical but most marked in the region of the macula where the retinopathy progresses to form a classic 'bull's eye' or 'doughnut' lesion (Figure 1). This consists of a central area of patchy pigmentation, surrounded by a clear zone and then a concentric ring of hyperpigmentation. In the advanced stages, narrowing of the retinal vessels, optic atrophy and diffuse depigmentation of the peripheral retina occurs.

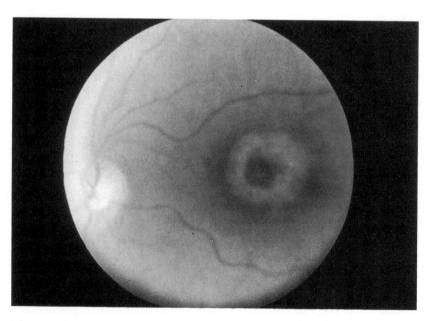

Figure 1. Advanced chloroquine retinopathy showing pigment cell drop-out and choroidal fluorescence (courtesy of Dr Michael Easterbrook).

With early lesions the retinopathy may be asymptomatic, but eventually a paracentral scotoma develops. Peripheral vision is initially unaffected but becomes constricted, with enlargement of the scotoma, as the lesion progresses. If the antimalarial drug is continued, permanent loss of vision may result.

Dose relationship

In several studies, chloroquine retinopathy was associated with high cumulative doses of the drug (Marks and Power, 1979; Finbloom et al, 1985). On this basis, maximum total doses of between 300 and 600 grams of chloroquine, or a maximum of three years on antimalarial drugs, were recommended in order to avoid toxicity (Butler, 1965; Arden and Kolb, 1966; Carr et al, 1966; Nylander, 1967). However, these data (as well as most published incidence reports) were gathered during a period when the daily dose of chloroquine used was between 250 and 500 mg, far exceeding those being prescribed today.

Recent evidence indicates that the retinopathy associated with antimalarial drugs is more closely related to the daily rather than the total dose. Bernstein (1983) in his review of 65 cases of retinopathy found that none of these patients took less than 250 mg of chloroquine per day. Scherbel and Mackenzie (Scherbel et al, 1965; Mackenzie and Scherbel, 1980; Mackenzie, 1970, 1983) followed more than 900 patients with rheumatoid arthritis for an average duration of seven years and did not observe ocular toxicity in those receiving daily doses of 3.5 mg/kg (body weight) of chloroquine or 6.5 mg/kg of hydroxychloroquine. Patients developing retinopathy took an average of 5.11 mg/kg per day of chloroquine or 7.77 mg/kg per day of hydroxy-chloroquine. These data indicate that ocular toxicity may be avoided, even with long-term treatment, provided that patients are kept within a safe daily dosage range. The safe dosage zone was thus considered to be less than 4.0 mg/kg per day for chloroquine and less than 6.5 mg/kg per day for hydroxychloroquine (Mackenzie, 1983).

Previously, 250 mg of chloroquine per day was regarded as an effective and safe dose but body mass of the patient was seldom taken into account. Easterbrook (1987) found that 21 of 35 patients with retinopathy had received 250 mg per day while 9 had taken less than this dose. In fact, 9 patients with irreversible scotomas had taken less than the recommended maximum daily chloroquine dose of 4.0 mg/kg. An additional 21 patients with retinopathy only exceeded this dose by an average of 9%. On this basis Easterbrook (1987) suggested that the maximum daily dose of chloroquine should be adjusted downwards. This author is now using 3.0 mg/kg per day for chloroquine and 6.0 mg/kg per day for hydroxychloroquine.

Human serum concentrations of chloroquine and hydroxychloroquine have been studied (Berliner et al, 1948; Laaksonen et al, 1974; Wollheim et al, 1978). A plateau in serum levels is reached after several weeks of dosing. While there is a clear relationship between the dose taken and serum levels achieved, the role of serum antimalarial drug concentrations in the prediction of toxicity has not been determined.

Other risk factors

Other factors that may contribute to retinal toxicity from antimalarial drugs include age, obesity, renal insufficiency and hepatic dysfunction.

Older patients were found to be more likely to develop chloroquine retinopathy (Elman et al, 1976; Finbloom et al, 1985). In one study, the mean age of patients with retinopathy was 55 years compared to 40 years in those without eye toxicity (Finbloom et al, 1985). Because of macular pigmentation associated with degenerative changes, older patients can also be more difficult to monitor for chloroquine-related retinopathy.

There is very little accumulation of chloroquine in fat (Mackenzie, 1983). In obese patients, dosages based on actual body weight may be excessive and contribute to toxicity. Dosage of antimalarial drugs should therefore be based on lean (ideal) body weight.

Following absorption, 30–50% of antimalarial drug is biotransformed in the liver and other tissues while the remainder is excreted unchanged: 40% in the urine, 8–12% in the faeces and 5% through the skin (Mackenzie, 1983). Patients with renal insufficiency and impaired hepatic function may therefore be at greater risk of retinopathy with these drugs, and in these patients antimalarials should be avoided or their dose reduced appropriately.

Monitoring for retinopathy

Apart from routine funduscopic retinal examination, a number of tests have been advocated for the detection of chloroquine retinopathy. These have been reviewed by Easterbrook (1988) and include colour vision testing, the macular dazzle test, fluorescein angiography, electro-oculogram, electro-retinogram, critical flicker frequency, visual field testing, and automated, static and kinetic perimetry. The object of these investigations is to detect evidence of retinopathy, preferably at an early stage before any permanent damage has been done.

Of these procedures, the use of the Amsler grid (Figure 2) to test for visual field defects has been found to be the most sensitive, as well as being simple, inexpensive, reproducible and rapid in performance (Carr et al, 1966). It takes the patient only a few seconds to perform. The test will readily detect shallow, relative paracentral scotomas and there is good correlation with the findings on static and kinetic perimetry (Easterbrook, 1984, 1988). The major advantage of the Amsler grid is its ability to pick up very small, early scotomas before they are apparent on static and kinetic field testing and at a stage when they are potentially reversible. Patients are asked to check their visual fields every two weeks, looking for 'faded' squares. Any abnormalities are then further investigated with static and kinetic perimetry (Easterbrook, 1988).

Fluorescein angiography, electro-oculogram and electroretinogram testing are not only time-consuming and tedious to perform but are positive only in the later stages of toxicity. However, in older patients visual field testing may not be very reliable and further difficulties arise from coexisting macular degenerative changes. In this situation colour testing with Ishihara

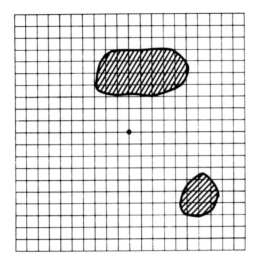

Figure 2. The Amsler grid. 'Faded' squares indicate relative scotomas with good prognosis, while 'absent' squares imply absolute scotomas and probable progressive visual loss (courtesy of Dr Michael Easterbrook).

plates and fluorescein angiography may help distinguish chloroquine retinopathy from such age-related abnormalities (Easterbrook, 1988).

Prognosis

The prognosis of chloroquine retinopathy was previously very guarded and there are several reports of the lesions progressing after discontinuation of the drug (Okun et al, 1963; Nozik et al, 1964; Krill et al, 1971) or presenting after cessation of treatment (Sataline and Farmer, 1962; Ehrenfeld et al, 1986). Prognosis now appears much more favourable because of the lower doses of chloroquine used and the early detection of toxicity with more effective monitoring. In patients presenting with early retinopathy the condition appears not to progress over a five-year period if the paracentral scotoma are relative and associated with normal visual acuity, colour vision and fluorescein angiogram. On the other hand, progression will occur in about 50% of cases with reduced visual acuity, abnormal colour vision, positive fluorescein angiogram and absolute scotoma (Easterbrook, 1988). Experience with currently used antimalarial regimens indicates that retinal toxicity in the form of severe visual loss is a very uncommon event. In Easterbrook's series of 46 cases, one patient is legally blind and there is only one other with vision worse than 20/40. The majority are asymptomatic and have relative scotomas which are only apparent on visual field testing.

Chloroquine versus hydroxychloroquine

Taken in the present recommended doses, retinopathy has been reported much more frequently with chloroquine than with hydroxychloroquine, suggesting that the latter is safer (Tobin et al, 1982; Rynes, 1983; Finbloom et al, 1985; Easterbook, 1987). This could be explained by the fact that 400 mg of hydroxychloroquine might not be therapeutically equivalent to 250 mg of chloroquine. Mackenzie (1983) presented data indicating similar toxic thresholds when optimal doses of the two drugs were compared. Furthermore, Easterbrook (1987) observed that fewer than 10% of patients treated with hydroxychloroquine had visible corneal deposits on slit-lamp examination, compared with 95% of those treated with chloroquine. These findings suggest that the tissue levels of chloroquine and hydroxychloroquine are very different with the currently recommended doses. Retinopathy with hydroxychloroquine is likely to be more frequent with daily doses of greater than 400 mg. In fact, the few cases of well-documented hydroxychloroquine-related retinopathy with visual loss all occurred with doses of more than 750 mg daily (Shearer and Dubois, 1967; Crews, 1961).

In summary, with the use of proper daily doses of chloroquine and hydroxychloroquine based on body weight, and careful monitoring using the Amsler grid, retinopathy associated with these drugs is largely a preventable condition.

AZATHIOPRINE AND MALIGNANCY IN RHEUMATOID ARTHRITIS

To evaluate the potential role of azathioprine in inducing malignancy in rheumatoid arthritis, the incidence of malignancy *de novo* in rheumatoid arthritis must first be investigated. The potential additive effect of azathioprine in possibly contributing to an increased incidence can then be analysed.

A review of the literature regarding the incidence of malignancy in rheumatoid arthritis is confusing as the methodologic approaches to this question have varied significantly. This has led to an equivocal conclusion regarding a possible relationship.

Proportional mortality studies in five centres (Isomaki et al, 1975; Monson and Hall, 1976; Koota et al, 1977; Allenbeck et al, 1981; Vanderbroucke et al, 1984) which examined the percentage distribution of deaths from malignancy in patients with rheumatoid arthritis and normal controls revealed no difference or a decreased incidence of malignancy in patients with rheumatoid arthritis. Cohort mortality studies (Monson and Hall, 1976; Lewis et al, 1980; Prior et al, 1984), which examined the excess of observed numbers of deaths in patients with rheumatoid arthritis as compared with expected numbers of deaths from malignancy in normal controls, revealed no increase or a slight increase in malignancy in patients with rheumatoid arthritis. The results from proportional mortality studies may be distorted if patients die from causes other than malignancy such as rheumatoid arthritis itself, and this is certainly the case. Cohort mortality studies depend on the reliability of the underlying cause of death as given on the death certificate, which must be used in conjunction with mortality rates of the general population. Thus each of these methods may result in unreliable conclusions.

The best methodological approach to this issue is a cohort morbidity study where all new diagnoses of malignancy are included in the observed numbers, whether a patient is alive or dead at the end of the study or died from a cause other than the malignancy itself. There are two major studies of this variety, one by Isomaki from Finland (Isomaki et al, 1978; Hakulinen et al, 1985) and the other by Prior (Prior et al, 1984) from England. The Finnish data are derived from the Finland Registry for patients with rheumatoid arthritis and malignancy and included 46 101 patients with rheumatoid arthritis and 1202 cases of rheumatoid arthritis and malignancy. This study revealed an excess risk of lymphoma, leukaemia and myeloma in patients with rheumatoid arthritis. Non-Hodgkin's lymphoma rate in the Finnish population was 0.31 cases per 1000 population, compared with 0.82 cases per 1000 rheumatoid arthritis patients.

The study from Birmingham (Prior et al, 1984) involved 489 patients with rheumatoid arthritis, revealing a slight increase in overall malignancy, but a significant increase in non-Hodgkin's lymphoma (14.31 cases per 1000 rheumatoid patients compared with 0.59 per 1000 population). There was also a tendency toward increasing relative risk of such a lymphoma with time.

It is important to stress that both the Finnish and Birmingham studies involved patients who had not received cytotoxic drugs of any type. Therefore, it must be assumed that the increased incidence of lymphoproliferative malignancies was associated with rheumatoid arthritis.

Although the oncogenic potential of cytotoxic drugs became evident relatively early in the experience of transplantation, no such clear relationship has been demonstrated in rheumatoid arthritis patients treated with azathioprine. In long-term recall studies of patients who were treated with azathioprine for rheumatoid arthritis, chromosomal abnormalities have been demonstrated (Hunter et al, 1975; Urowitz et al, 1982). There is a suggestion that these abnormalities are reversible when azathioprine is discontinued. A number of studies have reported the occurrence of a single case of malignancy in single patients treated with azathioprine for rheumatoid arthritis, and other studies have documented larger numbers of patients in any one series (Tilson and Whisnant, 1985).

Kinlen in 1985 reviewed 470 patients with rheumatoid arthritis treated with azathioprine (Kinlen, 1985). These patients were followed in a prospective study of 1634 patients who did not receive transplants but who were treated with immunosuppressive drugs. In the subset of rheumatoid patients treated with azathioprine there was a slight increase in non-Hodgkin's lymphoma, 6.38 cases per 1000 rheumatoids as compared to 0.47 cases per 1000 population. However, the incidence was lower than that in the other UK study by Prior (14.31 cases per 1000 rheumatoids), although it is higher than the Finnish study by Isomaki (0.82 cases per 1000 rheumatoids) (Isomaki et al, 1978). It is not clear at this time why the rate of non-Hodgkin's lymphoma appears to be higher in England than in Finland.

In an extension of the Finnish study, Laakso et al (1986), examined mortality due to malignancy in patients with rheumatoid arthritis. This study comprised a 10-year prospective follow-up assessing cause of death in a cohort of 1000 subjects with rheumatoid arthritis and 1000 controls without rheumatoid arthritis. The conclusions of this study revealed that the overall mortality was significantly higher in both men and women with rheumatoid arthritis than in controls, but the mortality due to malignancy in general was not statistically different between the two groups. However, there was a significant excess of deaths from neoplasms of the haematopoietic system in patients with rheumatoid arthritis, again emphasizing the significance of these malignancies both in morbidity and mortality in rheumatoid arthritis.

In conclusion, cohort morbidity studies in rheumatoid arthritis reveal an excess in lymphoproliferative malignancies in patients with rheumatoid arthritis receiving no cytotoxic therapy. Patients treated with azathioprine also show an increase in lymphoproliferative malignancies, but it is not clear that this is greater than the incidence in patients without such medications. Only a long-term follow-up in a large number of such patients, as is occurring in the Rheumatoid Arthritis Azathioprine Registry in Toronto (Tilson and Whisnant, 1985), will be able to answer this question definitively. When the true incidence is appreciated, one may then decide whether the risk–benefit ratio is appropriate for the use of this agent in rheumatoid arthritis.

METHOTREXATE LIVER TOXICITY

Although folate antagonists have been suggested for the treatment of rheumatoid arthritis since the early 1950s, it is only in the past decade that the use of methotrexate has been widely adopted as a useful treatment for patients with rheumatoid arthritis (Weinblatt et al, 1985; Andersen et al, 1985; Williams et al, 1985; Thompson et al, 1984; Tugwell et al, 1987). However, much of the early experience with methotrexate in non-malignant disease derived from studies in patients with psoriasis, as this drug had been used for 25 years for the treatment of psoriasis and psoriatic arthritis. This experience taught that methotrexate is best given in pulses, either orally or parenterally, generally on a weekly basis. The drug was usually well tolerated. Liver toxicity included abnormal liver function tests and in some instances hepatic fibrosis. There did not seem to be a definite relationship between abnormal liver function tests and the subsequent development of liver fibrosis.

As the use of methotrexate in rheumatoid arthritis became more commonplace, it became apparent that the drug's toxicity could not be extrapolated from psoriasis or psoriatic arthritis to rheumatoid arthritis. Obviously the two diseases are different, the hosts in which these diseases occur are different and the mean dose of drug used in rheumatoid arthritis is generally lower than the dose used in psoriasis, although the total duration of drug ingestion may be longer in rheumatoid arthritis. In addition, patients with rheumatoid arthritis were generally advised to take the medication in one dose rather than to split the doses over a 12-hour to 24-hour period weekly.

Addressing the issue of hepatic toxicity secondary to methotrexate requires an understanding of the nature of liver histology in patients with rheumatoid arthritis not on methotrexate. Three authors have addressed this issue (Kremer and Lee, 1986; Kremer et al, 1989; Rau et al, 1989; Brick et al, 1989). Kremer (Kremer et al, 1986) initially reported on 29 patients followed prospectively with oral methotrexate treatment for refractory rheumatoid arthritis. The patients all had liver biopsies at baseline, after two years and annually thereafter. In the first evaluation, 28 of 29 baseline biopsies were read as normal (Roenigk class I) (Roenigk et al, 1982). One biopsy showed moderate to severe fatty infiltration and portal tract inflammation and necrosis (Roenigk class II). Rau et al (1989) evaluated 60 liver biopsies from patients with rheumatoid arthritis before initiating methotrexate and later compared them to 40 biopsies taken from patients on methotrexate treatment. They also demonstrated abnormalities of fatty infiltration, portal tract inflammation and necrosis in the untreated patients. Similar findings were reported by Brick et al (1989).

Liver biopsy studies on patients receiving long-term methotrexate treatment have been reported by a number of authors (Kremer and Lee, 1986; Kremer et al, 1989; Shergy et al, 1988; Aponte and Petrelli, 1988; Weinblatt et al, 1988; Alarcon et al, 1989; Rau et al, 1989; Brick et al, 1989). In the long-term prospective biopsy study by Kremer (Kremer et al, 1986) similar changes of fatty infiltration, portal tract inflammation and portal fibrosis were seen in patients taking methotrexate. A very small number of patients showed some progression in fatty infiltration and one patient in this study had actually shown reversion from class II to class I despite remaining on methotrexate for three years. A later, longer-term follow-up in the same group of patients (Kremer et al, 1989) revealed some deterioration of histologic grade in 25 of 29 patients. Fibrosis—although mild in extent and not affecting hepatic architecture—occurred in 14 of 27 patients (52%) and correlated with total cumulative dose and duration of methotrexate therapy as well as with body weight. Aponte (Aponte and Petrelli, 1988) reported the longest follow-up of patients treated with methotrexate for more than ten years. Although changes of classes II and III were found in some biopsies, none of the biopsies showed cirrhosis. Repeat biopsies in 5 patients with class III changes in this study showed no progression of fibrosis.

In 1988, Shergy reported a retrospective analysis of methotrexate-associated hepatic toxicity in 210 patients with rheumatoid arthritis, and in this study hepatic fibrosis was reported in 6 patients with rheumatoid arthritis—a prevalence of 2.9% (Shergy et al, 1988). No specific risk factor was delineated for these 6 patients, including alcoholism, obesity or diabetes. Similar findings of minimal change in liver biopsies were reported by Weinblatt et al (1988), Alarcon et al (1989), Rau et al (1989) and Brick et al (1989). Although Brick et al (1989) reported that fatty changes and triaditis were significantly more common after treatment when both pre-treatment and post-treatment biopsies were available, Rau et al (1989) in their pre-treatment and post-treatment biopsies could find no difference between rheumatoid arthritis patients not on methotrexate and those patients using this medication, including the finding of periportal fibrosis.

In a study specifically examining the hepatic ultrastructure after metho-trexate therapy for rheumatoid arthritis, Bjorkman et al (1988) reported that the morphologic findings unique to patients treated with methotrexate were increased collagen deposition and electron-dense material in the space of Disse, prominence of the Ito cells (fat-storing cells that may be harbingers of cirrhosis) and an increase in hepatocyte lysosomes. The study of Brick et al (1989) revealed no increase in the number of Ito cells. Thus, although evidence of collagen deposition in the space of Disse has been reported, the natural history and clinical significance of this potential for fibrosis is not yet clear. It should be noted that there is still no case report of methotrexate-induced cirrhosis, again throwing into question the clinical significance of the ultrastructural changes noted.

Although most rheumatologists follow patients with rheumatoid arthritis on methotrexate with liver function tests, it appears from the evidence that elevated liver function tests are not good predictors of fibrosis and, on the other hand, normal liver function tests do not preclude this finding on liver biopsy. Two studies by Kremer and his colleagues (Kremer and Lee, 1986; Kremer et al, 1989) found no correlation between elevated transaminases and hepatic fibrosis in the early study, from months 1 to 29, but did find a correlation between the fibrosis and the number of elevated serum trans-aminases in the months from 29 to 53 of methotrexate therapy. Brick et al (1989) also found no correlation between elevations in transaminases, alkaline phosphatase and hepatic histology. They concluded that there was no laboratory index of liver function that can adequately assess the degree of methotrexate-induced damage.

An unusual acute, reversible form of hepatic failure was recently reported by Clegg et al (1989) in two patients treated with methotrexate for rheumatoid arthritis. One patient available for biopsy was shown to have chronic active hepatitis. This appears to be an unusual manifestation of methotrexate hepatic toxicity, and its prevalence in rheumatoid patients treated with methotrexate is probably very low.

Because cirrhosis developing on previous fibrosis occurred in patients with psoriasis treated with methotrexate, this problem has been investigated by rheumatologists. In the recent review by Brick et al (1989) of over 700 patients with rheumatoid arthritis treated with methotrexate, approximately 11% were found to have some evidence of fibrosis on biopsy but as yet there are no reported cases of cirrhosis.

The mechanism of hepatic toxicity in these patients is not clear. Kremer et al (1986) reported serum and red blood cell methotrexate levels as well as hepatic levels of methotrexate and folate in 24 patients receiving long-term oral methotrexate treatment for rheumatoid arthritis. In hepatic tissue obtained by liver biopsy, methotrexate was found predominantly in a poly-glutamated form with depleted hepatic folate stores when compared with baseline specimens. A brief period of treatment with oral folinic acid repleted hepatic folate. These authors suggested that methotrexate hepato-toxicity is related to reduced hepatic folate levels and the formation of methotrexate polyglutamates.

Morgan et al (1990) reported a reduced rate of methotrexate toxicity in patients treated for rheumatoid arthritis if they were also given a daily supplement of 1 mg of folic acid. Although most of the toxicity was not hepatic, with only 3 patients out of 32 developing elevated liver enzymes, these authors noted that patients receiving folate supplementation had less toxicity overall than did patients without the supplementation. They concluded that folic acid supplementation may allow earlier use of methotrexate in rheumatoid arthritis by diminishing potential toxicity. Whether this will have any further effect on the already low prevalence of significant liver disease induced by methotrexate is not yet clear.

In view of these facts, how useful is liver biopsy in patients with rheumatoid arthritis treated with methotrexate? Although liver biopsy is frequently a simple procedure, there is a definite risk associated and some degree of inconvenience to the patient and to outpatient care facilities. Since patients with rheumatoid arthritis are at low risk for liver disease, and since liver histology at onset is not predictive for the development of significant liver disease later, there is no indication for a pre-treatment biopsy. In addition, none of the long-term biopsy studies has indicated any morphologic abnormalities associated with significant functional liver disease. Therefore there is no indication to perform routine follow-up biopsies. This was also the conclusion of a recent editorial in the *Journal of Rheumatology* (Bridges et al, 1989). Biopsies should be reserved for patients who have chronically significantly elevated liver enzyme studies, especially patients using alcohol or those with signs of hepatic impairment. These indications will arise very infrequently.

REFERENCES

Alarcon GS, Tracy IC & Blackburn WD (1989) Methotrexate in rheumatoid arthritis; toxic effects as the major factor in limiting long-term treatment. *Arthritis and Rheumatism* **32:** 671–676.

Allenbeck P, Ahlbom A & Allender E (1981) Increased mortality among persons with rheumatoid arthritis, but where rheumatoid arthritis does not appear on the death certificate. *Scandinavian Journal of Rheumatology* **10:** 301–306.

Andersen PA, West SG, O'Dell JR (1985) Weekly pulse methotrexate in rheumatoid arthritis: clinical and immunologic effects in a randomized double-blind study. *Annals of Internal Medicine* **103:** 489–496.

Aponte J & Petrelli M (1988) Histopathologic findings in the liver of rheumatoid arthritis patients treated with long-term bolus methotrexate. *Arthritis and Rheumatism* **31:** 1457–1464.

Arden GB & Kolb H (1966) Antimalarial therapy and early retinal changes in patients with rheumatoid arthritis. *British Medical Journal* **1:** 270–273.

Berliner RW, Earle DP, Taggart JV et al (1948) Studies on the chemotherapy of the human malarias. VI. The physiological disposition, antimalarial activity and toxicity of several derivatives of 4-aminoquinoline. *Journal of Clinical Investigation* **27:** 98–107.

Bernstein HN (1983) Ophthalmologic considerations and testing in patients receiving long-term antimalarial therapy. *American Journal of Medicine* **75 (supplement):** 25–34.

Bernstein H & Ginsberg J (1964) The ocular pathology of chloroquine retinopathy. *Archives of Ophthalmology* **71:** 238.

Bjorkman DJ, Hammond EH, Leer G, Clegg DO & Tolman KG (1988) Hepatic ultrastructure after methotrexate therapy for rheumatoid arthritis. *Arthritis and Rheumatism* **31:** 1465–1472.

Brick JE, Moreland LW, Al-Kawas F et al (1989) Prospective analysis of liver biopsies before and after methotrexate therapy in rheumatoid patients. *Seminars in Arthritis and Rheumatism* **19:** 31–44.

Bridges SC, Alarcon GS & Koopman WJ (1989) Methotrexate-induced liver abnormalities in rheumatoid arthritis. *Journal of Rheumatology* **16:** 1180–1183.

Butler I (1965) Retinopathy following the use of chloroquine and allied substances. *Ophthalmologica* **149:** 204–208.

Cambioggi A (1957) Unusual ocular lesions in a case of systemic lupus erythematosus. *Archives of Ophthalmology* **57:** 451–453.

Carr RE, Gouras P & Gunkel RD (1966) Chloroquine retinopathy. Early detection by retinal threshold test. *Archives of Ophthalmology* **75:** 171–178.

Clegg DO, Furst DE, Tolman KG & Pogue R (1989) Acute, reversible hepatic failure associated with methotrexate treatment of rheumatoid arthritis. *Journal of Rheumatology* **16:** 1123–1126.

Crews SJ (1961) Chloroquine retinopathy with recovery in early stages. *Lancet* **ii:** 436–441.

Easterbrook M (1984) The use of Amsler grids in early chloroquine retinopathy. *Ophthalmology* **91:** 1368–1372.

Easterbrook M (1987) Dose relationships in patients with early chloroquine retinopathy. *Journal of Rheumatology* **14:** 472–475.

Easterbrook M (1988) Ocular effects and safety of antimalarial agents. *American Journal of Medicine* **85 (supplement):** 23–29.

Ehrenfeld M, Nesher R & Merins S (1986) Delayed-onset chloroquine retinopathy. *British Journal of Ophthalmology* **70:** 281–283.

Elman A, Gullberg R, Nilssen E et al (1976) Chloroquine retinopathy in patients with rheumatoid arthritis. *Scandinavian Journal of Rheumatology* **5:** 161–166.

Elner V, Schaffner T, Taylor K & Glagov S (1981) Immunophagocytic properties of retinal pigment epithelium cells. *Science* **211:** 74–76.

Fedorko M (1967) Effects of chloroquine on morphology of cytoplasmic granules in maturing leukocytes—an ultrastructural study. *Journal of Clinical Investigation* **46:** 1932–1942.

Finbloom DS, Silver K, Newsome DA & Gunkel R (1985) Comparison of hydroxychloroquine and chloroquine use and the development of retinal toxicity. *Journal of Rheumatology* **12:** 692–694.

Francois J & Maudgal MC (1967) Experimentally induced chloroquine retinopathy in rabbits. *American Journal of Ophthalmology* **64:** 886.

Fuld H (1959) Retinopathy following chloroquine therapy. *Lancet* **ii:** 617–618.

Hakulinen T, Isomaki H & Knekt P (1985) Rheumatoid arthritis and cancer studies based on linking nationwide registries in Finland. *American Journal of Medicine* **78 (supplement 1A):** 29–32.

Henkind P & Rothfield NF (1963) Ocular abnormalities in patients treated with synthetic antimalarial drugs. *New England Journal of Medicine* **269:** 433–439.

Hobbs H & Calnan C (1958) The ocular complications of chloroquine therapy. *Lancet* **i:** 1207–1209.

Hunter T, Urowitz MB, Gordon DA et al (1975) Azathioprine in rheumatoid arthritis. A long-term follow-up study. *Arthritis and Rheumatism* **18:** 15–20.

Isomaki HA, Mutru O & Koota K (1975) Death rate and causes of death in patients with rheumatoid arthritis. *Scandinavian Journal of Rheumatology* **4:** 205–208.

Isomaki HA, Hakulinen T & Joutsenlahti U (1978) Excess risk of lymphomas, leukemia and myeloma in patients with rheumatoid arthritis. *Journal of Chronic Disease* **31:** 691–696.

Kinlen LJ (1985) Incidence of cancer in rheumatoid arthritis and other disorders after immunosuppressive treatment. *American Journal of Medicine* **78 (supplement 1A):** 44–49.

Koota K, Isomaki H & Mutru O (1977) Death rate and causes of death in rheumatoid arthritis patients during a period of five years. *Scandinavian Journal of Rheumatology* **6:** 241–244.

Kremer JM & Lee JK (1986) The safety and efficacy of the use of methotrexate in long-term therapy for rheumatoid arthritis. *Arthritis and Rheumatism* **29:** 822–831.

Kremer JM, Galivan J, Streckfuss A & Kamen B (1986) Methotrexate metabolism analysis in blood and liver of rheumatoid arthritis patients. Association with hepatic folate deficiency and formation of polyglutamates. *Arthritis and Rheumatism* **29:** 832–835.

Kremer JM, Lee RG & Tolman KG (1989) Liver histology in rheumatoid arthritis patients receiving long-term methotrexate therapy. A prospective study with baseline and sequential biopsy samples. *Arthritis and Rheumatism* **32:** 121–127.

Krill AE, Potts AM & Johanson CE (1971) Chloroquine retinopathy. Investigation of discrepancy between dark adaptation and electroretinographic findings in advanced stages. *American Journal of Ophthalmology* **71**: 530–543.

Laakso M, Mutru O, Isomaki H & Koota K (1986) Cancer mortality in patients with rheumatoid arthritis. *Journal of Rheumatology* **13**: 522–526.

Laaksonen AL, Koskiahde V & Juva K (1974) Dosage of antimalarial drugs for children with juvenile rheumatoid arthritis and systemic lupus erythematosus. *Scandinavian Journal of Rheumatology* **3**: 103–108.

Lewis P, Hazleman BL, Hanka R & Roberts S (1980) Causes of death in patients with rheumatoid arthritis with particular reference to azathioprine. *Annals of the Rheumatic Diseases* **39**: 457–461.

Mackenzie AH (1970) An appraisal of chloroquine. *Arthritis and Rheumatism* **13**: 280–291.

Mackenzie AH (1983) Dose refinements in long-term therapy of rheumatoid arthritis with antimalarials. *American Journal of Medicine* **75** (supplement): 40–45.

Mackenzie AH & Scherbel AL (1980) Chloroquine and hydroxychloroquine in rheumatological therapy. *Clinics in Rheumatic Diseases* **6**: 545–566.

Mackenzie AH & Szilagyi PJ (1968) Light may provide energy for retinal damage during chloroquine therapy. *Arthritis and Rheumatism* **11**: 496–497.

Marks JS & Power BJ (1979) Is chloroquine obsolete in treatment of rheumatic diseases? *Lancet* **i**: 371–373.

Monson RR & Hall AP (1976) Mortality among arthritics. *Journal of Chronic Disease* **29**: 459–467.

Morgan SL, Baggott JE, Vaughn WH et al (1990) The effect of folic acid supplementation on the toxicity of low dose methotrexate in patients with rheumatoid arthritis. *Arthritis and Rheumatism* **33**: 9–18.

Nozik RA, Weinstock F & Vigros P (1964) Ocular complications of chloroquine. *American Journal of Ophthalmology* **58**: 774–778.

Nylander U (1967) Ocular damage in chloroquine therapy. *Acta Ophthalmologica* **92** (supplement): 5–71.

Okun G, Gouras P, Bernstein H & von Sallmann L (1963) Chloroquine retinopathy: a report of eight cases with ERG and dark-adaptation findings. *Archives of Ophthalmology* **69**: 59–71.

Percival SPB & Behrman J (1969) Ophthalmological safety of chloroquine. *British Journal of Ophthalmology* **53**: 101–109.

Prior P, Symmons DPM, Hawkins CF & Scott DL (1984) Cause of death in rheumatoid arthritis. *British Journal of Rheumatology* **23**: 92–99.

Rau R, Karger T, Herborn G & Frenzel H (1989) Liver biopsy findings in patients with rheumatoid arthritis undergoing long-term treatment with methotrexate. *Journal of Rheumatology* **16**: 489–493.

Roenigk HH, Averback R, Maibach HI & Weinstein GD (1982) Methotrexate guidelines revisited. *Journal of the American Academy of Dermatology* **6**: 145–155.

Rubin M (1968) The antimalarials and tranquilizers. *Diseases of the Nervous System* **29** (supplement): 67–76.

Rubin M & Slonicki A (1966) A mechanism for the toxicity of chloroquine. *Arthritis and Rheumatism* **9**: 537.

Rynes RI (1983) Ophthalmologic safety of long-term hydroxychloroquine sulfate treatment. *American Journal of Medicine* **75** (supplement): 35–39.

Sataline L & Farmer H (1962) Impaired vision after prolonged CQ therapy. *New England Journal of Medicine* **265**: 346.

Scherbel AL, Mackenzie AH, Nousek JE & Atdjian M (1965) Ocular lesions in rheumatoid arthritis and related disorders with particular reference to retinopathy. *New England Journal of Medicine* **273**: 360–366.

Shearer RV & Dubois EL (1967) Ocular changes induced by long-term hydroxychloroquine (Plaquenil) therapy. *American Journal of Ophthalmology* **64**: 245–252.

Shergy WJ, Polisson RP & Caldwell DS (1988) Methotrexate-associated hepatotoxicity: retrospective analysis of 210 patients with rheumatoid arthritis. *American Journal of Medicine* **85**: 771–774.

Thompson RN, Watts C, Edelman J, Esdaile J & Russel AS (1984) A controlled two-centre trial of parenteral methotrexate therapy for refractory rheumatoid arthritis. *Journal of Rheumatology* **11**: 760–763.

Tilson HH & Whisnant J (1985) Pharmaco-epidemiology—drugs, arthritis, and neoplasms:

industry contribution to the data. *American Journal of Medicine* **78** (supplement 1A): 69–76.

Tobin DR, Krohel GB & Rynes RI (1982) Hydroxychloroquine. Seven-year experience. *Archives of Ophthalmology* **100:** 81–83.

Tugwell P, Bennett K & Gent M (1987) Methotrexate in rheumatoid arthritis. *Annals of Internal Medicine* **107:** 358–366.

Urowitz MB, Smythe HA, Able T, Norman CS & Travis C (1982) Long-term effects of azathioprine in rheumatoid arthritis. *Annals of Rheumatic Disease* **41 (supplement):** 18–22.

Vanderbroucke JP, Hazevoet HM & Cats A (1984) Survival and cause of death in rheumatoid arthritis. *Journal of Rheumatology* **11:** 158–161.

Weinblatt ME, Coblyn JS, Fox DA et al (1985) Efficacy of low-dose methotrexate in rheumatoid arthritis. *New England Journal of Medicine* **312:** 818–822.

Weinblatt ME, Trentham DE, Fraser PA et al (1988) Long-term prospective trial of low-dose methotrexate in rheumatoid arthritis. *Arthritis and Rheumatism* **31:** 167–175.

Williams HJ, Willkens RF, Samuelson CO et al (1985) Comparison of low-dose oral pulses of methotrexate and placebo in the treatment of rheumatoid arthritis: a controlled clinical trial. *Arthritis and Rheumatism* **28:** 721–730.

Wollheim FA, Hanson A & Laurell CB (1978) Chloroquine treatment in rheumatoid arthritis. *Scandinavian Journal of Rheumatology* **7:** 161–176.

3

The risk of upper gastrointestinal haemorrhage during steroidal and non-steroidal anti-inflammatory therapy

PATRICK J. ROONEY
RICHARD H. HUNT

Mucosal damage to the upper gastrointestinal tract is a side-effect common to all the non-steroidal anti-inflammatory drugs (NSAIDs) in current use. These are among the most commonly used drugs throughout the world. It has been estimated that up to 20 billion aspirin tablets alone are consumed each year in the USA (Domschke and Domschke, 1984), and non-salicylate NSAIDs represent over a billion dollars in pharmaceutical company sales in one year (Baum et al, 1985). Upper gastrointestinal haemorrhage, as a complication of the use of NSAIDs, is now considered a major health-care problem and compulsory labelled warnings were required by the US Food and Drug Administration (FDA) from 1987 (Paulus, 1987; CSM, 1986).

Salicylates were first implicated as a cause of gastrointestinal bleeding in 1905 by Dreschfeld (cited by Bourne, 1961), but this causal relationship has remained controversial ever since (Langman, 1976; Belcon et al, 1985; Langman, 1988a). A similar debate has been evident regarding the non-salicylate NSAIDs (Eliakim et al, 1987; Belcon et al, 1985). Although less evident in the literature, the role of corticosteroids in gastrointestinal haemorrhage is also disputed (Spiro, 1977; Conn and Blitzer, 1976; Messer et al, 1983). The purpose of this review is to consider the evidence implicating each class of anti-inflammatory agents in the causation of major gastrointestinal bleeding; and to assess whether these risks justify the continued use of these agents in the clinic within different population groups.

A major difficulty in reaching valid conclusions about the relationship between anti-inflammatory drugs and gastroduodenal mucosal injury is caused by the likelihood that the incidence of such injury varies for each class of anti-inflammatory agent.

Aspirin acts on the mucosa of the upper digestive tract in more than one adverse way, and at least one of these effects is additional to that of non-acetylated salicylates (Davenport, 1966; Johnson and Overholt, 1967); the non-salicylate NSAIDs may act differently again (Rossi et al, 1987; Caruso and Bianchi-Porro, 1980), and corticosteroids probably have yet another mode of action.

Baillière's Clinical Rheumatology—
Vol. 4, No. 2, August 1990
ISBN 0–7020–1480–X

Similarly, there is no consistent relationship between drug ingestion, symptoms and the various types of injury recognized endoscopically. Dyspeptic symptoms are commonly reported by patients taking any of these agents (Upadhyay et al, 1990; Bijlsma, 1988); but such symptoms do not correlate with transient mucosal ulceration, with gastroduodenal microbleeding (Ivey, 1986), with chronic iron deficiency anaemia (Upadhyay, 1990), with major gastroduodenal haemorrhage (Husby et al, 1986), nor with peptic ulceration of the stomach (Giercksky, 1986; Husby et al, 1986) or duodenum (Jorde and Burhol, 1987). The relationship between each of these more objective entities is equally tenuous (Table 1).

Table 1. 24 potentially separate patient populations exist and to date have not received separate study.

	ASA	Other salicylate	Nonsalicylate NSAIDs	Steroids
Dyspepsia				
Transient mucosal ulceration				
Gastroduodenal microbleeding				
Major G.I. bleed				
Gastric ulcer				
Duodenal ulcer				

Thus the study of this problem is complicated by the fact that there are potentially 24 different populations involved. Much of the literature and previous research in this area fails to distinguish between these groups. This review attempts to do this in relation to the problem of major gastrointestinal bleeding.

DYSPEPSIA

That dyspepsia is caused by aspirin (acetylsalicylic acid) is not in doubt, although this drug was originally introduced in the hope of diminishing the dyspepsia caused by other salicylates (Gum, 1976; Dreser, 1989). Up to 40% of patients report dyspepsia with prolonged use of aspirin (Dick and Buchanan, 1971; Blechman et al, 1975) and there is some evidence that this effect is dose-related (Graham et al, 1988). Non-aspirin salicylates also cause dyspepsia. The acetyl group certainly changes the pharmacological properties of salicylic acid. Aspirin has a much greater inhibitory action on cyclo-oxygenase than non-acetylated salicylates (Vane, 1971; Estes and

Kaplan, 1980). Thus it would be expected that non-aspirin salicylates would have much fewer adverse effects on the gastroduodenal mucosa. Despite this, the clinical therapeutic response in rheumatoid arthritis patients is comparable (Singleton, 1980; Fazarinc and Steen, 1980; Multicenter Salsalate/Aspirin Comparison Study Group, 1989).

The newer, chemically esterified salicylates diflunisal (Hannah et al, 1977), benorylate (Liss and Palme, 1969) and salsalate (Aberg and Larsson, 1970) are not free from the problem of gastrointestinal bleeding but may be better tolerated from the point of view of dyspepsia (Huskisson et al, 1978). Cohen (1978) has indicated that the loss of chromium in the faeces from labelled red cells is much lower when salsalate is used rather than aspirin, and it has been suggested that there may be a lower incidence of gastrointestinal bleeding using this drug (Multicenter Salsalate/Aspirin Comparison Study Group, 1989). However, in view of the small numbers of reported studies such a conclusion can only be very tentative to date.

Dyspepsia is also a major side-effect of all non-salicylate NSAIDs (Coles et al, 1983; Ehsanullah et al, 1988; Caruso and Bianchi-Porro, 1980), although in most studies where direct comparison has been made, the incidence of dyspeptic symptoms is lower than that occurring with aspirin (Blechman et al, 1975; Gum, 1976; Cooperative Multicenter Canadian Trial, 1985; Multicenter Salsalate/Aspirin Comparison Study Group, 1989).

Different incidence rates of dyspepsia have been reported with different NSAIDs (Royer et al, 1975; Calin et al, 1977; Bower et al, 1979), but recent studies have challenged this (Giercksky, 1986; Duhamel et al, 1989), and no NSAID that has effective anti-inflammatory activity on the joints is free from this adverse effect (Eliakim et al, 1987). Many investigators are of the opinion that this NSAID side-effect is mediated solely through prostaglandin mechanisms (Hawkey and Rampton, 1985; Guth, 1986; Steel and Whittle, 1978) but evidence of this is lacking (Hawkey, 1988), although the pharmaceutical industry has spent a great deal of money developing therapeutic prostaglandins on the basis of this hypothesis (Hillman and Bloom, 1989).

MUCOSAL ULCERATION

While there is no doubt that dyspepsia forms one of the major obstacles to the use of NSAIDs in clinical practice, these drug-induced symptoms are, by themselves, of little concern as a major health-care problem, and it is the pathological lesions that develop in the mucosa of the gastrointestinal tract that concern rheumatologists and gastroenterologists alike. A large number of studies of the short-term and long-term effects of aspirin and NSAIDs on the gastric mucosa have been carried out using modern endoscopic techniques. Subjects who are on placebo medication tend to have a very low incidence of gastric mucosal injury (Lanza, 1984; Chernish et al, 1979; Lanza et al, 1981; Silvoso et al, 1979). However, up to 27% of normal subjects may have mucosal ulceration before any trial medication has been given (Akdamar et al, 1986), and very few trials are controlled for major confounding factors such as smoking, alcohol use, emotional stress, diet or drugs of other classes. From the major studies to date it seems likely that all NSAIDs increase gastric mucosal injury as observed at endoscopy, with aspirin proving in most studies to be the most ulcerogenic, although enteric coated preparations diminish this effect (Loebl et al, 1977; Cernish et al, 1979; Lanza et al, 1984; Rahbek, 1976; Kilander and Doterall, 1983; Lanza et al, 1989; Scheiman et al, 1989). After long-term use of NSAIDs for three months or more, up to 40% of subjects show mucosal lesions (Silvoso et al, 1979; Caruso and Bianchi-Porro, 1980). These results are disconcerting, since in neither short-term nor long-term studies was there any good correlation between dyspeptic symptoms and the endoscopic findings. Ehsanullah et al (1988) found no lesions in 18% of patients with dyspepsia caused by NSAIDs, while more than 50% of those with mucosal ulceration did not admit to any upper gastrointestinal symptoms. Many studies testify to a direct ulcerogenic effect of aspirin and NSAIDs on the gastric mucosa, both in the laboratory (Steel and Whittle, 1978) and in clinical practice (O'Laughlin et al, 1981; Hawkey, 1990). The balance of the evidence indicates a direct effect of the drugs on the mucosa, with aspirin being especially well documented in this regard because of its ionization characteristics and subsequent concentration within gastric epithelial cells (Davenport, 1966). Available studies indicate that the incidence of mucosal ulceration with aspirin on first ingestion is of the order of 80–100% (O'Laughlin et al, 1981; Lanza et al, 1980; Konturek et al, 1981; Smith et al, 1981). Although with continued exposure this incidence is known to fall (O'Laughlin et al, 1981)—a phenomenon termed mucosal adaptation (Graham and Smith, 1986)—about 30% of patients show such mucosal ulceration at any time during ingestion of aspirin or NSAIDs (Silvoso et al, 1979; Caruso and Bianchi-Porro, 1980).

GASTRODUODENAL BLEEDING

The identification of gastrointestinal haemorrhage is easy when sufficient bleeding occurs to cause red blood to appear in vomitus or faeces, or when bleeding is of sufficient severity to have major effects on cardiovascular homeostasis, causing hypotension, tachycardia and cardiovascular collapse. However, the identification of lesser degrees of haemorrhage are more controversial and this problem has been well reviewed by Belcon et al (1985).

Haemorrhage from the upper gastrointestinal tract is the most serious side-effect of NSAIDs. The literature in this area is very difficult to evaluate properly because it fails to distinguish between a number of different clinical problems, each of which may represent a distinct pathology.

Microbleeding

Increased faecal excretion of radiochromium label from tagged erythrocytes in the circulation is a consistent feature of both aspirin and non-salicylate

NSAID ingestion in normal subjects, as well as in patients with chronic rheumatic diseases (Croft and Wood, 1967; Hooper et al, 1984; Graham and Smith, 1986). The pharmaceutical industry spends a great deal of money comparing the amount of chromium excretion caused by any putative new NSAID and that caused by aspirin or other NSAIDS in current use. However, even where the excretion has been considerably reduced there is no evidence that the incidence of major gastrointestinal bleeding in clinical use of the drug will be any lower (Collins and Dutoit, 1987; Semble and Wu, 1987; Del Favero and Patoia, 1989). Nor is the source of this increased loss of label certain (Belcon et al, 1985). It has been stated that if the excretion of radiochromium exceeds the equivalent of 10 ml of blood per day, anaemia is likely to result (Domschke and Domschke, 1984). In studies of large groups of patients with rheumatoid arthritis the mean haemoglobin rises with time during the exhibition of aspirin (Barager and Duthie, 1960; New Zealand Rheumatism Study, 1974), although 80% of subjects using aspirin have increased excretion of label and of these a quarter exceed the 10-ml threshold (Grossman et al, 1961; Croft and Wood, 1967; Hooper et al, 1984; Graham and Smith, 1986).

Thus to date there is little evidence that this phenomenon of 'micro-bleeding' bears any direct relationship to the life-threatening major gastrointestinal bleeding which is the great concern of both rheumatologists and gastroenterologists alike, especially in the elderly female population (Langman, 1988b).

Major gastrointestinal bleeding

Major gastrointestinal bleeding has been the chief issue of concern relating to the use of aspirin and NSAIDs over the past fifty years. From the time of Dreschfeld (Bourne, 1961) until very recently, despite heated debate, the evidence for a causative relationship has been inconclusive (Belcon et al, 1985; Langman, 1976; Chalmers et al, 1988). Hawkey (1990), in a very thoughtful review, has laid out very clearly the evidence implicating NSAIDs in the causation of peptid ulceration of the gastroduodenal mucosa. Even this review fails to separate clearly the issues of uncompli-cated mucosal ulceration from the more life-threatening risk of major gastrointestinal haemorrhage. One careful study (Levy et al, 1988) has shown that the risk of major gastrointestinal bleeding after aspirin use is increased. The risk is also much enhanced in elderly females taking non-salicylate NSAIDs. As much as 20% of the major gastrointestinal bleeds in this group may be attributable to this cause (Langman, 1989). However, the evidence that endoscopic mucosal ulceration is the pathological lesion leading to these major haemorrhages is less clear (Soll et al, 1989; Langman, 1989). The large majority of major bleeds are due to peptic ulceration, but it is among those patients who do not have evidence of a chronic ulcer crater that there is evidence of an increased incidence of aspirin or NSAID use (Langman, 1970; Devine et al, 1979). Perhaps there is an excess of peptic ulceration due to NSAIDs as well, but this may be lost in the large number of ulcers from other causes.

Gastric peptic ulceration

It is now abundantly clear that chronic ingestion of aspirin is directly causative of gastric peptic ulcers. The studies from the literature are consistent in reaching this conclusion (Gillies and Skyring, 1968; Levy, 1974; Piper et al, 1981; Duggan et al, 1986; Chapman and Duggan, 1969; Henry et al, 1987), although the strength of the association has been extremely variable. Hawkey (1990) in a careful meta-analysis using some of the above studies, has shown a relative risk for aspirin causing gastric ulceration of 4.67. A similar relative risk (4.03) is demonstrated for non-salicylate NSAIDS (Cooke and Thomson, 1980; McIntosh et al, 1985; Duggan et al, 1986; Griffin et al, 1988). While there are clearly many instances where major gastrointestinal bleeding caused by NSAIDs is due to haemorrhage from chronic gastric peptic ulcer (Petersen, 1990), this is not the most common pathological lesion causing upper gastrointestinal bleeding in patients taking aspirin or NSAIDs (Graham, 1990).

Duodenal peptic ulcer

The evidence implicating aspirin or NSAIDs in the causation of duodenal peptic ulcer is more tenuous. The studies of aspirin by and large have failed to show any association (Gillies and Skyring, 1968; Levy, 1974; Cooke and Thompson, 1980; Clinch et al, 1983), but some studies have implicated other NSAIDs (Griffin et al, 1988) especially in the more serious complications of perforation and haemorrhage (Griffin et al, 1988; Quader and Logan, 1988; Smedley et al, 1988). Certainly there has been endoscopic evidence of mucosal damage in the duodenum (Eliakim et al, 1987), but the relationship between these two entities remains unclear.

STEROIDS

It remains uncertain whether corticosteroids *per se* are toxic to the upper gastrointestinal mucosa. There is no doubt these agents have a trophic effect on the gastric oxyntic cells (Crean, 1963). Steroids are generally not a cause of dyspepsia. Indeed, the major risk of the use of these drugs in relation to the gastrointestinal tract has been their tendency to mask gastrointestinal symptoms, especially those of major crises such as peptic ulcer perforation (Debas and Mulholland, 1989). Over the past twenty years a number of investigators have reviewed the evidence that steroids are ulcerogenic (Conn and Blitzer, 1976; Messer et al, 1983; Conn and Poynard, 1985). While Messer et al (1983) considered it likely that there was a direct causative association between peptic ulceration and the clinical use of steroids, the fallacies in their study were clearly exposed in the critical review by Conn and Poynard (1985).

Thus, at the present time, although the belief that steroids contribute to the causation of peptic ulcer remains widespread, the level of risk is of little concern in clinical practice (Jick and Porter, 1978; Conn and Poynard,

1985). On the other hand, whether the risk of NSAIDs to the upper gastroduodenal mucosa is enhanced by the concomitant use of steroids remains an unaddressed question.

CONCLUSION

Although aspirin and NSAIDs do cause upper gastrointestinal haemorrhage the overall risk is small; however, the risk is enhanced in elderly females where the use of NSAIDs is likely to be at its highest (Langman, 1988b). Current evidence from the FDA data on new NSAID and aspirin preparations suggests that after one year of treatment the incidence of clinically significant major gastrointestinal bleeding may be between 3% and 6% in this high-risk group (Temple, 1986).

Thus, although many thousands of patients benefit safely from these drugs, the risks are real. Conflicts in patient management between rheumatologist and gastroenterologist will remain because of contrasting impressions of the problem. The rheumatologist sees a long-time friend with increasing pain and discomfort and with deterioration in function and independence for whom any relief of symptoms is valuable. The gastroenterologist sees an elderly patient, otherwise well, whose life is threatened or lost by devastating haemorrhage caused by a medication that is not essential.

REFERENCES

Aberg G & Larsson RS (1970) Pharmacological properties of some antirheumatic salicylates. *Acta Pharmacologica et Toxicologica* **28:** 249–257.

Akdamar K, Ertan A, Agarwal NM, McMahon PG & Ryan J (1986) Upper gastrointestinal endoscopy in normal asymptomatic volunteers. *Gastrointestinal Endoscopy* **32:** 78–80.

Barager FD & Duthie JJR (1960) Importance of aspirin as a cause of anaemia and peptic ulcer in rheumatoid arthritis. *British Medical Journal* **1:** 1106–1108.

Baum C, Kennedy DL & Forbes MB (1985) Utilization of nonsteroidal antiinflammatory drugs. *Arthritis and Rheumatism* **28:** 686–692.

Belcon M, Rooney PJ & Tugwell P (1985) Aspirin and gastrointestinal haemorrhage. A methodologic assessment. *Journal of Chronic Disease* **38:** 101–111.

Bijlsma JWJ (1988) Treatment of endoscopy-negative NSAID-induced upper gastrointestinal symptoms with cimetidine: an international multicentre collaborative study. *Alimentary Pharmacology and Therapeutics* **25:** 75–83.

Blechman WJ, Schmid FR, April PA et al (1975) Ibuprofen or aspirin in rheumatoid arthritis therapy. *Journal of the American Medical Association* **233:** 336–340.

Bower RJ, Umbenhauer ER & Hercus V (1979) Clinical evaluation of sulindac; a new nonsteroidal antiinflammatory drug. In Weissman G, Samuelson B & Paolett R (eds) *Advances in Inflammation Research*, vol. 1, pp 559–567. New York: Raven Press.

Burne JC (1961) Drug induced gastrointestinal bleeding. *Lancet* **ii:** 599.

Calin A, Bennett RM, Sukhupunyarakssa S et al (1977) Double blind multicentre parallel trial of ketoprofen and ibuprofen in the treatment of rheumatoid arthritis. *Journal of Rheumatology* **4:** 153–157.

Caruso I & Bianchi-Porro G (1980) Gastroscopic evaluation of antiinflammatory agents. *British Medical Journal* **280:** 75–78.

Chalmers TC, Berrier J, Hewitt P et al (1988) Meta analysis of randomised controlled trials as a method of estimating rare complications of nonsteroidal antiinflammatory drug therapy. *Alimentary Pharmacology and Therapeutics* **25:** 9–26.

Chapman HL & Duggan JM (1969) Aspirin and uncomplicated peptic ulcer. *Gut* **10**: 443–450.

Chernish S, Rosenak BD, Brunelle RL & Crabtree R (1979) Comparison of gastrointestinal effects of aspirin and fenoprofen. A double blind crossover study. *Arthritis and Rheumatism* **22**: 76–83.

Clinch D, Banerjee AK, Ostick G & Levy DW (1983) Nonsteroidal antiinflammatory drugs and gastrointestinal adverse effects. *Journal of the Royal College of Physicians* **17**: 228–230.

Cohen A (1978) Faecal blood loss and plasma salicylate study of salicylsalicylic acid and aspirin. *Journal of Clinical Pharmacology* **19**: 242–247.

Coles LS, Fries JF, Draines RG et al (1983) From experiment to experience. Side effect of nonsteroidal antiinflammatory drugs. *American Journal of Medicine* **74**: 820–828.

Collins AJ & Dutoit JA (1987) Upper gastrointestinal findings and faecal occult blood in patients with rheumatic diseases taking nonsteroidal antiinflammatory drugs. *British Journal of Rheumatology* **26**: 295–298.

CSM (1986) Committee on Safety of Medicines Update. Nonsteroidal anti-inflammatory drugs and serious gastrointestinal reactions. *British Medical Journal* **292**: 614, 1190–1191.

Conn HO & Blitzer BL (1976) Nonassociation of adrenocorticosteroid therapy and peptic ulcer. *New England Journal of Medicine* **294**: 473–479.

Conn HO & Poynard T (1985) Adrenocorticosteroid administration and peptic ulcer: a critical analysis. *Journal of Chronic Disease* **38**: 457–468.

Cooke P & Thompson MR (1980) Old ladies, drugs and gastric ulceration. *Gut* **23**: A430.

Cooperative Multicenter Canadian Trial (1985) A double-blind comparison of piroxicam and enteric coated aspirin in rheumatoid arthritis. *Journal of Rheumatology* **12**: 68–77.

Crean GP (1963) The endocrine system and the stomach. *Vitamins and Hormones* **21**: 215–280.

Croft DN & Wood PHN (1967) Gastric mucosa and susceptibility to occult gastrointestinal bleeding caused by aspirin. *British Medical Journal* **1**: 137–141.

Davenport HW (1966) Fluid produced by the gastric mucosa during damage by acetic and salicylic acids. *Gastroenterology* **50**: 487–499.

Debas HT & Mulholland MW (1989) Approach to the patient with the acute abdomen. In Kelly WN (ed.) *Textbook of Internal Medicine*, pp 657–666. Philadelphia: J.B. Lippincott.

Del Favero A & Patoia L (1989) Nonsteroidal antiinflammatory drugs: seven years experience in preparing an annual review. *Clinical Experimental Rheumatology* **7(S3)**: 171–175.

Devine BL, Carmichael HA, Atherton ST, MacKenzie JF & Russell RI (1979) Aspirin, alcohol and acute gastrointestinal haemorrhage: an endoscopic study. *Gut* **20** (Supplement A): 433.

Dick WC & Buchanan WW (1971) Advances in the treatment of rheumatic disorders. *Practitioner* **207**: 483–491.

Domschke S & Domschke W (1984) Gastroduodenal damage due to drugs, alcohol and smoking. *Clinical Gastroenterology* **13**: 405–436.

Dreser H (1989) Pharmacologisches uber aspirin (acetylsalicylsaure). *Pfluger's Archiv* **76**: 306.

Duggan JM, Dobson AJ, Johnson H & Fahey P (1986) Peptic ulcer and nonsteroidal anti-inflammatory agents. *Gut* **27**: 929–933.

Duhamel C, Czernichow P, Dechelotte P, Ducrotte P, Lelrebours E & Colin R (1989) Hemorragies digestives hautes sous anti-inflammatoires. *Gastroenterologie Clinique et Biologique* **13**: 239–244.

Ehsanullah RSB, Page MC, Tildesley G & Wood JR (1988) Prevention of gastroduodenal damage induced by nonsteroidal antiinflammatory drugs: controlled trial of ranitide. *British Medical Journal* **297**: 1017–1021.

Eliakim R, Ophir M & Rachmilewitz D (1987) Duodenal mucosal injury with nonsteroidal antiinflammatory drugs. *Journal of Clinical Gastroenterology* **9(4)**: 395–399.

Estes D & Kaplan K (1980) Lack of platelet effect with the aspirin analog salsalate. *Arthritis and Rheumatism* **23**: 1303–1307.

Fazarinc F & Steen SN (1980) Long term management of rheumatoid arthritis with disalcid. *Journal of International Medical Research* **8**: 339–342.

Giercksky KE (1986) Piroxicam and gastrointestinal bleeding. *American Journal of Medicine* **81** (supplement 5B): 2–6.

Gillies M & Skyring A (1968) Gastric ulcer, duodenal ulcer and gastric carcinoma: a case controlled study of certain social and environmental factors. *Medical Journal of Australia* **2**: 1132–1136.

Graham DY (1990) The relationship between nonsteroidal antiinflammatory drug use and peptic ulcer disease. *Gastroenterology Clinics of North America* **19:** 171–182.

Graham DY & Smith JL (1986) Aspirin and the stomach. *Annals of Internal Medicine* **104:** 390–398.

Graham DY, Smith JL, Spjut HJ & Torres E (1988) Gastric adaptation studies in humans during continuous aspirin administration. *Gastroenterology* **95:** 327–333.

Griffin MR, Ray WA & Schaffner W (1988) Nonsteroidal antiinflammatory drug use and death from peptic ulcer in elderly persons. *Annals of Internal Medicine* **109:** 359–363.

Grossman M, Matsumoto KK & Lichter R (1961) Faecal blood loss produced by oral and intravenous administration of various salicylates. *Gastroenterology* **40:** 383–388.

Gum OB (1976) Fenoprofen in rheumatoid arthritis: a controlled crossover multicentre study. *Journal of Rheumatology* **3** (supplement 2): 26–31.

Guth PH (1986) Gastric blood flow and prostaglandin cytoprotection. *Scandinavian Journal of Gastroenterology* **21** (supplement 125): 86–91.

Hannah J, Royle WV, Jones H, Matzuk AR et al (1977) Discovery of diflunisal. *British Journal of Clinical Pharmacology* **4:** 7–13.

Hawkey CJ (1988) Nonsteroidal antiinflammatory drugs and the gastric mucosa: mechanisms of damage and protection. *Alimentary Pharmacology and Therapeutics* **25:** 57–64.

Hawkey CJ (1990) Non-steroidal anti-inflammatory drugs and peptic ulcers. Facts and figures multiply, but do they add up? *British Medical Journal* **300:** 278–284.

Hawkey CJ & Rampton DS (1985) Prostaglandins and the gastrointestinal mucosa: are they important in function, disease or treatment. *Gastroenterology* **89:** 1162–1188.

Henry DA, Johnston A, Dobson A & Duggan J (1987) Fatal peptic ulcer complications and the use of nonsteroidal anti-inflammatory drugs, aspirin and corticosteroids. *British Medical Journal* **295:** 1227–1229.

Hillman AL & Bloom BS (1989) Economic effects of prophylactic use of misoprostol to prevent gastric ulcer in patients taking nonsteroidal antiinflammatory drugs. *Archives of Internal Medicine* **149:** 2061–2065.

Hooper JW, Anslow JA, Martin WS et al (1984) Faecal blood loss during izoxicam and piroxicam administration for 28 days. *Clinical Pharmacology and Therapeutics* **38:** 533–537.

Husby G, Holme I, Rugstad HE, Herland OB & Giercksky KE (1986) A double blind multicentre trial of piroxicam and naproxen in osteoarthritis. *Clinical Rheumatology* **5:** 84–91.

Huskisson EC, Williams TN, Shaw LD et al (1978) Diflunisal in general practice. *Current Medical Research and Opinion* **5:** 589–592.

Ivey KJ (1986) Gastrointestinal intolerance and bleeding with non-narcotic analgesics. *Drugs* **32** (supplement 4): 71–89.

Jick H & Porter J (1978) Drug induced gastrointestinal bleeding. *Lancet* **ii:** 87–89.

Johnson LR & Overholt BF (1967) Release of histamine into gastric venous blood following injury by acetic and salicylic acid. *Gastroenterology* **52:** 505–509.

Jorde R & Burhol PG (1987) Asymptomatic peptic ulcer disease. *Scandinavian Journal of Gastroenterology* **22:** 129–134.

Kilander A & Doterall G (1983) Endoscopic evaluation of the comparative effects of acetylsalicylic acid and choline magnesium trisalicylate on human gastric and duodenal mucosa. *British Journal of Rheumatology* **22:** 36–40.

Konturek SJ, Obtulowicz W, Sito E et al (1981) Distribution of prostaglandins in gastric and duodenal mucosa of healthy subjects and duodenal ulcer patients: effect of aspirin and paracetamol. *Gut* **22:** 283–289.

Langman MJS (1970) Epidemiological evidence for the association of aspirin and acute gastrointestinal bleeding. *Gut* **11:** 627–634.

Langman MJS (1976) Aspirin is not a major cause of acute gastrointestinal bleeding. In Ingelfinger FJ, Ebert RV, Finland M & Relman AS (eds) *Controversy in Internal Medicine*, vol. 2, pp 493–499. Philadelphia: WB Saunders.

Langman MJS (1988a) Ulcer and ulcer complications from nonsteroidal anti-inflammatory drugs. What is the risk? *Alimentary Pharmacology and Therapeutics* **25:** 27–31.

Langman MJS (1988b) Ulcer complications and nonsteroidal antiinflammatory drugs. *American Journal of Medicine* **84** (supplement 2A): 15–19.

Langman MJS (1989) Epidemiologic evidence on the association between peptic ulceration and antiinflammatory drug use. *Gastroenterology* **96:** 640–646.

Lanza FL (1984) Endoscopic studies of gastric and duodenal injury after the use of ibuprofen, aspirin, and other nonsteroidal antiinflammatory agents. *American Journal of Medicine* **77**: 19–24.

Lanza FL, Royer GL, Nelson RS et al (1979) The effects of ibuprofen, indomethacin, aspirin, naproxen and placebo on the gastric mucosa of normal volunteers. A gastroscopic and photographic study. *Digestive Diseases and Sciences* **24**: 823–828.

Lanza FL, Royer GL & Nelson RS (1980) Endoscopic evaluation of the effects of aspirin, buffered aspirin, and enteric coated aspirin on the gastric and duodenal mucosa. *New England Journal of Medicine* **303**: 136–138.

Lanza F, Royer GL, Nelson RS et al (1981) A comparative endoscopic evaluation of the damaging effects of non steroidal antiinflammatory agents in the gastric and duodenal mucosa. *American Journal of Gastroenterology* **75**: 17–21.

Lanza FL, Nelson RS & Rack MF (1984) A controlled endoscopic study comparing the toxic effects of sulindac, naproxen, aspirin and placebo on the gastric mucosa of healthy volunteers. *Journal of Clinical Pharmacology* **24**: 89–95.

Lanza F, Rack MF, Doucette M, Ekholm B, Goldlust B & Wilson R (1989) An endoscopic comparison of the gastroduodenal injury seen with salsalate and naproxen. *Journal of Rheumatology* **16**: 1570–1574.

Levy M (1974) Aspirin use in patients with major upper gastrointestinal bleeding and peptic ulcer disease. *New England Journal of Medicine* **290**: 1158–1162.

Levy M, Miller DR, Kaufman DW et al (1988) Major upper gastrointestinal tract bleeding. Relation to the use of aspirin and other non narcotic analgesics. *Archives of Internal Medicine* **109**: 359–363.

Liss E & Palme G (1969) The pharmacokinetic behaviour of the new acetylsalicylic derivative 4-(acetamido) phenyl 2 acetoxybenzolite in animal tests. *Arzneimittel Forschung* (Aulendorf) **19**: 1177–1180.

Loebl DH, Craig RM, Culic DD et al (1977) Gastrointestinal blood loss, effect of aspirin, fenoprofen, and acetaminophen in rheumatoid arthritis as determined by segmental gastroscopy and radioactive faecal markers. *Journal of the American Medical Association* **237**: 976–981.

McIntosh JH, Byth K & Piper DW (1985) Environmental factors in the aetiology of chronic gastric ulcer; a case control study of exposure variables before the first. *Gut* **26**: 789–798.

Messer J, Reitman D, Sacks HS et al (1983) Association of adrenocorticosteroid therapy and peptic-ulcer disease. *New England Journal of Medicine* **309**: 21–24.

Multicenter Salsalate/Aspirin Comparison Study Group (1989) Does the acetyl group of aspirin contribute to the antiinflammatory efficacy of salicylic acid in the treatment of rheumatoid arthritis. *Journal of Rheumatology* **16**: 321–327.

New Zealand Rheumatism Study (1974) Aspirin and the kidney. *British Medical Journal* **1**: 593–600.

O'Laughlin JC, Hofteizer JW & Ivey KJ (1981) Effect of aspirin in the stomach in normals: endoscopic evaluation of damage produced one hour, 24 hours and 2 weeks after administration. *Scandinavian Journal of Gastroenterology* **16** (supplement): 211–214.

Paulus H (1987) FDA Arthritis Advisory Committee Meeting: Risks of agranulocytosis/aplastic anaemia, flank pain, and adverse gastrointestinal effects with the use of nonsteroidal antiinflammatory drugs. *Arthritis and Rheumatism* **30**: 593–595.

Peterson WL (1990) Bleeding peptic ulcer epidemiology and nonsurgical management. *Gastroenterology Clinics of North America* **19**: 155–170.

Piper DW, McIntosh JH, Ariotti DE, Fenton BH & MacLennan R (1981) Analgesic ingestion and chronic peptic ulcer. *Gastroenterology* **80**: 427–432.

Quader K & Logan RFA (1988) Peptic ulcer (PV) deaths: how many occur at home or after nonsteroidal antiinflammatory drug (NSAID) prescribing (abstract). *Gut* **29**: A1443.

Rahbek I (1976) Gastroscopic evaluation of the effects of a new antirheumatic compound, ketoprofen on the human gastric mucosa. A double blind crossover trial against acetylsalicylic acid. *Scandinavian Journal of Rheumatology* **14**: 63–72.

Rossi AC, Hsu JP & Faich GA (1987) Ulcerogenicity of piroxicam: an analysis of spontaneously reported data. *British Medical Journal* **294**: 147–150.

Royer GL, Moxley TE, Hearron MS et al (1975) A six month double blind trial of ibuprofen and indomethacin in osteoarthritis. *Current Therapeutic Research* **17**: 234–238.

Scheiman JM, Behler EM, Berardi RR & Elta GH (1989) Salicylsalicylic acid causes less gastroduodenal mucosal damage than enteric coated aspirin—an endoscopic comparison. *Digestive Diseases and Sciences* **34:** 229–232.

Semble EL & Wu WC (1987) Antiinflammatory drugs and gastric mucosal damage. *Seminars in Arthritis and Rheumatism* **16:** 271–286.

Silvoso CR, Ivey KJ, Butt JH et al (1979) Incidence of gastric lesions in patients with rheumatic disease on chronic aspirin therapy. *Annals of Internal Medicine* **91:** 517–520.

Singleton PT (1980) Salsalate: its role in the management of rheumatic disease. *Clinical Therapeutics* **3:** 80–102.

Smedley FH, Taube M, Leach R & Wastell C (1988) Nonsteroidal antiinflammatory drugs: retrospective study of bleeding and perforated peptic ulcers (abstract). *Gut* **29:** A1443.

Smith JL, Graham DY & Dobbs SM (1981) The course, extent and duration of acute aspirin injury to the stomach of man. *Gastrointestinal Endoscopy* **27:** 129.

Soll AH, Kurata J & McGuigan JE (1989) Ulcers, nonsteroidal antiinflammatory drugs and related matters. *Gastroenterology* **96:** 561–568.

Spiro HM (1977) *Clinical Gastroenterology*, 2nd edn. New York: Macmillan.

Steel G & Whittle BJR (1978) Gastric damage induced by topical salicylate can be potentiated by aspirin or indomethacin. *British Journal of Pharmacology* **81:** 78.

Temple R (1986) FDA's NSAID GI warning. *Scrip* **1163:** 11.

Upadhyay R, Torley HI, McKinlay AW, Sturrock RD & Russell RL (1990) Iron deficiency anaemia in patients with rheumatic disease receiving nonsteroidal anti-inflammatory drugs: the role of upper gastrointestinal lesions. *Annals of the Rheumatic Diseases* **49:** 359–362.

Vane JR (1971) Inhibition of prostaglandin synthesis as a mechanism of action for aspirin-like drugs. *Nature* **231:** 232–235.

4

Intramuscular versus oral gold therapy

W. F. KEAN

The element gold has been known to humans since the earliest civilizations. The presumed magical qualities of gold and its resemblance to the 'essence' of the sun made it a natural choice by priests, healers and shamans. The medical use of gold was known to the Chinese circa 2500 BC (Wiegleb, 1965). The dramatic Biblical account of Moses burning the golden calf, preparing a potion from the ashes, and forcing the Children of Israel to '. . . drink of it', is probably one of the earliest accounts of the practice of alchemy involving gold (Exodus 32:20). The Taoist philosophers of China circa 600 BC (Waley, 1956; Fung, 1952) used gold and silver to enhance the quality of their medicines; Pliny the Elder and Dioscorides in the first century AD recorded the use of gold as a medicinal agent (Garrison, 1966a,b). In the great Persian medical schools initiated by the Nestorian Christians, pharmacist–physicians such as Yabir, Avicenna and Rhazes all advocated the use of gold compounds as panaceas. Yabir is attributed with the discovery of the formulation of aqua regia. Medical knowledge from Arab culture spread into Europe and the British Isles by the eleventh and twelfth centuries. One of the first gold researchers in the British Isles was the Franciscan scholar Roger Bacon (circa 1214–1292 AD), who documented one of the first known descriptions of gold chloride (Pattison-Muir, 1972).

Paracelsus advocated the use of gold as a panacea, but the modern use of gold compounds in medicine occurred in the early nineteenth century through the work of Andre-Jean Chrestien and Pierre Figuier (1765–1817), two professors at the University of Montpellier (Hunt, 1979). Figuier, a pharmacist, provided the chemical formulation for the gold compounds, in particular gold sodium chloride, which Chrestien advocated as of value in the treatment of tuberculosis and syphilis.

It was the observation of Dr Robert Koch that gold cyanide was bactericidal in vitro to tubercle bacilli (Koch, 1890) that led European scientists and physicians over the next forty years to experiment with the use of gold complexes in the treatment of human and bovine tuberculosis. The erroneous but serendipitous assumption by Dr Jacques Forestier that rheumatoid disease was an infectious disease analogous to tuberculosis led him to use gold thiopropanol sodium sulphonate on 15 patients with inflammatory rheumatoid disease (Forestier, 1929). The success of this initial experiment was the seed that led researchers over the next fifty years

Baillière's Clinical Rheumatology—
Vol. 4, No. 2, August 1990
ISBN 0–7020–1480–X

to investigate both the beneficial and the toxic effects of antiarthritic gold complexes.

CHEMISTRY

Gold is a soft, yellow, lustrous metal, with a unique stability since it is not attacked by either oxygen or sulphur at any temperature (Puddephatt, 1978). Gold is present at approximately 0.004 parts per million in the Earth's crust. Gold deposits on Earth exist as the metallic form or in mineral form, either as tellurides such as calaverite and krennerite (different crystalline forms of $AuTe_2$), montbrayite (Au_2Te_3) and mixed gold–silver tellurides such as sylvanite ($AuAgTe_4$) (Puddephatt, 1978). To a lesser extent mineral forms of auriferous sulphides also exist (Mohide, 1981). Metallic gold and silver–gold mixtures also exist, perhaps the most well-known being electrum, which contains 20% silver.

Gold is classified as a Group IB metal in the period table. The most commonly recognized oxidation states are I, II, III and V, although metal–metal bonds do exist in complexes in which it is difficult to assign a formal oxidation state to the gold atom. The true salts of Au(I) such as the halides are unstable in the presence of water and disproportionate to Au^o (metallic gold) and Au(III). However, Au(I) can be stabilized by the formation of complexes with 'soft' ligands (Pearson, 1963) such as the thiolates and phosphines. All currently used antiarthritic gold complexes exist as Au(I) thiol or phosphine compounds (Sadler, 1982). The high toxicity of the Au(III) complexes such as chlorauric acid ($HAuCl_4$), makes them unsuitable for human use. Elder and colleagues have shown that if sodium aurothiomalate (gold sodium thiomalate) is administered to laboratory animals, the gold recovered from the tissue and urine exists in the Au(I) oxidation state—i.e. the same oxidation state as the gold in sodium aurothiomalate—and not the Au(III) oxidation state (Elder et al, 1983). Further, if $Au(III)Cl_3$ is administered to laboratory animals, gold recovered in tissues and urine exists only in the Au(I) oxidation state. The Au(I) oxidation state therefore appears to be the primary oxidation state in a biological milieu.

A common misconception among members of the medical profession is the idea that D-penicillamine may be used as a chelating agent for gold, if a toxic reaction occurs during or following the administration of the antiarthritic gold complexes. There is no theoretical nor biochemical evidence that D-penicillamine chelates Au(I) in vivo. Au(I) compounds normally have a linear geometry in which the Au(I) atom is attached to only two ligand atoms (X) such that the X–Au(I)–X angle is 180°. Less frequently, and only for rather specific ligands, Au(I) binds to three or four ligand atoms. Thus one would expect D-penicillamine to bind to Au(I) only through the sulphydryl site. As supported by the studies of Davis and Barraclough (1977), there is no theoretical reason why D-penicillamine should chelate Au(I) (Kean and Lock, 1983).

The antiarthritic gold complexes and related structures

The current commonly used gold complexes in the treatment of rheumatoid arthritis and in related research work are illustrated in Figure 1.

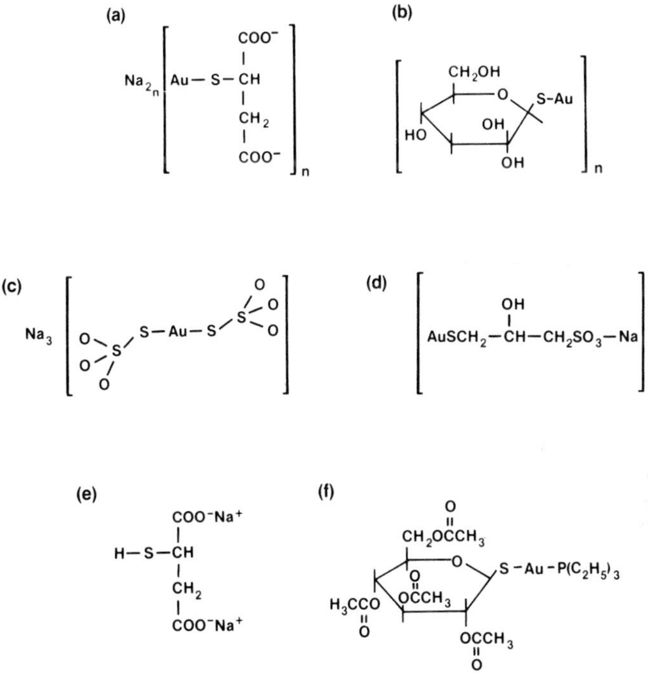

Figure 1. Structures of commonly used gold complexes: (a) sodium aurothiomalate; (b) aurothioglucose; (c) sodium aurothiosulphate; (d) sodium auro-3-thio-2-propanol-1-sulphonate; (e) disodium thiomalate; (f) 2,3,4,6-tetra-o-acetyl-1-thio-β-D-glucopyranosato-S(triethylphosphine) gold.

Sodium aurothiomalate has been used in the treatment of rheumatoid arthritis since the early 1930s. It is marketed by May & Baker (UK), Rhône-Poulenc (Canada) and Merck Sharp & Dohme (USA) as vials of 50 mg/ml of compound suspended in sterile water for use as an intramuscular injection. The compound contains approximately 51% gold and 0.3 mol of glycerol per mol of thiomalate. During the manufacturing process glycerol is used in the final purification step. The vials of compound marketed for human use also contain the following preservatives: phenylmercuric nitrate 0.002% (May & Baker preparation); chlorocresol 0.05% (Rhône-Poulenc preparation); benzyl alcohol 0.5% (Merck Sharp & Dohme preparation). The currently assumed molecular weight of sodium aurothiomalate is 390.12. This value is based on the empirical formula of the compound but clearly this structure is incompatible with the known chemical properties of

Au(I) and a more likely explanation of the structure is that of a polymer or oligomer (Shaw et al, 1979; Sadler, 1976; Isab and Sadler, 1976, 1981).

Aurothioglucose (gold thioglucose) (Figure 1b) was manufactured in the USA by Merck Sharp & Dohme in the early 1930s and is currently manufactured under the brand name Solganal by the Schering Corporation of New Jersey. It is administered as an intramuscular injection. Although it is water soluble, it is marketed as 50 mg/ml of aurothioglucose in sterile sesame oil with 2% aluminium monostearate; 1 mg of propyl p-hydroxybenzoate is added as a preservative. Gold content is approximately 50.25% and the molecular weight based on the empirical formula is 392.18, but as with sodium aurothiomalate, the structural formulation of aurothioglucose based on the known chemistry of gold is most likely an oligomer (Figure 1).

Sodium aurothiosulphate (Figure 1c) is marketed as Sanochrysine in Europe by Nordiske in Denmark, in vials of 100 mg/ml of compound for use as an intravenous injection. It has been available since 1924 when it was first introduced by Möllgard. The compound has a molecular weight of 490.21 and contains 40.19% gold. The anion contains two thiosulphate moieties bound to gold through the sulphur atoms. Sodium aurothiosulphate is one of the few Au(I) compounds whose structure is known and which has been studied crystallographically.

Sodium auro-3-thio-2-propanol-1-sulphonate (Figure 1d) is marketed in Europe as Allochrysine lumiere by Laboratoires de Therapeutique Moderne France. The manufacturer lists the gold content as being 30%, but some analysts place the value as high as 52.9%. This variation may be dependent upon associated H_2O molecules or variations in the structural formulation of the gold compound during the manufacturing process (see discussion on sodium aurothiomalate). This compound, like sodium aurothiomalate, is most probably a small polymer. It was the original compound used by Forestier in 1928–9 and is still widely used in France, Switzerland and other parts of Europe.

The compound 2,3,4,6-tetra-o-acetyl-1-thio-β-D-glucopyranosato-S(triethylphosphine) gold (Figure 1f) is manufactured as auranofin by Smith Kline & French in the USA. It is a monomeric species with a gold phosphine bond as well as a gold thiol bond. It is marketed as a 3-mg tablet administered orally. The compound is a white, odourless, crystalline solid which is insoluble in water. The powder is unstable and must be protected from light and heat. On a weight basis it contains approximately 29% gold and has a molecular weight of 678.5 with a melting point of 112–115°C.

Gold keratinate is manufactured in Germany as Aurodetoxin by Beecham-Walfing. It is basically a gold thiol structure attached to a polypeptide with the graphic representation of Au-S-R where R represents the polypeptide. The compound contains approximately 13% of Au(I). Gold distribution studies indicate that the gold from this compound binds predominantly to albumin (90%) with approximately 5% bound to macroglobulins. It is still widely used in Germany as an antiarthritic agent.

Many other active Au(I) thiol antiarthritic agents have been developed in this century, but the majority of research (both basic scientific and clinical), has been carried out on the gold compounds listed above.

PHARMACOKINETICS

Injectable gold compounds

The chemical structures of the commonly used injectable gold complexes, such as sodium aurothiomalate and aurothioglucose, are not known. Knowledge of their pharmacokinetic profiles is therefore largely centred on the measurement of the gold molecule. These compounds are not monomeric Au(I) salts but are most probably small polymeric structures. For these reasons extrapolation of the pharmacokinetics of the gold molecule as an interpretation of drug activity is not useful.

The Au moiety of the injectable gold complex is rapidly absorbed into the circulation after intramuscular injection. After each 50-mg injection, peak serum levels of 700–1000 µg% are achieved in 2–6 hours. In the succeeding 6 days the serum levels fall to around 300 µg%. Approximately 75% of the gold is excreted via the kidney and the remainder in the faeces. More than 95% of the administered gold is bound to albumin and the remainder of the gold is bound to the macroglobulins (Herrlinger, 1983; Rudge et al, 1983).

The gold from injectable gold compounds is widely distributed throughout the reticuloendothelial system, particularly in the phagocytic cells of the liver, bone marrow, lymph nodes, spleen, and also in the synovium (Kean et al, 1984a). Gold deposition in the skin is predominantly in the dermal area and there is a quantitative correlation between the amount of gold in the dermis and the total dose given (Aaron et al, 1984). Electron-dense deposits of gold are also seen in the tubular cells of the kidney, another site rich in sulphydryl-containing enzymes, but the presence of gold associated with the glomerulus is extremely uncommon (Nagi et al, 1971).

Gold levels have also been detected in the milk of lactating mothers and in the serum and red blood cells of the nursing infant. The presence of the gold in the serum and red blood cells of the infant indicate that the chemical composition or binding of the Au as presented to the infant is in an orally absorbable form (Blau, 1973).

Auranofin

Like the gold thiol compounds, auranofin only contains Au(I) and also binds predominantly to albumin (Shaw, 1979).

Following administration of [195]Au-labelled auranofin, approximately 25% of the administered dose is detected in plasma and peak concentrations of 6–9 µg/100 mL are reached in 1–2 hours (Giannini et al, 1984; Walz et al, 1983). The plasma half-life is in the order of 15–25 days with a total body elimination of 55–80 days (Blocka, 1983). Only about 1% of [195]Au is detectable by 180 days, whereas up to 30% of [195]Au from sodium aurothiomalate may be detected at this time (Gottlieb et al, 1974).

MECHANISM OF ACTION

Injectable gold compounds

The definitive mechanism of action of the injectable gold compounds is unknown. In vitro, these gold thiol compounds have been shown to inhibit prostaglandin synthesis (Penneys et al, 1974), to modulate phagocytic cells (Davis et al, 1979a) and to have the capacity to either kill or inhibit the growth of tubercle bacilli (Koch, 1890). The gold thiol compounds are also known to inactivate the first component of complement (C1) (Schultz et al, 1974) and to inhibit lysosomal enzymes such as acid phosphates, β-glucuronidase (Ennis et al, 1968), elastase (Janoff, 1970) and cathepsin G (Starkey and Barrett, 1976). In our own laboratories we have shown that sodium aurothiomalate—but no other gold compound—inhibits the action of the serine esterase enzyme thrombin, both in vitro and in vivo (Kean et al, 1984a,b; 1986).

An extensive literature exists on the action of gold compounds in vivo and in vitro on immune response. With regards to effect on humoral immunity, studies have shown that sodium aurothiomalate treatment causes a fall in all classes of immunoglobulin and also rheumatoid factor titre (Persellin et al, 1967; Strong et al, 1973; Gottlieb et al, 1975; Lorber et al, 1978). Sodium aurothiomalate has been shown to have a significant effect on cell-mediated immune responses in vitro (Rosenberg and Lipsky, 1979). The addition of sodium aurothiomalate on day one of lymphocyte culture will inhibit lymphocyte transformation to the mitogen phytohaemagglutinin (Cahill, 1977) and Concanavlin A (Lipsky and Ziff, 1977). It has been shown by Lipsky and Ziff that the direct effect of the gold compound was on the monocyte, thus inhibiting the helper function of the macrophages (Lipsky and Ziff, 1977). A similar effect is seen with mixed lymphocyte culture in which sodium aurothiomalate will inhibit the mixed lymphocyte reaction if it is added on day one (Harth et al, 1977; Davis et al, 1979a; Russell et al, 1982).

Sodium aurothiomalate has an indirect effect on human B-cell function both in vitro and in vivo, probably due to inhibition of the human monocyte. This latter effect may be mediated through some inhibition of interleukin-I production and/or function (Rischke et al, 1984; Goto et al, 1981).

There are no known interactions between the injectable antiarthritic gold compounds and other drugs, although it is advisable to avoid using drugs that are potential marrow suppressants (e.g. phenylbutazone) when using gold. Several centres are at present claiming less toxicity and equal benefit when hydroxychloroquine and sodium aurothiomalate are given together.

Auranofin

Chemical structure, biological actions and pharmacokinetic studies indicate that the oral compound auranofin differs from the injectable gold thiol compounds (Walz et al, 1983). Walz and colleagues showed that auranofin inhibited carrageenan-induced oedema in rats in a dose-related fashion in concentrations of 40, 20 and 10 mg/kg, with maximum inhibition of 86% at the highest dose, and a serum gold level of approximately 10 µg/mL. The two basic ligands of auranofin, namely triethylphosphine oxide and 2,3,4,6-tetra-o-acetyl-1-thio-β-D-glucopyranosato, were without biological activity, and sodium aurothiomalate, aurothioglucose and the thiomalic acid did not significantly affect rat paw oedema (Walz et al, 1971). Auranofin was shown to significantly suppress adjuvant arthritis, whereas the ligands were without any effect. Auranofin inhibits antibody-dependent complement lysis, whereas antibody-dependent complement lysis is enhanced in the serum of rats treated with sodium aurothiomalate (Walz et al, 1983).

The gold thiol compounds, particularly sodium aurothiomalate, are ubiquitous inhibitors of cellular enzymes, particularly the serine esterase enzymes such as elastase and cathepsin G (Kean et al, 1984a,b). No specific inhibitory effect of auranofin on these enzymes has been recorded, but auranofin has been shown to inhibit the release of lysosomal enzymes such as β-glucuronidase and lysozyme from stimulated polymorphs (Walz et al, 1983). Aurothioglucose has no apparent effect on extracellular release of lysosomal enzymes. Similarly the ligands of the above gold complexes have no effect on either release or enzyme inhibition. Auranofin is a potent inhibitor of antibody-dependent cellular cytotoxicity exhibited by polymorphs from adjuvant arthritic rats. In contrast, sodium aurothiomalate, aurothioglucose and the ligands of auranofin had no significant effect on polymorphonuclear antibody-dependent cellular cytotoxicity. Depending on the system used to study superoxide production, auranofin is a much more potent inhibitor of superoxide production than sodium aurothiomalate. In certain systems such as an immune phagocytosis system, sodium aurothiomalate was devoid of inhibitory activity at a concentration 40 times that of auranofin, which had produced marked inhibition (Walz et al, 1983). Walz and colleagues postulated that auranofin has also been shown to be more potent than sodium aurothiomalate in the inhibition of cutaneous migration, chemotaxis and phagocytosis by peripheral blood monocytes.

Lipsky and colleagues have shown that auranofin, like sodium auro-thiomalate, inhibits lymphoblastogenesis in vitro by direct inhibition of mononuclear phagocyte function, but also has an inhibitory effect on lymphocyte function not seen with sodium aurothiomalate. The inhibitory action on monocytes is achieved with concentrations of auranofin that are 10–20 times lower than those of the sodium aurothiomalate (Salmerton and Lipsky, 1983). The above findings suggest that auranofin has immunosuppressive activity. In general, patients with active rheumatoid disease have a decreased capacity for either mitogen-stimulated lymphoblastogenesis or for lymphoblastogenesis produced by the mixed lymphocyte reaction. Although patients initially treated with sodium aurothiomalate exhibit suppression of mitogen-stimulated lymphoblastogenesis, those who eventually respond to the drug will have normalization of lymphocyte responsiveness in vitro (Percy et al, 1978). In contrast, within a few weeks of patients receiving auranofin, lymphocyte responsiveness is markedly inhibited (Lorber et al, 1977). Thus auranofin has powerful immunosuppressant effects in vitro and acts at concentrations an order of magnitude lower than the injectable gold compounds. This may reflect major differences in the pharmacological properties of the oral compounds versus the injectable gold thiol compounds. Indeed it has been proposed that auranofin could have potential in cancer therapy (Simon et al, 1979) because of its potent immunosuppressive properties (Crooke, 1982). No data are yet available on the safety of long-term auranofin treatment with respect to the dangers of long-term immunosuppression. In contrast, sodium aurothiomalate can be given with safety for prolonged periods of time with no recorded evidence of increased mitotic disease.

INDICATIONS FOR GOLD THERAPY

Injectable gold compounds

Injectable gold therapy is indicated in the treatment of rheumatoid arthritis, Felty's syndrome, polyarticular juvenile rheumatism, psoriatic arthritis and palindromic rheumatism. Patients with prior serious blood, liver or renal disease should be reviewed by a specialist before being given gold therapy (Kean and Anastassiades, 1979). Gold therapy should be avoided during pregnancy, although there are numerous reports of the drug being administered during pregnancy without any major adverse reactions being recorded (Tarp et al, 1983). The drug administration dosage schedule for injectable gold was derived empirically from Forestier's original use of these compounds (Forestier, 1929). Gold compound injections are started in patients who have failed to respond to an unhurried trial of non-steroidal anti-inflammatory drugs (NSAIDs) (Kean and Anastassiades, 1979). An initial test dose of 10 mg is given in the first week, followed by 25 mg intramuscularly in the second week. In subsequent weeks 50 mg intramuscularly is given for 20 weeks, followed by maintenance therapy every 2–4 weeks. Maintenance therapy is given for an indefinite time if there are no instances of any serious side-effects related to the administration of gold.

Discontinuing gold therapy is usually considered on the basis of no response, toxicity or the development of a complete remission. Patients who have not responded to the drug after at least 20 months of therapy probably will not benefit. If a patient develops remission it is recommended that the NSAID be slowly discontinued initially, then the interval between injections of the gold compound be increased gradually prior to completely stopping the gold drug. Should clinical symptoms recur, the NSAID therapy should be reviewed and restarted at maximum tolerable anti-inflammatory dose, and injectable gold therapy should be restarted or increased to weekly injections until the previously achieved clinical response is obtained (Kean and Anastassiades, 1979). When patients are being treated with injectable gold therapy it is recommended that a clinic monitoring chart be used to record the efficacy, toxicity and haematological and urinary test results.

The general response to injectable gold therapy is that 65–70% of patients improve clinically. The majority of these patients have what is known as a partial remission, although complete remission with no evidence of disease activity occurs in approximately 10% of all patients treated with the drug (Kean and Anastassiades, 1979). A response to therapy usually occurs after a period of 10–12 weeks. Approximately 20–30% of patients have to discontinue therapy because of no response. In the studies that have been done there is no clinical evidence to suggest that the drug should be withheld from the elderly rheumatoid patient. In this age group the injectable compound has been shown to be as effective as for young people at any time period examined after three months of therapy (Kean et al, 1983).

Auranofin

Auranofin, the oral gold compound, is indicated in all of the conditions tested above for injectable gold. It is available in 3-mg capsules. The usual initiating dose is 3 mg twice daily, and this can be increased to 3 mg three times daily. In clinical studies of rheumatoid arthritis it has been shown that the oral gold compound is better than placebo and similar in efficacy to the injectable gold compounds (Ward et al, 1983). The time of onset of benefit with the oral gold compound is again about 5–10 weeks. Claims of complete disease suppression have not been reported.

ADVERSE EFFECTS

Injectable gold compounds

Adverse reactions are the major limiting factor to the use of injectable gold compounds. Approximately 30–50% of patients who receive the injectable gold compound will develop some form of toxicity (Kean and Anastassiades, 1979).

Skin rash is the most common side-effect and occurs in approximately 30% of patients. The rash is usually a dry, itchy area, approximately 1–10 cm in diameter. Most lesions are slightly erythematous with scaly patches resembling a seborrhoeic rash. The most common distribution is on the hands, forearm, trunk and shins, and occasionally the face. The drug should be discontinued following the development of skin rash and should not be reintroduced until the rash has completely resolved. The drug should then be administered in low doses of 10 mg or 25 mg intramuscularly. Severe skin rash problems in the form of nummular eczema, total exfoliation and intense pruritus have been known to develop. Exfoliation constitutes a medical emergency and appropriate support measures (such as observation of electrolytes) should be undertaken. Problems are less common when a strict monitoring system is in force.

Oral ulceration occurs in approximately 20% of patients who receive injectable gold therapy. The ulcers may or may not be painful and in appearance resemble the aphthous ulcer. The most common site of occurrence of these ulcers is the mucous membrane in the vestibule of the mouth. Occasionally the lesion is present on the tongue or the hard palate. The development of a mouth ulcer is a definite contraindication to gold therapy until the ulcer has resolved. On occasion, oral ulceration has preceded the development of pemphigoid-like bullous skin lesions.

There is a wide variation (0–40%) in the reported frequency of protein-uria (Cooperating Clinics Committee, 1973; Furst et al, 1977; Kean and Anastassiades, 1979; Kean et al, 1983; Ward et al, 1983). One reason for this discrepancy in the literature has been a considerable variation in the definition of what constitutes proteinuria (Kean and Anastassiades, 1979). Most authors agree that persistent spillage of protein in urine in amounts of 1+ by dipstick over two to three weeks warrants a 24-hour urine protein examination. If proteinuria is less than 500 mg for 24 hours the drug should be continued. Between 500 and 3000 mg for 24 hours, gold therapy should be withheld until it is established that renal function is normal. Patients whose proteinuria is greater than 3000 mg for 24 hours should have the gold therapy stopped until the proteinuria resolves. There are no well-documented cases of any long-term serious or permanent renal damage due to gold therapy. The most common histological lesion is that of a membranous glomerulo-nephritis (Tornrot and Skrifvars, 1974), although heavy metal tubular damage does occur during injectable gold therapy (Merle et al, 1980). Proteinuria secondary to oral gold is extremely uncommon (Ward et al, 1983). If microscopic haematuria develops gold therapy should be stopped immediately and a cause for the haematuria sought. Once proteinuria has reduced in quantity or the haematuria has resolved gold therapy may be reinstated at a reduced dosage.

Most laboratories now specify a value of $150\,000\,10^6/l$ as a lower level of normal for the platelet count. Physicians monitoring gold therapy, however, should observe a platelet count of less than $200\,000\,10^6/l$ as an indication to withhold gold therapy. A falling platelet count even within the normal range may be equally ominous. A sudden change in a weekly platelet count which has been steady at $400\,000\,10^6/l$ to $210\,000\,10^6/l$ makes it advisable to with-hold gold therapy until a repeat platelet count confirms a stable value above $200\,000\,10^6/l$ on at least two occasions one week apart. If a fall in platelet count results in a value that is persistently less than $200\,000\,10^6/l$ extreme caution is advised, and where facilities are available, blood should be tested for the presence of platelet surface associated IgG autoantibodies (Kelton et al, 1984). Platelet antibodies do not appear to be present with the much rarer gold-induced thrombocytopenia secondary to bone marrow suppression. Although it has been stated that thrombocytopenia secondary to injectable gold therapy may occur precipitously, close observation of changes in platelet count even within the normal range should result in earlier identifi-cation of some patients who may potentially develop a sudden thrombo-cytopenia. The development of thrombocytopenia secondary to injectable gold therapy is an absolute contraindication to the further use of the gold compound. Over the past five years many studies report that the presence of HLA-DR3 may be indicative of an increased risk of a patient developing thrombocytopenia associated with platelet surface antibodies (Ford, 1984).

Bone marrow suppression secondary to the gold compounds is rare, but is a sufficiently serious complication to warrant strict monitoring on a weekly basis (Kean and Anastassiades, 1979). The marrow suppression secondary to either injectable gold therapy or oral gold therapy appears to be due to direct action of the drug on the marrow cells (Howell et al, 1975). A fall in platelet count as recorded above, a fall in haemoglobin below 100 mmol/l or a fall in total white count below $4000\,10^6/l$ requires immediate discon-tinuation of therapy until cause and effect have been established. A reversal of the white cell differential ratio or a rise in monocyte count above 0.1 are also indications for immediate discontinuation of the gold drug until at least two normal values, one week apart, have been recorded. If any of the above indicators of haemopoiesis remain abnormal a bone marrow examination and investigation for autoantibodies to white cells, red cells and platelets are essential before gold therapy can be reintroduced. Bone marrow suppression secondary to gold compounds is an absolute contraindication to further continuation of therapy.

Despite this potential for the rare side-effect of bone marrow suppression it should be noted that during routine gold therapy for rheumatoid disease return to normal of the haemoglobin is one of the first indications of clinical improvement. Recent work in our laboratory by Dr Andrew Harvey has shown that some forms of rheumatoid anaemia have a humoral basis and it can be postulated that modulation of the humoral mechanisms by injectable gold compounds may result in improvement of rheumatoid anaemia (Harvey et al, 1983). In spite of the potential for gold compounds to induce marrow suppression, injectable gold compounds are now recognized as the treatment of choice for Felty's syndrome (Gowans and Salami, 1973). The drug should be administered in exactly the same manner as described for rheumatoid disease. The recommended starting dose is 10 mg or 25 mg weekly until an observed rise in the absolute white count takes place. Physicians without facilities for the assessment of bone marrow tissue should avoid using gold compounds in the treatment of Felty's syndrome.

The nitritoid reaction or immediate allergic reaction appears to be unique to sodium aurothiomalate. Affected patients experience flushing, sweating, headache, joint pain, hypertension or hypotension and, on occasion, chest pain which has led to myocardial infarction in one reported case (Harris, 1977). The variable chemical structure of sodium aurothiomalate may be implicated in precipitating this toxic reaction. The nitritoid reaction is not seen with any other gold compound, and is usually mild and self-limiting. Patients need only be switched to either aurothioglucose or the oral gold compound if they find the nitritoid reaction intolerable.

Pulmonary injury associated with gold therapy has been reported in the form of a diffuse interstitial lung disease, usually with radiologically visible infiltrates (Winterbauer et al, 1976; McCormick et al, 1980; Scott et al, 1981). Fortunately pulmonary toxicity is rare and usually responds to the withdrawal of the injectable gold compound. Idiopathic toxicity in the form of cholestatic jaundice (Favreau et al, 1977) and also acute enterocolitis (Stein and Urowitz, 1976) has also been reported secondary to the injectable gold compounds, particularly sodium aurothiomalate. Hepatic toxicity is rare but appears to be predominantly of the cholestatic type either with frank jaundice or with elevated bilirubin, alkaline phosphatase, aspartate aminotransferase and alanine aminotransferase. The drug should be stopped immediately. The condition may appear early or late in the treatment regimen. No specific mechanism of action has been determined. In general the condition is self-limiting but in 1937 Hartfall and colleagues in a review of 900 patients treated with injectable gold compounds recorded 85 cases of toxic jaundice, 2 of which resulted in death from subacute necrosis of the liver (Hartfall, 1937). This incidence is not observed in any modern study and it is not possible to determine from Hartfall's paper what associated factors may have been present. In view of the rare association of hepatic toxicity with the injectable gold compounds all other causes of jaundice should be excluded before assuming a cause and effect relationship with the gold compound.

Deposition of gold in the lens of the eye (Gottlieb and Major, 1978) and in the cornea (Panayi et al, 1978) has been reported, but this does not seem to result in any specific damage to visual acuity.

Elderly patients do not appear to be at increased risk from gold therapy (Kean et al, 1983), although specific caution should be taken with regard to haematological toxicities, since bone marrow aplasia secondary to any drug is more commonly recorded in the elderly than in the young. In one study in 1983 (Kean et al, 1983) it was shown that the elderly responded to sodium aurothiomalate just as well as young adults and that the drop-out rate for no response and toxicity was the same in both groups. However, it was noted that serious haematological toxicity only occurred in patients over 42 years old and nephrotic syndrome only occurred in patients over 52 years old in that study. The elderly should not be denied injectable gold therapy in the treatment of rheumatoid disease.

Over the past nine years numerous reports have observed the possible association of toxicity to injectable gold compounds (and D-penicillamine) and the patient's human leucocyte antigen (HLA) types (Ford, 1984). HLA-D4 and HLA-DR4 are present in 25–30% of normals but are found in rheumatoid patients in a ratio of 2:1 over controls, although this is less apparent in Jewish and East Indian groups. However, patients with HLA-DR3 (also claimed to be associated with increased levels of rheumatoid factor) have been shown to be at increased risk of developing toxic reactions to injectable gold sodium thiomalate and also to D-penicillamine. In 1978 Panayi and colleagues reported on 95 patients with rheumatoid arthritis and noted that although there was no increase in HLA-DR3 over controls, 14 out of 18 with DR3 had a toxic reaction to gold or D-penicillamine and that 7 of 8 patients with HLA-DR2 had a toxic reaction (Panayi et al, 1978). HLA-DR2 has been reported to be associated with mouth ulcers (Panayi et al, 1979) but the association between HLA-DR2 and toxicity in general has been disputed. Several reports suggest that HLA-DR2 and also HLA-DR7 may be protective against the development of toxicity and, like HLA-DR4, the HLA-DR2 group may be a disease modifier (Repice et al, 1979). In a follow-up report Panayi and colleagues reported that 79% of patients with HLA-DR3/B8 developed proteinuria while on gold (14 out of 15) or on D-penicillamine (9 out of 13) (Wooley et al, 1980). Subsequent reports reviewed by Ford have claimed an association with HLA-DR3 and thrombocytopenia, HLA-DR3/B8 and proteinuria and HLA-DR3 alone for skin rash (Ford, 1984). The last association is unusual in view of the known linkage disequilibrium between HLA-DR3 and B8 (Ford, 1984). DeQueker and colleagues found no association between gold thiopropanol sodium sulphonate use and HLA groups, but they did find an association between HLA-B8 (but not DR3) and proteinuria (DeQueker et al, 1984); again, an unusual outcome in view of the linkage disequilibrium between DR3 and

B8. Dr Ford pointed out that most studies, if not retrospective, only looked at the first 6 months of therapy, when clearly side-effects due to gold or penicillamine can occur at any time (Kean and Anastassiades, 1979; Ford, 1984). In particular it is our experience and that of others that proteinuria occurs predominantly between 6 and 15 months (Kean and Anastassiades, 1979; Kean et al, 1983; Ward et al, 1983; Cooperating Clinics Committee, 1973; Furst et al, 1977). It is of interest that HLA-DR3 and B8 are rare in Japanese people, and that in a large Japanese trial of D-penicillamine, proteinuria occurred in only 2.2% of patients (Shiokana et al, 1977).

Most investigators agree that HLA-DR3 and HLA-B8 are associated with drug toxicity, particularly proteinuria in association with injectable gold therapy and D-penicillamine. However, patients with these antigens should not be denied therapy with these agents since the relative risk does not outweigh the clinical benefit.

Auranofin

Change in stool pattern, with the development of loose, soft stools, is the most common side-effect of auranofin therapy and may occur in over 40% of treated patients (Van Riel et al, 1983a; Bandilla et al, 1983). The frequency of this side-effect is highest in the first month of treatment. It should be noted that the lower incidence of altered stool pattern in later months may be directly related to the drop-out of patients susceptible to the diarrhoea. The development of frank, watery diarrhoea occurs in 2–5% of patients and is dose related, but some patients are totally intolerant of even 3 mg per day. The postulated mechanism is an elevation in cyclic AMP in the gut mucosal cell with a resultant outpouring of intracellular contents (Van Riel et al, 1983a).

Rash is another common side-effect of auranofin therapy, occurring in up to 20% of patients. Half of these patients also experience pruritus. Rash is most common in the first year of therapy but can occur at any time. When rash develops, the drug should be withheld until the condition resolves. Approximately 2–3% of patients have to discontinue therapy because of severe skin rash (Ward et al, 1983).

Stomatitis occurs in 1–12% of patients and may be concomitant with skin rash. The occurrence is greatest in the first month but, like other side-effects, may occur at any time (Ward et al, 1983).

Non-specific digestive system complaints account for approximately 20% of all side-effects and 2% of all withdrawals (Morris et al, 1984).

Conjunctivitis occurs in 4% of patients and occurs with equal frequency at any time period throughout treatment.

Although less common than with injectable gold therapy, proteinuria occurs in up to 5% of patients treated with auranofin. The drug should be withheld and assessments of renal function made in a manner similar to that for injectable gold toxicity to the kidney.

Rarely thrombocytopenia and bone marrow suppression may occur as a result of auranofin treatment. This type of thrombocytopenia (unlike the more common type seen with sodium aurothiomalate) does not have platelet surface associated autoantibodies. The treatment of choice is immediate withdrawal of drug therapy. The development of thrombocytopenia or a low white blood cell count is an absolute contraindication to therapy.

Despite the apparent overall lower number of side-effects occurring with auranofin compared with injectable gold compounds, auranofin should not be considered a benign drug. A strict monitoring system as for injectable gold compounds should be undertaken for each patient. Insufficient data are available at present to determine whether there will be any long-term side-effects related to auranofin therapy. Particular attention should be paid to effects on immune functions related to long-term therapy.

CLINICAL STUDIES

Injectable gold compounds

In 1928 Dr Jacques Forestier hypothesized that since the manifestations of rheumatoid arthritis were similar to those of tuberculosis, gold compounds (shown to be of benefit against the dreaded bacillus) could be effectively employed against chronic rheumatoid arthritis (Kean et al, 1985). In his original series, Forestier treated 11 women and 4 men (mean age 42 years) with 250 mg of gold thiopropanol sodium sulphonate given as weekly intramuscular injections. Five patients had an excellent response, 5 patients were much improved and 2 were recorded as having a minimal response. In 3 patients insufficient knowledge of outcome was available, but according to the author, none of them was worse (Forestier, 1929). Significant improvement was thus recorded in local and general features of a hitherto progressive, destructive disease.

In February 1930 Jacques Forestier supported his initial findings by reporting the outcome of a further 33 patients with symmetrical inflammatory polyarthritis which he believed to be consistent with rheumatoid arthritis. The outcome of this second study confirmed the efficacy and toxicity data of the first, and also showed that the use of 100 mg of gold thiopropanol sodium sulphonate weekly was probably less toxic and equally effective compared with the original higher dose of 250 mg weekly (Forestier, 1930).

In 1934, at the Hunterian Address (Forestier, 1934), Forestier presented the results of 50 patients with rheumatoid arthritis treated with gold compounds. He recorded a 70–80% success rate. Fifty per cent of patients treated early in the disease state were permanently improved, compared with only 25% of patients with disease of two or more years' duration. In his discussion of gold compounds Forestier stated that sodium aurothiomalate and aurothioglucose were the most useful agents. In this publication, Forestier recorded a fatal case of agranulocytosis, which was his first reported death due to gold therapy.

Over the next ten years numerous descriptive analyses of gold therapy in rheumatoid disease appeared in the literature. In a series of publications between 1935 and 1937 (Hartfall and Garland, 1935, 1937; Hartfall et al,

1937), Hartfall and colleagues recorded their observations of benefit and toxicity due to gold therapy in patients with rheumatoid arthritis. The final article described the outcome of 900 patients (750 of whom were rheumatoid patients) treated with gold compounds. Striking improvement was noted in approximately 70% of patients and toxicity occurred in 42% of cases, although only 6% were severe. The relapse rate was 21% and the authors stated that relapse was less common if two courses of gold therapy were given.

Hartfall and colleagues also stated that gold therapy was of doubtful value in other forms of arthritis. This has never been challenged by a series of controlled clinical trials, although in 1978 Dorwart et al (1978) reported a comparative trial of gold therapy with either sodium aurothiomalate or sodium aurothioglucose in patients with psoriatic arthritis compared with patients with rheumatoid arthritis. The authors recorded that the 14 patients with psoriatic arthritis had greater benefit and less toxicity than the 42 patients with rheumatoid arthritis. Except for this study and that of Brewer et al (1980) on the use of gold therapy in juvenile rheumatism, no other controlled study of injectable gold therapy has been done to examine efficacy and toxicity in the other rheumatic diseases.

Uncontrolled studies on the use of gold therapy in rheumatoid disease suggested that the drugs were of benefit to between 50% and 80% (Snyder et al, 1939; Rawls, 1944) of patients given these compounds, but that a wide range of adverse effects occurred which could be serious and even fatal.

In 1939 Sir Stanley Davidson, chairman of the Scientific Advisory Committee of the Empire Rheumatism Council, proposed a multicentre, controlled, double-blind trial to investigate the compound sodium aurothiomalate in rheumatoid arthritis. World War II disrupted the success of this initial proposal, but the late Dr Thomas N. Fraser of Glasgow completed his section of the multicentre trial at the Western Infirmary of Glasgow and published his results in 1945 (Fraser, 1945). Fraser's trial was the first published double-blind, controlled trial of any antirheumatic drug. It confirmed Forestier's original findings and demonstrated an efficacy rate of 82% in the treated group compared to 45% in the control patients. Fraser emphasized that the results should only be interpreted within the confines of the study group. The control group had a marked improvement rate which was apparently unexpected. He explained firstly that all study patients received physiotherapy, and secondly, that some spontaneous remissions might have occurred. If this also accounted for some improvement in the group receiving sodium aurothiomalate, improvement attributable to gold therapy would be reduced to 42%. It is important to note that 72% of the control group recorded a subjective improvement, although for the purpose of the study improvement was only recorded for the 45% who showed objective improvement. This suggests that a considerable psychological factor might have been operative.

In 1947 Waine and colleagues reported on 58 patients treated with either sodium aurothiomalate or aurothiosulphate. All patients received a minimum of 500 mg with an average total dose of 1600 mg. The authors reported a significant improvement in 57% of the treated group compared with 29%

of controls. However, the controls were a group of 62 rheumatoid arthritis patients who were treated only with 'supportive' therapy and who did not receive a placebo injection (Waine et al, 1943).

In 1950 Adams and Cecil reported on 106 patients with rheumatoid disease who received either sodium aurothiomalate or aurothioglucose during the first year of their disease (Adams and Cecil, 1950). The total dose of compound given was between 1000 mg and 1500 mg. These authors recorded a 66% rate of remission (by their definition) in the group treated with gold, compared with a remission rate of only 24.1% in the control group. These figures were not comparable, since the control group only received conventional therapy and no placebo injection. Remission occurred on average 10 months later in the control group than in the gold-treated group (17 months and 7 months respectively). The average time from remission to relapse was 27 months. The authors concluded that gold therapy increases the incidence and accelerates the appearance of remission if given during the first year of the disease.

In contrast to the beneficial effects of injectable gold therapy over conventional therapy so far cited, Merliss and colleagues found that aurothioglycolanilide (Lauron) given over six months to 27 patients was no better than saline or serum injections given to 44 control patients over a similar period of time (Merliss et al, 1951).

The largest series of data recorded to date is the 47 years of clinical experience with injectable gold therapy documented by Dr Maxwell Lockie of Buffalo and reported at the Pan-American Congress of Rheumatology in Washington, DC in 1982. Dr Lockie recorded the outcome of 1019 patients with classical or definite rheumatoid disease treated with injectable gold between 1933 and 1980. There were 317 males and 702 females of mean age 46 and 47 years respectively. His patients were assessed as having 'mild', 'moderate' or 'severe' disease. At the discontinuation of therapy the 'mild' group had increased by 95% and the 'moderate' and 'severe' groups had decreased by 35% and 37% respectively. Thirty-eight patients discontinued therapy because of disease remission and 589 (59%) patients discontinued therapy because of a serious side-effect (Lockie et al, 1982).

The need for hard scientific evidence as to the usefulness of injectable gold compounds led the Empire Rheumatism Council in 1957 to plan a second multicentre trial in 24 centres throughout the UK. Ninety-nine patients in the treated group received 1000 mg of sodium aurothiomalate as 50 mg injections weekly over 20 weeks. One hundred control patients were given 0.01 mg of sodium aurothiomalate as 0.5 µg weekly over a 20-week period (i.e. they received 1×10^{-6} the quantity of gold compound received by the controls). It was unequivocally demonstrated that in most patients given the 50 mg weekly dose of sodium aurothiomalate, there was progressive improvement in a number of objective variables, including the number of joints clinically inflamed, grip strength and sedimentation rate. Although gold therapy was stopped after 20 weeks (1000 mg of compound), improvement persisted for up to 12 months in many patients and was generally maintained up to 18 months. However, by the 30th month (i.e. 24 months after gold therapy had been discontinued), little if any advantage was recorded in the original gold treatment group compared with controls (Empire Rheumatism Council, 1960). In 1973 the Cooperating Clinics Committee of the American Rheumatism Association reported their double-blind trial of 68 patients with definite or classical rheumatoid arthritis (Cooperating Clinics Committee, 1973). The initial phase of this study compared 36 patients who received sodium aurothiomalate 50 mg weekly for six months and a control group of 32 patients who received sterile water vehicle over the same period. Twelve patients in the group treated with gold dropped out because of adverse effects, and 8 patients in the placebo group dropped out because of no benefit. The gold-treated group showed slight but definite improvement in all parameters measured, although only the change in sedimentation rate was statistically significant. In the second phase of the study, designed to compare the results of maintenance therapy, patients received six 50-mg doses at two-week intervals until a total of two years of treatment had been given. Control patients received the sterile water vehicle. In this phase the group receiving gold showed no increase in the number of involved joints, improved their grip strength and demonstrated a fall in sedimentation rate, but the control group deteriorated in all of these measurements. The results of the Co-operating Clinics Committee trial confirmed the results of the Empire Rheumatism Council trial and suggested that the larger sample size of the latter allowed the differences recorded for grip strength and number of active joints to reach statistical significance as had been achieved by the sedimentation rate. The two trials were comparable in almost all respects but there were marked differences in the duration of disease prior to therapy. The majority of patients in the Empire Rheumatism Council trial had disease of less than three years' duration and a maximum duration of five years; whereas patients in the Cooperating Clinics Committee trial had no disease duration limit, and almost one-third of the patients had had rheumatoid arthritis for longer than five years. If injectable gold works better when given early in the disease process, this would explain the greater demonstrable benefit in the Empire Rheumatic Council trial results.

Sigler and colleagues reported a two-year double-blind study of 13 patients who received sodium aurothiomalate compared with 14 patients who received placebo identical in appearance to the gold compound (Sigler et al, 1974). Significant improvements in relation to global measurement, ring size and grip strength were recorded in the gold-treated group. The most striking finding was the claim by the authors that radiological examination showed arrest of bone and cartilage destruction in several patients, and that the mean progression rate of destruction was significantly slowed for the treated group. In the Cooperating Clinics Committee trial, posteroanterior radiographs of the hands were taken at the beginning and end of phase one (0–27 weeks). The results obtained by a single-blinded observer indicated deterioration in nine of 19 controls and 3 of 20 gold-treated patients. This difference was not significant ($P = 0.06$) but favoured gold therapy as being possibly beneficial. In the Empire Rheumatism Council trial no significant radiological differences were detected between the gold-treated group and the control group in terms of joint narrowing, development of new erosions or extension of new erosions in any period of the trial. The minimal differences that did occur were in favour of the gold-treated group. The apparent arrest or even regression of radiological changes recorded by Sigler et al has also been recorded in a much larger but uncontrolled study by Luukhainen et al (1977).

Thus double-blind trials have confirmed that injectable gold therapy is of value in the treatment of rheumatoid disease. The dosage schedule, however, has been achieved by empirical means based on descriptive analyses and poorly controlled comparative studies. Furst and colleagues questioned whether 50 mg of sodium aurothiomalate weekly was equally efficacious and less toxic than higher doses, by comparing the outcome in 23 patients who were given 50 mg of sodium aurothiomalate weekly, with a group of 24 patients who were given 150 mg weekly (Furst et al, 1977). Drug administration and evaluations were carried out double-blind. Serum gold concentrations were recorded but did not correlate with efficacy or toxicity. The conventional dose—50 mg weekly—was just as efficacious as the high dose—150 mg weekly. However, side-effects were more frequent and severe in the high-dose group. These findings are identical to those observed by Forestier in his second publication on the use of gold thiopropanol sodium sulphonate (Forestier, 1930).

Since the results of Fraser's trial and subsequent confirmation by the Empire Rheumatism Council trial, sodium aurothiomalate has become the most widely used injectable gold compound in the treatment of rheumatoid arthritis. However, aurothioglucose is used in the USA and aurothiosulphate is still used in Europe. In 1972 Sutton and colleagues reported that orally administered alkylphosphine gold coordination complexes exhibited anti-inflammatory properties when administered to adjuvant arthritic rats (Sutton et al, 1972), and in the same year the same group reported that triethylphosphine gold chloride was equipotent to parenterally administered sodium aurothiomalate in suppressing the inflammatory lesions of adjuvant arthritis (Walz et al, 1972). Triethylphosphine gold chloride is extremely toxic in humans and further studies were not evaluated. However, a related compound auranofin, 2,3,4,6-tetra-o-acetyl-1-thio-β-D-glucopyranosato-S(triethylphosphine) gold, was shown to exhibit anti-arthritic properties (Walz et al, 1976). Subsequent studies have shown that this compound is beneficial in the treatment of rheumatoid arthritis (Ward et al, 1983; Finkelstein et al, 1976).

Auranofin

The first clinical study of auranofin by Finkelstein et al (1976) described eight patients with rheumatoid arthritis treated for 12 weeks followed by a 12-week period on placebo. During the treatment period the total number of active joints fell from 60 to 17 at week 12 and to 9 at week 15. Clinical improvement was recorded at 5 weeks and in general the drug was well tolerated. Rheumatoid factor titre, IgG levels and α_2-macroglobulin levels fell during the treatment period. During the following 12-week placebo period, IgG levels rose and patients experienced a flare-up in disease activity, suggestive of a cause and effect action of the drug.

Calin and colleagues reported on 137 patients given either 1 mg or 9 mg of auranofin in a double-blind fashion (Calin et al, 1982). At the first 12-week period approximately 60% of the 1-mg group and 33% of the 9-mg group broke the code because of insufficient therapeutic effect. It was also noted that reduction in immunoglobulins IgM and IgG and reduction in ESR were greater for patients receiving the 9-mg dose. Conclusions from this interim assessment were that 1 mg was insufficient for therapeutic effect but 9 mg caused sufficient diarrhoea to make this dosage unsuitable. The majority of studies since conducted have involved the use of either 3 mg or 6 mg per day. Most investigators have found that a dosage of 6 mg per day is significantly better than placebo, although a higher frequency of diarrhoea is noted with this dosage than at the 3-mg dosage.

A multicentre, double-blind, controlled trial of auranofin versus sodium aurothiomalate has been reported (Rau et al, 1983). All patients were given appropriate placebo injections or placebo tablets. In a 1983 interim report 121 patients were assessed, 59 on auranofin and 62 on sodium aurothiomalate. There was an equal distribution between the groups for age, duration of disease, age at onset of disease, American Rheumatism Association anatomical stage (majority stage II) and functional class. There were slightly more patients in the higher functional class (class III) in the auranofin group. After 12 weeks of therapy improvement in pain score was greater for the sodium aurothiomalate group compared with the auranofin group, although the scores were approximately the same by 24 weeks. In a group of 46 patients who had received 48 weeks of therapy, pain scores were better in the sodium aurothiomalate group at both 12 and 24 weeks, but had equalized to the auranofin group by week 48. The authors concluded that sodium auro-thiomalate influenced pain more rapidly than auranofin. Similarly the decrease in Lansbury Articular Index and Lansbury Activity Index was more rapid and more pronounced in the sodium aurothiomalate group. Improvement in ESR values was better for the sodium aurothiomalate group at both 24 and 48 weeks. Improvement in grip strength was faster with sodium auro-thiomalate, but better in the auranofin group at 24 weeks. The overall benefit in grip strength was the same at 24 weeks. Morning stiffness reduction was faster in the sodium aurothiomalate group at 24 weeks but the overall reduction in duration was equal at 48 weeks. Twenty-one patients in the sodium aurothiomalate group—but none of the auranofine group—were able to reduce the dosage of the drug at 24 weeks because of 'striking improve-ment'.

Patients on auranofin experienced 192 adverse reactions, 34% being diarrhoea and a further 34% other gastrointestinal side-effects. Aphthous ulcers, skin rash and pruritus accounted for 22%, 12% and 25% respectively of all side-effects. Conjunctivitis occurred in 9% and alopecia occurred in 9%. Nine of the 59 patients on auranofin dropped out of the study because of adverse reactions. Seven had serious mucocutaneous reactions, 1 had herpes zoster and 1 had a haemorrhagic cystitis. There were 177 side-effects recorded in the 62 patients who received sodium aurothiomalate. Diarrhoea ($n = 11$) and other gastrointestinal side-effects ($n = 11$) accounted for 34% of all side-effects. This is an unusually high incidence for diarrhoea or gastro-intestinal upset, and has not been recorded with such frequency in any other double-blind controlled trial of the drug. Rash, pruritus, alopecia and conjunctivitis occurred in 42%, 7% and 11% respectively. Again it should be noted that alopecia and conjunctivitis are rarely recorded in other studies of sodium aurothiomalate. Eleven patients dropped out of the sodium aurothiomalate group because of severe adverse reactions: 4 had skin rash; 1 had eosinophilia; 3 had injection reaction; 1 had abnormal liver function; 1 had dysuria and 1 had osteomyelosclerosis. Dysuria and osteomyelo-sclerosis are not recognized side-effects of sodium aurothiomalate and are most likely incidental findings.

The authors suggested that sodium aurothiomalate acts faster than auranofin and may be clinically superior in overall outcome.

In 1982 Katz and colleagues reported a randomized, double-blind, con-trolled study of 242 patients who received three months of therapy and 144 patients who received six months of therapy with 3 mg twice daily of auranofin or with placebo (Katz et al, 1982). Significant improvement in the treated group was recorded for the number of tender joints at three months and six months and for the number of swollen joints and increase in grip strength at six months. The investigators' global assessment of efficacy was recorded as significantly improved at three months and six months in the auranofin group for those patients recorded as having a marked improve-ment. The authors concluded that the addition of auranofin to NSAID therapy added to the benefit derived from the latter in the treatment of rheumatoid arthritis (Katz et al, 1982).

In 1983 Van Riel and colleagues reported a single-blind trial of 26 patients treated with auranofin compared with 26 patients treated with aurothio-glucose (Van Riel et al, 1983). The authors felt that aurothioglucose was superior to auranofin in that the index of disease activity measured showed a clinically significant benefit of aurothioglucose over auranofin at four months and nine months. The 10 patients who dropped out of therapy because of lack of response to auranofin developed a beneficial clinical response when started on D-penicillamine. More side-effects were recorded for aurothio-glucose ($n = 21$) than auranofin ($n = 14$). Adverse response was the major reason (20% of total) for drop-out from therapy from aurothioglucose.

In 1983 Ward and colleagues who comprised the Cooperative Systematic Studies of Rheumatic Diseases group reported a prospective, controlled, double-blind multicentre trial which compared placebo, auranofin and sodium aurothiomalate (Ward et al, 1983). Of the 208 patients who fulfilled entry criteria, 193 were eligible for study, and 161 patients completed 20 weeks of therapy. When sodium aurothiomalate was compared with placebo, there was a significant improvement over placebo for number of tender joints, joint tenderness score, joint swelling score, increase in haemoglobin, fall in ESR and fall in platelet count. Skin rash was the most common cause for withdrawal from therapy (10%) followed by stomatitis (5%), nitritoid reactions (4%), abnormal liver enzymes (4%), thrombo-cytopenia (2%), proteinuria (2%) and individual patients with diarrhoea, leucopenia and pneumonitis. Three patients had rash plus either thrombocytopenia, leucopenia or stomatitis.

When auranofin was compared to placebo significant improvement was recorded for number of tender joints, pain tenderness score, physician's global assessment of disease activity and decrease in ESR. Adverse reactions accounted for the withdrawal of 6% of patients from the auranofin group due to single cases of rash, diarrhoea, stomatitis, eosinophilia and leucopenia.

A comparison of auranofin with sodium aurothiomalate in the above study by Ward and colleagues demonstrated that the injectable sodium aurothiomalate was superior to the oral gold drug for improvement in anaemia and thrombocytosis. Both auranofin and sodium aurothiomalate were superior to placebo for improvement in number of tender joints, joint pain and tenderness score, physician's overall assessment and ESR. Although statistical significance was not achieved, the authors indicated that sodium aurothiomalate produced a 12% greater improvement in the joint pain and tenderness score and a 32% advantage relative to joint swelling score. The authors concluded that type II error was possible with the small sample sizes, thus masking a significant indicator of benefit of sodium aurothiomalate over auranofin for these variables.

Ward and colleagues concluded that sodium aurothiomalate does have a therapeutic advantage over auranofin, although the oral gold preparation has fewer side-effects leading to cessation of therapy. An overall assessment of trials of auranofin versus placebo and auranofin versus injectable gold compounds would support these conclusions by Ward and colleagues. In many patients treated with injectable gold, individual observers will discontinue the drug following the development of rash, mouth ulcer or proteinuria less than 1000 mg per 24 hours. In contrast, many observers will merely temporarily withhold the gold drug until the side-effect has cleared or modified and then reintroduce the drug. Thus variations between observers and clinical variations have to be considered, especially in multicentre studies of toxicity and when two or more trials are compared. It may therefore be a false conclusion that there are more adverse effects resulting in withdrawal in patients treated with sodium aurothiomalate than in the auranofin patients.

In an open study by Giannini and colleagues in 1983, 21 children aged 1–17 years were treated with 0.1–0.2 mg/kg daily of auranofin (Giannini et al, 1983). The authors claimed a significant clinical improvement (25%) in more than half of the children. This included number and severity of joints with swelling, pain on motion and tenderness. Beneficial response was greater in children taking the higher doses. Only 2 of 21 had to discontinue therapy, 1 because of headaches and 1 because of haematuria, anaemia and a flare in disease activity. Three other children had side-effects which required dose reduction. These were proteinuria, diarrhoea and one with haematuria and anaemia.

SUMMARY OF CLINICAL GUIDELINES

Oral gold therapy in children should be under the supervision of a physician with in-depth knowledge of paediatrics and gold therapy. Treatment with gold compounds should be commenced as early as possible after the diagnosis of rheumatoid disease, once it has been established that the disease symptoms are not responsive to adequate treatment with NSAIDs. In view of the potential for toxicity, a strict monitoring system should be applied. Therapy should be conducted as outlined above with the use of a flexible regimen, e.g. if a patient is on monthly maintenance therapy and appears to be developing a flare-up in symptoms, the NSAID regimen should be altered if need be, and the frequency of gold injections increased to weekly.

The long-term outcome of patients treated with gold compounds, or indeed any of the antiarthritic agents, is unknown. Only a large cohort prospective study will answer the question as to whether disease-modifying agents do modify the long-term outcome of the arthritis. The weight of evidence to date suggests that gold therapy does beneficially modify the disease process and possibly the clinical and functional outcome.

INTRAMUSCULAR OR ORAL GOLD?

Injectable gold compound 50 mg weekly is similar in cost to auranofin 3 mg twice daily. When maintenance therapy is started at approximately five or six months, the injectable gold is usually given as 50 mg intramuscular monthly whereas maintenance with auranofin is continued at 3 mg once or twice daily. Thus oral auranofin is a more expensive maintenance programme. Fortunately for the majority of patients, cost is not a major issue.

Drug effectiveness is one of the principal factors influencing decision-making in drug administration. If auranofin is given in high enough dosage of 9 mg per day, its immunosuppressive actions should result in faster onset of action than the injectable gold compounds, but toxicity in the form of diarrhoea generally precludes the use of this dosage (Calin et al, 1982; Rangachari and Kean, 1989). Auranofin in a dosage of 3–6 mg per day does not appear to have a faster onset of action than the injectable gold compounds (Van Riel et al, 1983b; Ward et al, 1983) and indeed the reverse is true—a faster, more meaningful and clinically measured response is achieved with the injectable gold compounds when compared with the oral auranofin (Rau et al, 1983; Van Riel et al, 1983b; Ward et al, 1983). The convenience of oral medication is a much-discussed topic, especially in relation to compliance, but the compliance issue is best reserved for non-symptom driven usage, such as blood pressure control or oral contraception. Patients with pain are usually compliant; those who are not will never be, irrespective of the route of administration. The convenience of the oral auranofin is a small concession which is outweighed by the benefits accruing from injectable gold therapy. The process of the patient attending the 'gold clinic' to receive the injection ensures that someone with medical expertise will question the patient regarding drug benefit and adverse effects, and will test blood and urine for potential abnormalities. Thus patients are more likely to have a regular 'hands-on' management of their treatment, and will perhaps also benefit from the additional placebo effect recorded by Dr Thomas Fraser (Fraser, 1945). Patient compliance with gold injection treatment is reinforced by physicians and staff keeping a weekly record of the drug administration, clinical response and blood and urine measurements. Patients are provided with a copy of these results and will thus be more intimately involved in their own care, leading to increased compliance. Toxicity monitoring of auranofin is usually carried out only on a monthly basis.

Clinical studies have documented a greater quantity of adverse reactions for injectable gold compounds compared to auranofin (Rau et al, 1983; Van Riel et al, 1983b; Ward et al, 1983), but the quality and relevance of these side-effects have to be considered. The most common side-effect of injectable gold is rash, and in the context of a clinical trial this is recorded in approximately 30–50% of those treated. However, in clinical practice the majority of cases of rash are extremely mild and patients merely require a reduction in dosage or a temporary discontinuation of therapy without major interference or termination of treatment. The most common side-effect of auranofin is diarrhoea (Calin et al, 1982; Rau et al, 1983; Van Riel et al, 1983a; Ward et al, 1983; Rangachari and Kean, 1989), which is also dose related. Patients with severe rheumatoid arthritis, like gout sufferers treated with colchicine, do not thank their clinicians for the diarrhoea caused by auranofin. Reduction in dose of auranofin to reduce the potential for diarrhoea reduces efficacy (Calin et al, 1982). Haematological side-effects are uncommon with both injectable compounds and auranofin. The total quantity of adverse haematological effects is probably less with auranofin than with the injectable gold compounds. The mechanism of auranofin-induced thrombocytopenia is probably central, whereas the most common type of injectable gold-induced thrombocytopenia is peripheral and associated with IgG surface autoantibodies (Kelton et al, 1984). Central induced thrombocytopenia from injectable gold compounds is commonly a precursor of aplastic anaemia and is fortunately rare. The renal side-effects of auranofin are less common than those of injectable compounds (Rau et al, 1983; Van Riel et al, 1983b; Ward et al, 1983), but since the consequences of gold compound-induced proteinuria are rarely serious, the difference in frequency of this side-effect is not relevant.

When the decision is made to treat a rheumatoid arthritis patient with a gold compound, the greater effectiveness of the injectable compound can therefore take precedence over the fewer side-effects experienced with auranofin.

REFERENCES

Aaron S, Davis P & Biggs D (1984) D-penicillamine does not chelate skin gold. *Journal of Rheumatology* **11:** 869–870.
Adams CH & Cecil RL (1950) Gold therapy in early rheumatoid arthritis. *Annals of Internal Medicine* **33:** 163–173.
Bandilla KK, Delattre M, Rahn B & Missler B (1983) Long-term treatment of rheumatoid

arthritis with auranofin: clinical results with auranofin from German and international studies which included a comparison of once and twice daily treatment. In Capell HA, Cole DS, Manghani KK & Morris RW (eds) *Auranofin*, pp 97–114. Amsterdam: Excerpta Medica.

Blau S (1973) Metabolism of gold during lactation. *Arthritis and Rheumatism* 16: 777–778.

Blocka AK (1983) Auranofin versus injectable gold. Comparison of pharmacokinetic properties. *American Journal of Medicine* 75: 114–122.

Brewer EJ, Giannini EH & Barkley E (1980) Gold therapy in the management of juvenile rheumatoid arthritis. *Arthritis and Rheumatism* 23: 404–411.

Cahill RN (1977) Effect of sodium aurothiomalate (Myocrisin) on DNA synthesis in phytohaemagglutinin stimulated cultures of sheep lymphocytes. *Experientia* 27: 913–914.

Calin A, Saunders D, Bennett R et al (1982) Auranofin 1 mg or 9 mg. The search for appropriate dose. *Journal of Rheumatology* 9: 146–148.

Cooperating Clinics Committee (1973) A controlled trial of gold salt therapy in rheumatoid arthritis. *Arthritis and Rheumatism* 16: 353–358.

Crooke ST (1982) A comparison on the molecular pharmacology of gold and platinum complexes. *Journal of Rheumatology* 9: 61–70.

Davis P & Barraclough D (1977) Interaction of D-penicillamine with gold salts. *Arthritis and Rheumatism* 20: 1413–1418.

Davis P, Percy JS & Russell AS (1979a) In vivo and in vitro effects of gold salts on lymphocyte transformation responses and antibody dependent cell-mediated cytotoxicity. *Journal of Rheumatology* 6: 527–533.

Davis P, Miller CL & Johnston CA (1979b) Effect of gold salts on adherent mononuclear cells in tissue culture. *Journal of Rheumatology* 6: 98–102.

DeQueker J, Van Wanghe P & Verdict WA (1984) Systematic survey of HLA ABC and D antigens and drug toxicity in rheumatoid arthritis. *Journal of Rheumatology* 11: 282–290.

Dorwart BB, Gall EP, Schumacher HR & Krauser RE (1978) Chrysotherapy in psoriatic arthritis. Efficacy and toxicity compared to rheumatoid arthritis. *Arthritis and Rheumatism* 21: 513–515.

Elder RC, Eidsness MK, Heeg MJ, Tepperman KG, Shaw CF & Schaeffer N (1983) Gold-based antiarthritic drugs and metabolites. *American Chemical Society Symposium Series* 209: 385–390.

Empire Rheumatism Council (1960) Gold therapy in rheumatoid arthritis: report of a multicentre controlled trial. *Annals of the Rheumatic Diseases* 19: 95–119.

Empire Rheumatism Council (1961) Gold therapy in rheumatoid arthritis: final report of a multicentre controlled trial. *Annals of the Rheumatic Diseases* 20: 315–344.

Ennis RS, Granda JL & Posner AS (1968) Effect of gold salts and other drugs in the release and activity of lysosomal hydrolases. *Arthritis and Rheumatism* 11: 756–776.

Favreau M, Tannenbaum H & Louch J (1977) Hepatic toxicity associated with gold therapy. *Annals of Internal Medicine* 87: 717–719.

Finkelstein AE, Walz DT, Batista V et al (1976) Auranofin. New oral gold compound for the treatment of rheumatoid arthritis. *Annals of the Rheumatic Diseases* 35: 251–257.

Ford PM (1984) HLA antigens and drug toxicity in rheumatoid arthritis (editorial). *Journal of Rheumatology* 11: 259–261.

Forestier J (1929) L'Aurothérapie dans les rhumatismes chroniques. *Bulletin et Mémoires de la Société Médicale des Hôpitaux de Paris* 53: 323–327.

Forestier J (1930) Le traitement des polyarthries chroniques par les sels d'or. Résultats cliniques et contrôles hematologiques. *Bulletin et Mémoires de la Société Médicale des Hôpitaux de Paris* 54: 272–280.

Forestier J (1934) Rheumatoid arthritis and its treatment by gold salts. *Lancet* ii: 646–648.

Fraser TN (1945) Gold treatment in rheumatoid arthritis. *Annals of the Rheumatic Diseases* 4: 71–75.

Fung YL (1952) *A History of Chinese Philosophy*, translated by Derk Bodde, ch. 8. Yu-Lan.

Furst D, Levine S, Srinivasan R et al (1977) A double-blind trial of high versus conventional dosages of gold salts for rheumatoid arthritis. *Arthritis and Rheumatism* 20: 1473–1480.

Garrison FH (1966a) Dioscorides: De Materia Medica. In *Introduction to the History of Medicine*, 4th edn, pp 109–110. Philadelphia: W.B. Saunders.

Garrison FH (1966b) Pliny: Historia Naturalis. In *Introduction to the History of Medicine*, 4th edn, p 112. Philadelphia: W.B. Saunders.

Giannini EH, Brewer EJ & Person DA (1983) Auranofin in the treatment of juvenile rheumatoid arthritis. *Journal of Rheumatology* 102: 138–141.

Giannini EH, Brewer EJ & Person DA (1984) Blood gold concentrations in children with juvenile rheumatoid arthritis undergoing long term oral gold. *Annals of Rheumatic Diseases* 43: 228–231.

Goto M, Tanimoto K, Chihara R & Horiuchi Y (1981) Natural cell-mediated cytotoxicity in Sjögren's syndrome and rheumatoid arthritis. *Arthritis and Rheumatism* 24: 1377–1382.

Gottlieb NL & Major JC (1978) Ocular chrysiasis—a clinical study correlated with gold concentrations in the crystalline lens during chrysotherapy. *Arthritis and Rheumatism* 21: 704–708.

Gottlieb NL, Smith PM & Smith EM (1974) Pharmacodynamics of [195]Au-labelled aurothiomalate in blood. *Arthritis and Rheumatism* 17: 171–183.

Gottlieb NL, Kiem IM, Penneys NS & Schultz DR (1975) The influence of chrysotherapy on serum protein and immunoglobulin levels, rheumatoid factor and antiepithelial antibody titres. *Journal of Laboratory and Clinical Medicine* 86: 962–972.

Gowans JDC & Salami M (1973) Response of rheumatoid arthritis and leukopenia to gold salts. *New England Journal of Medicine* 288: 1007–1008.

Haris BK (1977) Myocardial infarction after a gold-induced nitritoid reaction (letter). *Arthritis and Rheumatism* 20: 1561.

Hartfall SJ & Garland HG (1935) Gold treatment of rheumatoid arthritis. *Lancet* ii: 8–11.

Hartfall SJ & Garland HG (1937) Gold treatment of rheumatoid arthritis. *Lancet* ii: 838–842.

Hartfall SJ, Garland HG & Goldie W (1937) Gold treatment of arthritis. A review of 900 cases. *Lancet* ii: 1459–1463.

Harth M, Stiller CR, Sinclair NR et al (1977) Effects of gold salt on lymphocyte responses. *Clinical and Experimental Immunology* 27: 357–364.

Harvey AR, Clarke B, Chui D, Kean WF & Buchanan WW (1983) Anaemia associated with rheumatoid disease: inverse correlation between erythropoiesis, and both IgM and rheumatoid factor levels. *Arthritis and Rheumatism* 26: 28–34.

Hashimoto A, Maeda Y, Ito H et al (1972) Corneal chrysiasis—a clinical study in rheumatoid arthritis patients receiving gold therapy. *Arthritis and Rheumatism* 15: 309–312.

Herrlinger JD (1983) Difference in the pharmacokinetics, protein binding and cellular distribution of gold when different gold compounds are used. In Schattenkirchner M & Muller W (eds) *Modern Aspects of Gold Therapy*. Basel: Karger.

Howell A, Gumpel JM & Watts RWE (1975) Depression of bone marrow colony formation in gold induced neutropenia. *British Medical Journal* 1: 432–434.

Hunt LB (1979) The Figuiers of Montpellier. *Ambix* 26: 221–223.

Isab AA & Sadler PJ (1976) ^{13}C nuclear magnetic resonance detection of thiol exchange in gold(I): significance in chemotherapy. *Journal of the Chemical Society Communications* 1051–1052.

Isab AA & Sadler PJ (1981) Hydrogen-I and carbon-13 nuclear magnetic resonance studies of gold(I) thiomalate (Myocrisin) in aqueous solution: dependence of the solution structure on pH and ionic strength. *Journal of the Chemical Society* 1657–1663.

Janoff A (1970) Inhibition of human granulocyte elastase by gold sodium thiomalate. *Biochemical Pharmacology* 19: 626–628.

Katz WA, Alexander S, Bland JH et al (1982) Efficacy and safety of auranofin compared to placebo. *Journal of Rheumatology* 9: 173–178.

Kean WF & Anastassiades TP (1979) Long term chrysotherapy. Incidence of toxicity and efficacy during sequential time periods. *Arthritis and Rheumatism* 22: 495–501.

Kean WF & Lock CJL (1983) Penicillamine does not chelate gold(I). *Journal of Rheumatology* 10: 527–530.

Kean WF, Bellamy N & Brooks PM (1983) Gold therapy in the elderly rheumatoid patient. *Arthritis and Rheumatism* 26: 705–711.

Kean WF, Lock CJL, Kassam YB et al (1984a) A biological effect on platelets by the minor component of gold sodium thiomalate—a by-product of heat sterilization and exposure to light. *Clinical and Experimental Rheumatology* 2: 321–328.

Kean WF, Kassam YB, Lock CJL et al (1984b) Antithrombin activity of gold sodium thiomalate. *Clinical Pharmacology and Therapeutics* 35: 627–632.

Kean WF, Forestier F, Kassam YB et al (1985) The history of gold therapy in rheumatoid disease. *Seminars in Arthritis and Rheumatism* 14: 180–186.

Kean WF, Somers D, Kassam YB et al (1990) The action of gold sodium thiomalate on experimental thrombosis in vivo. *Journal of Pharmaceutical Sciences* (in press).

Kelton JG, Carter CJ, Rodger C et al (1984) The relationship between platelet-associated IgG, platelet life-form and reticuloendothelial cell function. *Blood* **63:** 1434–1438.

Koch R (1890) Uber bacteriologische Forschung. *Deutsche Medizinische Wochenschrift* **16:** 756–757.

Lipsky PE & Ziff M (1977) Inhibition of antigen and mitogen induced human lymphocyte proliferation by gold compounds. *Journal of Clinical Investigation* **59:** 455–466.

Lockie LM, Smith D, Kean WF et al (1982) Forty-seven years experience with gold therapy in the treatment of rheumatoid arthritis, Abstract C65. Pan-American Congress of Rheumatology, Washington, DC.

Lorber A, Jackson WH & Simon TM (1977) 6th Western Regional Meeting of the American Rheumatism Association, Scottsdale, Arizona.

Lorber A, Simon T, Leeb J et al (1978) Chrysotherapy. Suppression of immunoglobulin synthesis. *Arthritis and Rheumatism* **21:** 785–791.

Luukhainen R, Isomaki H & Kajander A (1977) Effect of gold treatment on progress of erosions in RA patients. *Scandinavian Journal of Rheumatology* **6:** 123–127.

McCormick J, Cole S, Lahirir B et al (1980) Pneumonitis caused by gold salt therapy. Evidence for the role of cell-mediated immunity in its pathogenesis. *American Review of Respiratory Diseases* **122:** 145–152.

Merle LJ, Reidenberg MM, Camacho MT, Jones BR & Drayer DE (1980) Renal injury in patients with rheumatoid arthritis treated with gold. *Clinical Pharmacology and Therapeutics* **28:** 216–222.

Merliss RR, Axelrod P, Fineberg J & Melnick M (1951) Clinical evaluation of aurothioglycolanilide (Lauron-Endo) in rheumatoid arthritis. *Annals of Internal Medicine* **35:** 352–357.

Mohide TP (1981) *Gold*. Mineral Policy Background Paper no. 12, ppp 246–252. Ontario: Ministry of Natural Resources.

Morris RW, Cole DS, Horton J, Hever MA & Pietrusko RG (1984) Worldwide clinical experience with auranofin. *Clinical Rheumatology* 3(supplement 10): 105–112.

Nagi AH, Alexander F & Barabas AZ (1971) Gold nephropathy in rats in light and electron microscopic studies. *Experimental Molecular Pathology* **15:** 354–362.

Panayi GS, Wooley PM & Batchelor JR (1978) Genetic basis of rheumatoid disease: HLA antigens, disease manifestations, and toxic reactions to drugs. *British Medical Journal* **2:** 1326–1328.

Panayi GS, Griffin AJ & Wooley PM (1979) Genetic predisposition to gold and penicillamine toxicity. *Arthritis and Rheumatism* **22:** 645.

Pattison-Muir MM (1972) Roger Bacon: his relations to alchemy and chemistry. In Little AG (ed.) *Roger Bacon Essays*, pp 285–320. New York: Russell & Russell.

Pearson RG (1963) Hard and soft acids and bases. *Journal of the American Chemical Society* **85:** 3533–3539.

Penneys SA, Zibow V, Gottlieb NL et al (1974) Inhibition of prostaglandin synthesis and human epidermal enzymes by aurothiomalate in vitro: possible action of gold. *Journal of Investigative Dermatology* **63:** 356–361.

Percy JS, Davis P, Russell AS & Brisson E (1978) A longitudinal study of in vitro tests for lymphocyte function in rheumatoid arthritis. *Annals of the Rheumatic Diseases* **37:** 416–420.

Persellin RH, Hess EV & Ziff M (1967) Effect of gold salt on the immune response. *Arthritis and Rheumatism* **10:** 99–106.

Puddephatt RJ (1978) *The Chemistry of Gold*. New York: Elsevier.

Rangachari PK & Kean WF (1989) Gold and D-penicillamine and the gastrointestinal tract. *Clinical Rheumatology* **3:** 411–423.

Rau R, Kaik B, Müller-Fassbender H et al (1983) Treatment of rheumatoid arthritis. In Schattenkirchner M & Müller W (eds) *Modern Aspects of Gold Therapy*, pp 162–174. Basel: Karger.

Rawls WB, Gruskin BJ, Ressa AA, Dworzan HJ & Schreiber D (1944) Analysis of results obtained with small doses of gold salts in the treatment of rheumatoid arthritis. *American Journal of Medical Science* **207:** 528–533.

Repice MM, Radvany RM & Schmid FR (1979) HLA, A, BC and DR locus antigens and gold toxicity in rheumatoid arthritis. *Clinical Research* 647A.

Rischke J, Rosenthal K, Nablo L et al (1984) Ridaura enhances natural killer cell activity in vitro. *Clinical Research* **32**: 665A.

Rosenberg SA & Lipsky PE (1979) Inhibition of pokeweed mitogen-induced immunoglobulin production in humans by gold compounds. *Journal of Rheumatology* **6**: 107–111.

Rudge SR, Perret D, Drury PL & Swannell AJ (1983) Determination of thiomalate in physiological fluids using high performance liquid chromatography and electrochemical detection. *Journal of Pharmacology and Biochemical Analysis* **1**: 205–210.

Russell AS, Davis P & Miller C (1982) The effect of a new anti-rheumatic drug triethyl-phosphine gold (auranofin) on lymphocyte and monocyte toxicity. *Journal of Rheumatology* **9**: 30–35.

Sadler PJ (1976) The biological chemistry of gold: a metallo-drug and heavy atom label with variable valency. *Structure and Bonding* **29**: 171–215.

Sadler PJ (1982) The comparative evaluation of the physical and chemical properties of gold compounds. *Journal of Rheumatology* **9**: 71–78.

Salmerton G & Lipsky PE (1983) Effect of gold compounds on human mononuclear phagocyte function. In Schattenkirchner M & Müller W (eds) *Modern Aspects of Gold Therapy*, pp 63–74. Basel: Karger.

Schultz DR, Volankis JE, Arnold PL et al (1974) Inactivation of C1 in rheumatoid synovial fluid, purified C1 and C1 esterase by gold compounds. *Clinical and Experimental Immunology* **17**: 395–406.

Scott DL, Bradby GVH, Aitman TJ et al (1981) Relationship of gold and penicillamine therapy to diffuse interstitial lung disease. *Annals of the Rheumatic Diseases* **40**: 136–141.

Shaw CF (1979) The mammalian biochemistry of gold: an inorganic perspective of chryso-therapy. *Inorganic Perspectives in Biology and Medicine* **2**: 287–355.

Shaw CF, Schmitz G, Thompson HO & Witkiewicz P (1979) Bis(L-cysteinato) gold(I): chemical characterization and identification in renal cortical cytoplasm. *Journal of Inorganic Biochemistry* **10**: 317–330.

Shiokano Y, Horiuchi Y, Homma M et al (1977) Clinical evaluation of D-penicillamine by multicentre double-blind comparative study in chronic rheumatoid arthritis. *Arthritis and Rheumatism* **20**: 1464–1472.

Sigler JW, Bluhm GB, Duncan H, Sharp JT, Ensign DC & McCrum WR (1974) Gold salts in the treatment of rheumatoid arthritis: a double-blind study. *Annals of Internal Medicine* **80**: 21–26.

Simon TM, Kunishmia DH, Biert GJ & Lorber A (1979) Inhibitory effects of a new oral gold compound on HeLa cells. *Cancer* **44**: 1865–1875.

Snyder RG, Traeger C & Kelly L (1939) Gold therapy in arthritis: observations in 100 cases treated with gold sodium thiosulphate and aurocein. *Annals of Internal Medicine* **12**: 1672–1681.

Starkey PM & Barrett AJ (1976) Human cathepsin G—catalytic and immunological properties. *Journal of Biochemistry* **155**: 273–278.

Stein HB & Urowitz MB (1976) Gold-induced enterocolitis. *Journal of Rheumatology* **3**: 21–26.

Strong JS, Bartholomew BA & Smyth CJ (1973) Immunoresponsiveness of patients with rheumatoid arthritis receiving cyclophosphamide or gold salts. *Annals of the Rheumatic Diseases* **32**: 233–237.

Sutton BM, McGustry E, Waltz DT & Dimartino MJ (1972) Oral gold. Antiarthritic properties of alkylphosphine gold coordination complexes. *Journal of Medical Chemistry* **15**: 1095–1098.

Tarp U, Graudal H, Moller-Madsen B & Danscher G (1983) A follow-up study of children exposed to gold salts in utero (abstract). European Congress of Rheumatology.

Tornrot T & Skrifvars B (1974) Gold nephropathy prototype of membranous glomerulo-nephritis. *American Journal of Pathology* **75**: 573–584.

Waine H, Baker F & Mettier SR (1943) Controlled evaluation of gold therapy in rheumatoid arthritis. *California Medical Journal* **66**: 295.

Waley A (1956) *The Way and its Power: A Study of the Tao Teaching and its Place in Chinese Thought*. London: Allen & Unwin.

Walz DT, Dimartino MJ, Juch JH & Zuccarello W (1971) Adjuvant-induced arthritis in rats. I. Temporal relationship of physiological, biochemical and haematological parameters. *Proceedings of the Society of Experimental Biology and Medicine* **136**: 907–910.

Walz DT, Dimartino MJ, Sutton BM & Misher A (1972) SK&F 36914—an agent for oral chrysotherapy. *Journal of Pharmacology and Experimental Therapeutics* **181:** 292–297.

Walz DT, Dimartino MJ, Chakrin LW, Sutton BM & Misher A (1976) Antiarthritic properties and unique pharmacologic profile of a potential chrysotherapeutic agent: SK&F D-39162. *Journal of Pharmacology and Experimental Therapeutics* **197:** 142–152.

Walz ET, Dimartino MJ, Griswold DE, Intoccia AP & Flanagan TL (1983) Biologic actions and pharmacokinetic studies of auranofin. *American Journal of Medicine* **75:** 90–108.

Ward JR, Williams NJ, Egger MJ et al (1983) Comparison of auranofin, gold sodium thiomalate, and placebo in the treatment of rheumatoid arthritis. *Arthritis and Rheumatism* **26:** 1303–1315.

Wiegleb JC (1965) *Historische-kritische Untersuchung der Alchemie*, 1777 (facsimile edition), p 185. Leipzig: Zentral-Antiquariat.

Winterbauer RH, Wilske KR & Wheelis RF (1976) Diffuse pulmonary injury associated with gold treatment. *New England Journal of Medicine* **17:** 919–921.

Wooley PM, Griffin J, Panay GS, Batchelor JR, Welsh KI & Gibson TS (1980) HLA-DR antigens and toxic reaction to sodium aurothiomalate and D-penicillamine in patients with rheumatoid arthritis. *New England Journal of Medicine* **303:** 300–303.

Van Riel PL, Gribnau FW, Van de Putte LB & Yap SH (1983a) Loose stools during auranofin treatment: clinical study and some pathogenic possibilities. *Journal of Rheumatology* **10:** 222–226.

Van Riel PL, Van de Putte LB, Gribnau FW et al (1983b) A single-blind comparative study of auranofin and gold thioglucose in patients with rheumatoid arthritis. In Capell HA, Cole DS, Monghoni KK & Morris RW (eds) *Auranofin*, pp 135–146. Amsterdam: Excerpta Medica.

5

Aspirin versus the non-acetylated salicylates

K. D. RAINSFORD
W. W. BUCHANAN

Bitter im Mund, gesund im Korper

German proverb (Strauss, 1968)

Historically, it was salicylate—as the acid, sodium salt, aldehyde alcohol or glucoside—that found application in the treatment of rheumatic conditions (for review see Rainsford, 1984). These forms were present in plant-derived extracts which were employed from ancient times until the middle of the last century. With the development of organic chemistry in Germany and France at that time came first the purified compounds, then later synthetic methods (chiefly the Kolbe and Lautermann procedure) for the synthesis of salicylic acid. While no clinical trials of the type and standard employed today were then undertaken to establish the efficacy of salicylic acid or its salts (collectively salicylates) in the relief of pain and soft tissue swelling in various rheumatic conditions, the mere fact that salicylates found such wide use and acceptance in the treatment of rheumatic fever, gout and other arthritides in the latter part of the last century is evidence of a kind for their efficacy.

Aspirin (acetylsalicylic acid) really only came into popular use through (a) recognition of the need to obtain a drug which was more palatable and less upsetting to the gastrointestinal tract than sodium salicylate, (b) the powerful competitive forces operating at the time, and (c) clever marketing approaches (Rainsford, 1984). Evidence supporting claims for the reduced gastric irritancy of aspirin over salicylate were initially based on a series of cleverly contrived experiments notably featuring a model of epithelial injury in fish tails immersed into acidic solutions of the two drugs (Rainsford, 1984). The biological relevance of this model with respect to mucosal injury in the gastrointestinal tract must be considered remote, let alone the deductive reasoning for the lack of injury from aspirin (Rainsford, 1984). These and other earlier studies were the basis upon which the marketing of aspirin and especially its claims for superiority over salicylate were based.

In contrast, it was less than a decade after aspirin was introduced that the first reports of gastric ulceration in dogs appeared (Chistoni and Lapresa, 1909). This was followed in 1912 by reports of 'gastralgia' from aspirin in humans not evident with sodium salicylate (Roch, 1912). Hurst and Lintott (1939) were the first to identify aspirin positively as a cause of gastric ulceration and haematemesis. Doubtless, the highly effective advertising in the early marketing of aspirin overwhelmed the populace and the medical profession alike. Moreover, it must be said that an appreciable amount of the medical application of the drug was probably for the relief of (a) fever and headaches accompanying colds and influenza (especially during the flu epidemic of the late 1910s to early 1920s), (b) *acute* painful conditions, and (c) rheumatic fever. In the first two of these conditions only fever has been shown to be more responsive in humans to aspirin than to salicylate. However, only in animal models has aspirin been proven to be more effective than salicylate (Rainsford, 1984; Higuchi et al, 1986). The use of aspirin for the treatment of chronic pain and soft tissue inflammatory reactions in rheumatoid arthritis (Seed, 1965) did not receive particular attention in the medical literature (Goodwin and Goodwin, 1981) until the famous British trials on gold thiomalate and oral corticosteroids in the late 1950s and early 1960s, where aspirin was employed as a comparative (positive) standard (Empire Rheumatism Council, 1950, 1955, 1957, 1960, 1961; Medical Research Council, 1954, 1957; Medical Research Council and Nuffield Foundation 1954, 1955, 1957a,b, 1959, 1960). Indeed, it was not until the mid 1960s that salicylates in high doses were definitively proven to have anti-inflammatory effect in rheumatoid arthritis (Fremont-Smith and Bayles, 1965).

Aspirin then became a comparative standard in a considerable number of trials in subjects with rheumatoid arthritis and osteoarthritis; many of these trials were sponsored by drug companies and were performed during the introduction of the newer non-steroidal anti-inflammatory drugs (NSAIDs) in the past two decades or so (Rosenbloom et al, 1985). Thus, the place of aspirin in the treatment of chronic pain and soft tissue inflammation became entrenched because of its use as a 'gold standard' and its historic recognition, especially in North America, as a 'drug of first choice' in the treatment of rheumatoid arthritis, osteoarthritis and other chronic arthritic conditions (Csuka and McCarty, 1989).

A few small studies in the past two decades have, however, challenged the traditional view (Lasagna, 1960; Levy, 1965; Martin, 1971; Anonymous, 1983) that aspirin is more potent than salicylate (Paulus, 1989), details of which are considered in the next section. Furthermore, clinical success of the salicylate diester, salsalate (Riker Laboratories; see Reynolds, 1989)—also known as salicylsalicylic acid and historically as diplosal—has been noted in extensive investigations (Singleton, 1980; McPherson, 1984). This drug hydrolyses to yield salicylate in vivo following oral ingestion. Salsalate is effective in the treatment of pain and soft tissue inflammation in rheumatoid arthritis, osteoarthritis and other chronic inflammatory conditions in some studies, and has been shown to be almost equipotent with aspirin on a weight or molar basis. Salsalate also has—in contrast to aspirin—an appreciably low propensity to cause ulcers and haemorrhage in the upper gastro-intestinal tract (Cohen, 1979; Mielants et al, 1981; Scheiman et al, 1989; Roth et al, 1989, 1990). While there are important chemical properties underlying these observations, it can be said that the evidence for the efficacy of both salicylate and salsalate in the relief of chronic pain and inflammation in rheumatoid arthritis and possibly other arthritides being approximately equivalent to that of aspirin has led to the view that the acetyl group of aspirin is not *ipso facto* necessary for the therapeutic actions of the drug in *chronic* inflammation (Graham et al, 1977; Whitehouse and Rainsford, 1982; Multicenter Salsalate/Aspirin Comparison Study Group, 1989; Paulus, 1989). There are also pharmacokinetic studies supporting the concept that it is the salicyl (salicoyl) of salicylate moiety of aspirin that is responsible for its pain-relieving and anti-inflammatory actions in chronic inflammation (Soren, 1975, 1977; Graham et al, 1977).

The term 'non-acetylated' salicylates used to embrace all non-aspirin salicylates, though widely used, can in fact be misleading if there is inadequate definition of what specific drugs are being discussed. Thus, diflunisal or 5-(4,5'-difluorophenyl)-salicylic acid (Reynolds, 1989) is strictly speaking a non-acetylated salicylate. For the purposes of the present discussion it is more appropriate to describe it as a 'fluorophenylsalicylate'.

USE OF NON-ACETYLATED SALICYLATES, DIFLUNISAL AND ASPIRIN IN RHEUMATOLOGY

Some idea of the relative use of various salicylate preparations in rheumatologic practice is a good guide to patient and prescriber acceptance of these drugs (Luggan et al, 1989). It is well known that different NSAIDs vary in clinical responses (Capell et al, 1979; Scott et al, 1982; Cox and Doherty, 1987), the incidence of adverse reactions and the occurrence of symptoms likely to influence withdrawal (Rainsford and Velo, 1987) or patient acceptance (Cox and Doherty, 1987).

A recent mail survey by Pincus and Callahan (1989) of 15 private rheumatology practices in 11 cities of 7 states in the USA compared use of NSAIDs and non-prescription salicylates by patients with rheumatoid arthritis. Multiple use of these drugs, which is frequent (Lee et al, 1974), was not identified, though up to 15 NSAIDs were used singly. A total of 33.8% of patients were reported to be taking non-prescription aspirin preparations. The percentages of prescribed salicylates were 'zero-order release' aspirin (Zorprin) 8.5%, salsalate 5.7%, choline magnesium trisalicylate (Trisilate) 2.4%, magnesium salicylate (Magan) 1.2% and diflunisal (Dolobid) 0.8%, totalling 20.5%. Non-salicylate NSAIDs totalled 46.2% of all the drugs surveyed.

These results show that salicylates represent an appreciable amount of all drugs consumed by patients with rheumatoid arthritis, and the non-acetylated salicylates total 90.3% of prescribed drugs; a considerable proportion, especially in relation to the total of aspirin consumed. While this is only one representative study, it shows that salicylate and aspirin use still dominate drug therapy in rheumatoid patients, in spite of strong competition from the numerous NSAIDs marketed in the USA. The dominance of these salicylates, despite competition, is recognition of their relative safety and efficacy. The extensive use of non-salicylate preparations alone, by comparison with aspirin and other NSAIDs, might be regarded in part as a recognition that these less ulcerogenic agents (cf. aspirin) (Cohen, 1979; Mielants et al, 1981; Scheiman et al, 1989; Roth et al, 1989, 1990) are possibly as therapeutically effective as aspirin and maybe even other NSAIDs (though there is some question about the latter).

PHARMACOLOGY OF NON-ACETYLATED AND ACETYLATED SALICYLATES

To understand the differing clinical effects of the various salicylates (pain relief, control of soft tissue inflammation and upper gastrointestinal ulcerogenicity) it is necessary to consider their modes of action. Much of the work on the pharmacology of the salicylates has been performed in laboratory animals and in vitro. The extrapolation of these results to human subjects with arthritic diseases is, therefore, subject to the obvious caveats that there may be species differences and drug–disease interactions, and that

Table 1. Comparison of the pharmacological properties of acetylated versus non-acetylated salicylates.

Property	Aspirin	Salicylate	Salsalate	Diflunisal
In vitro				
1. Inhibition of PG cyclo-oxygenase*	+++	±	0	++++
2. Inhibition of platelet aggregation*	+++ (IR)	0	0	++(R)
3. Inhibition of superoxide production	+	+++	? = SAL	NT
4. Inhibition of proteoglycan synthesis	+	++	? = SAL	NT
5. Inhibition of PMN cell migration	++	++		
6. Uncoupler of oxidative phosphorylation*	0	+++	? = SAL	NT
7. Inhibition of gastric mucus synthesis*	+++	++	? = SAL	NT
8. Labilization (L)/stabilization (S) of lysosomes	L/S	++ L/S	? = SAL	
In vivo				
9. Acute anti-inflammatory— carrageenan inflammation in rats	+++	++	? = SAL	++++
10. Chronic anti-inflammatory in adjuvant arthritis in rats	++	NT	NT	+++
11. Antipyretic effects in rats	++	+	NT	+++

Based on data in Stone et al (1977); Whitehouse et al (1977); Rainsford (1978a, 1981, 1984), Estes and Kaplan (1986); Morris et al (1985); Abramson and Weissman (1989); Pelletier et al (1989). Potency in various test systems graded on an arbitrary scale of 0 (no effect) to ++++ (most potent compared with other salicylates); NT not known to have been tested; R reversible; IR irreversible (inhibition); ? = SAL probably derived from salicylate though metabolism rate limiting.
* Also demonstrated in vivo or ex vivo.

part of the responses in vitro will not always represent the intact system in vivo. Some approximation to rationalization of the understanding of drug actions should include information on (a) expected plasma, synovial fluid or tissue concentrations of drugs or their metabolites (if these are pharmacologically active), and (b) what (if any) influence on drug plasma or tissue kinetics, biochemical or cellular functions may be attributed to a manifestation of an arthritic condition. Often much of this information is lacking so that the relation of the experimental results from animal or in vitro models to the arthritic patient can only be regarded as speculative. Given these provisos it is possible to summarize the main features of the acetylated compared with non-acetylated salicylates, the essential features of which are shown in Table 1.

Some important features are worth noting from this summary, especially with respect to the relative anti-inflammatory and analgesic potency of these drugs compared with aspirin, and also the lower gastrointestinal ulcerogenicity of salicylate and salsalate.

Anti-inflammatory effects

The *acute* anti-inflammatory effects of aspirin can in some animal models and in humans appear more potent than that of salicylate and salsalate (Whitehouse et al, 1977; Rainsford and Whitehouse, 1980a). It should be noted, however, that salsalate is metabolized to salicylate in both humans and laboratory animal species and the rate of this determines the bioefficacy of this drug (Rainsford and Whitehouse, 1980a; Droomgoole et al, 1983; Rainsford, 1984). However, in some studies of the acute anti-inflammatory effects of these drugs salicylate has been shown to be approximately equipotent to aspirin (Walker et al, 1976; Smith, 1978; Smith et al, 1979), though this may depend on the nature of the acute inflammation (Higgs et al, 1987). Moreover, careful analysis has been shown that only a negligible amount of aspirin actually reaches the *acutely* inflamed sites from the orally administered drug given to rats.

Thus, it appears that much of the acute anti-inflammatory action of aspirin actually resides in its metabolite, salicylate. The uptake of salicylate *vis-à-vis* aspirin into inflamed joints of arthritis subjects will determine the pharmacological actions at this site. Kinetic analysis of the amount of aspirin accumulating in synovial fluids of subjects with synovitis of traumatic origins or in those with rheumatoid arthritis or osteoarthritis receiving aspirin (0.6 g single dose) revealed that the peak aspirin concentrations in the fluids were about one-eighth of the total salicylates there and about two-thirds of the aspirin concentration in the blood (Soren, 1975, 1977). The latter peak concentration is about one-sixth that of total salicylates and decays very rapidly, whereas the accumulation of aspirin in synovial fluids follows that in blood and persists for 120 to 400 minutes after dosing. The areas under the curve for aspirin in the synovial fluid are appreciably small compared with total salicylates in plasma (Soren, 1977). It is clear that in the arthritic joint much less aspirin accumulates in the synovial compartment than salicylate. Our major interest should, therefore, be the accumulation of salicylate in the synovial compartment, whether it be from aspirin or derived by hydrolysis from salsalate.

Examination of Table 1 shows that the pharmacological actions of salicylate that distinguish it from aspirin include:

1. The lack of prostaglandin synthesis inhibition.
2. Inhibitory effects on superoxide anion production.
3. Uncoupling of oxidative phosphorylation.
4. Effects on lysosomal stability.

The lack of effects of salicylate on prostaglandin synthesis led to a search for other modes of action of salicylate. Its influence in preventing accumulation of leucocytes at inflamed sites, while unproven in the rheumatic patient, must be an important action of the drug. Recently, much interest has been shown in the superoxide radical scavenging effects of salicylate (Sagone and Husney, 1987; Grootveld and Halliwell, 1988). Furthermore, the growing importance of superoxide and other oxygen reactive species in inflammatory processes (Hurst, 1987; Lunec et al, 1981; Biemond et al, 1988; Suzuki et al, 1989), including those mediated by neutrophils (Ginsberg et al, 1981, 1985); the potential of superoxide ions to degrade hyaluronic acid (Betts and Cleland, 1982; Weitz et al, 1988) and other proteins (Kleinfeld et al, 1989); that interleukin-I and tumour necrosis factor (both important peptide inflammatory mediators of chronic inflammation) stimulate oxyradical production (Radeke et al, 1990); that superoxide is produced by an ion-dependent reaction in inflammatory diseases (Biemond et al, 1988); are all indicators of the importance of oxyradicals in inflammation. A variety of NSAIDs and disease-modifying antirheumatic drugs inhibit the production or actions of oxyradicals in a variety of in vitro model systems representative of components of the inflammatory processes (Oyanagui, 1978; Betts and Cleland, 1982; Van Dyke et al, 1982; Gay et al, 1984; Carlin et al, 1985; Arrigoni-Martelli, 1985; Biemond et al, 1986; Ginsburg et al, 1987; Rainsford et al, 1989; Zoschke and Kaja, 1989). Thus, on the basis of the potential pharmacological actions of salicylate principally on oxyradicals, leucocyte accumulation and enzyme release it is important to consider the actions of this drug alone and the fact that aspirin, like salsalate, may be a pro-drug of salicylate.

CLINICAL EFFICACY OF SALICYLATE AND SALSALATE

Comparisons with aspirin

Salicylate was used to control pain and swelling in inflammation long before the introduction of aspirin. Probably the first placebo-controlled study comparing the analgesic effects of salicylate versus aspirin in rheumatoid arthritis was reported by Graham et al (1977). They showed in 21 subjects with rheumatoid arthritis that the pain relief following a single oral dose of 1.07 g sodium salicylate was comparable with that from an equimolar dose of 1.2 g aspirin over a six-hour period; both were 3–4 times more effective than the placebo. A more extensive, randomized double-blind study of 18 subjects with rheumatoid arthritis was reported recently by Preston et al (1989) in which enteric coated sodium salicylate (4.8 g daily) was compared for pain relief, articular index of joint tenderness, increase in grip strength, decrease in digital joint circumference and patient's own assessment with that of an equal quantity *by weight* of aspirin in an enteric coated formulation. The study design involved an initial three-day washout period followed by a two-week period of salicylate or aspirin, then the two treatments were crossed over. Both drugs showed significant improvements in all parameters, and notably no significant or clinically relevant differences were observed between the two treatments; both produced the same plasma salicylate levels. Thus, these studies by Graham et al (1977) and Preston et al (1989) both show that acute and chronic pain relief and anti-inflammatory activity can be achieved by salicylate and seriously challenge the need to prescribe aspirin in rheumatoid arthritis where salicylate will do the pharmacological job.

Comparisons between salsalate and aspirin in the therapy of rheumatoid arthritis have been reported by the Multicenter Salsalate/Aspirin Comparison Study Group (1989) and April et al (1990). In a double-blind, randomized, parallel group of the Multicentre Salsalate/Aspirin Comparison Study Group (1989) investigation of 150 subjects (initially 233 started the trial) with rheumatoid arthritis, 83 took salsalate (starting dose 3 g daily) and 67 received aspirin (starting dose 3.6 g daily). Regrettably, the study design allowed for self-adjustment of dosage, as it did in the similarly designed study of April et al (1990) according to efficacy and tolerance, such that control over the comparative aspects was lost. Thus, the conclusions that both treatments were equally effective but that aspirin produced more severe gastrointestinal complications is in a sense invalid because of the adjustment of dosage in the study design. No information was provided on dosage ingested or on the plasma salicylate levels during therapy, which would have been ways of controlling for dosage adjustment. On the positive side it could be said that this represents more of a 'real world' study, but it is flawed because no critical analysis can be made of the relation to drug dosage ingested from plasma salicylate determination. Critics who suggest the literature shows that there is no relation of plasma salicylate levels to therapeutic efficacy should consider that the evidence for such conclusions is based on studies where the salicylate dosage has been fixed, not variable as in the above-mentioned study.

Regalado (1978) has reported the satisfactory use of salsalate for control of long-term musculoskeletal pain in an open non-comparative assessment.

Three double-blind, randomized, multicentre trials comparing the therapeutic efficacy in rheumatoid arthritis of aspirin with that of choline magnesium trisalicylate (Trisilate), both at the same dosage with respect to salicylate content, were reported by Lecher and Blechman (1978), Blechman and Lechner (1979) and Rothwell (1983). While some of the original data were notably lacking in one of the unpublished studies—that of Abeles quoted by Rothwell (1983)—the results of these trials showed that the numbers of swollen and painful joints were significantly and equivalently reduced over 1–7 or 1–11 weeks of therapy with the two preparations. In all the trials there was comparable efficacy of other parameters (articular index, duration of morning stiffness) with the two drugs, but the number of gastrointestinal side-effects reported was lower with the choline magnesium trisalicylate (CMT).

Liyanage and Tambar (1978) showed in a double-blind, placebo-controlled study that salsalate (3 g daily) was as effective as aspirin (3.6 g daily) during a two-week period of therapy for osteoarthritis of the hip or knee. The measurements included pain, stiffness determinations and sleep disturbances graded on a visual analogue scale. The plasma salicylate levels achieved were comparable with both therapies. The side-effects of the gastrointestinal tract and occult faecal blood loss assessed on both treatments were lower with salsalate than aspirin. Unfortunately, the availability of paracetamol as a 'rescue' analgesic in this study placed some restriction on its value for precise determination of analgesic response.

Comparisons with other NSAIDs

A number of studies have been reported over the past two decades comparing the therapeutic efficacy of salicylate with NSAIDs other than aspirin in the treatment of various rheumatic conditions. Dick et al (1969, 1970) were the first to employ xenon-133 clearance in the knee joints of patients with rheumatoid arthritis to study the local anti-inflammatory response of two NSAIDs, sodium salicylate and indomethacin. The response was identical in both cases. In general therapy of rheumatoid arthritis, studies reported by Deodhar et al (1973) and Lee et al (1974) showed that sodium salicylate was about equally effective in most parameters of pain response as other NSAIDs, and all were superior to placebo.

It has also been shown that CMT is equal to or slightly more effective than ibuprofen (Ehrlich et al, 1980) or naproxen (McLaughlin, 1982) for pain and joint swelling in rheumatoid arthritis. CMT has also been found to be equianalgesic with indomethacin in subjects with osteoarthritis (Goldenberg et al, 1978). The 'fishy' odour which develops in patients taking CMT is due to intestinal flora producing decomposition products of choline (Whitehouse and Rainsford, 1982) and this may be offensive to some.

Comparisons of salsalate with other NSAIDs have also been reported suggesting that the former is as effective in rheumatoid arthritis and other arthritides as most NSAIDs. Thus, Deodhar et al (1977) showed that salsalate (3 g daily) was as effective as indomethacin (75 mg daily) in a double-blind, placebo-controlled study of a small group of 15 subjects with rheumatoid arthritis. Patient preference was, however, in favour of indomethacin. The dosage of both drugs was low, and no doubt differences in reports of side-effects as well as therapeutic response would have been evident at the higher doses used in therapy with these agents today.

One of the most thorough comparisons of the effects of salicylate (CMT) with an NSAID (naproxen, 1.5 g daily) in the therapy of rheumatoid arthritis was reported by Furst et al (1987). These authors analysed the responses of a total of 12 joint, pain and activity parameters in a randomized, double-blind, placebo-controlled, cross-over study in 84 subjects who took the test drugs or placebo for four-week periods. The dose of CMT was initially started in a run-in period at 45 mg/kg daily, given in two doses 12 hours apart, and the period of dosage adjusted until the plasma salicylate concentrations were 150–300 mg/l at 1–2 hours after the morning dose. Plasma salicylate and naproxen levels were monitored throughout the study. There appeared to be no statistically significant differences in any of the pain, inflammation or activity parameters measured in subjects who received CMT compared with those on naproxen. Not surprisingly, tinnitus was most frequent in subjects who received CMT, whereas gastrointestinal complaints were more common with naproxen. Incidentally, a major objective of the authors of this study was to establish if the combination of CMT with naproxen conferred any benefits over the drugs given alone; this proved negative.

Hicklin (1978) showed in a cross-over study in osteoarthritis and rheumatoid arthritis patients that salsalate (3 g daily) was comparable to a low dose of 250 mg daily of diflunisal in pain relief. Symptoms of 'salicylism' (tinnitus) were also observed in an open study of salsalate by this author and were claimed to be related to high plasma salicylate levels, though in comparison with other studies the values obtained were not all that remarkable.

Miscellaneous reports with salsalate

Re (1979) reported results of a multicentre trial for a 'two-week efficacy and safety field' among 28 medical specialities, and noted that erythrocyte sedimentation rate (ESR) was reduced in some subjects, though this was not correlated with patient response to the drug. The results showed a 67% favourable clinical report in physician's global evaluation, a 60% improvement in pain, and the drug was well tolerated by 96% patients. While such an encompassing yet tenuous study is difficult to accept by present-day standards of conduct of clinical trials, the results can be interpreted as showing the drug works in that nebulous entity known as the 'real world'. The reduction in ESR in some subjects deserves more detailed investigation, especially to establish why this occurred in some but not all subjects.

Open-label (McPherson, 1984), small-scale studies (Fazarinc and Steen, 1980) and conclusions from the analysis of data (Paulus, 1989) attest the clinical efficacy of salsalate in a variety of arthritic conditions. An interesting favourable indication for salsalate has been suggested in haemophiliacs with arthritic conditions, where this drug, like ibuprofen and benoxaprofen (now discontinued), had no effect on platelet function, bleeding time coagulation or the frequency of bleeds when ingested by haemophiliacs compared with non-haemophiliac subjects (Steven et al, 1985).

Diflunisal and Flufenisal

These fluorophenylsalicylates are appreciably more potent as anti-inflammatory and analgesic agents than salicylate, salsalate or aspirin in various animal models (Stone et al, 1977; Rainsford and Whitehouse, 1980, 1976). Remarkably, their clinical utility in arthritic conditions has been limited, though diflunisal does find some place in the analgesic market for osteoarthritis, where it was initially and is still primarily indicated. The story with flufenisal (MK-835;4-fluoro-4-hydroxy-3-biphenylcarboxylic acid acetate; Merck, Sharp & Dohme), though its life was short, is interesting in relation to the toxicity of the acetyl ester moiety in this drug. It exhibited analgesic effects at doses of 300 mg and 600 mg comparable with that of aspirin (600 mg and 1200 mg respectively) in relief of episiotomy pain (Bloomfield et al, 1970). The duration of analgesia was about twice as long as that with aspirin, being correlated with its longer plasma half-life(7 hours) compared with aspirin (i.e. as salicylate metabolite, 3 hours). Regrettably, gastrointestinal and renal toxicity noted with this drug in humans and laboratory animal models (Rainsford and Whitehouse, unpublished results; Rainsford, 1984) forced its withdrawal (T. Y. Shen, personal communication). The recognition of the role of the acetyl moiety in toxicity in these organ systems led to the search for a more potent salicylate, as reflected by substitution of a second fluoro moiety in diflunisal (Rainsford, 1984). Various studies have attested to the analgesic efficacy of diflunisal in various pain models in human subjects (Forbes et al, 1982a,b) as well as in osteoarthritis (Essigman et al, 1979).

GASTROINTESTINAL SIDE-EFFECTS

Studies in human subjects

Grossman et al (1961) were the first to show that sodium salicylate, whether given orally or intravenously, caused appreciably less gastrointestinal blood loss (assessed by the chromium-51 red blood cell method) than aspirin given by the same routes to male volunteers. In these studies blood loss was measured over a three-day period with the drugs being given three times daily in the following doses: aspirin 3 g daily orally or intravenously (as the bicarbonate salt), sodium salicylate 3 g daily orally or 2 g daily intravenously. Interestingly, in subjects who had shown a tendency to bleed before drug treatment, it was found that salicylate could markedly enhance blood loss. Many of the subjects employed in these studies had a history of peptic ulcer disease and some had bled just before the study. It is, therefore, likely that salicylate could potentiate a pre-existing ulcer or tendency to bleed. The authors noted that though salicylate is a weaker agent than aspirin in provoking bleeding, this former drug 'may be as dangerous as aspirin as far as initiation of significant hemorrhage is concerned'. In retrospect, with some thirty years' knowledge of the actions of salicylate compared with aspirin in laboratory animals (see next section) and from clinical observations in humans (as noted in the previous section), these quantitative and qualitative observations and the comment are probably most apposite today.

Recent endoscopic studies have been reported which show that salsalate (3.5 g daily for 14 days) produced appreciably fewer gastroduodenal lesions than naproxen (750 mg daily for 14 days) in normal, healthy subjects ($n = 20$

per group) (Lanza et al, 1989). Of the subjects who received salsalate 10% developed mucosal lesions, whereas 55% of subjects on naproxen had damage, which was much more pronounced than in the former group. The authors noted that these differences in drug effects paralleled clinical observations of the incidence of gastrointestinal side-effects in subjects with rheumatoid arthritis (Roth et al, 1989, 1990). Salsalate has also been shown to produce appreciably less endoscopically observed gastroduodenal injury than aspirin (Scheiman et al, 1989). In subjects with rheumatoid arthritis 3.0 g daily of salsalate ($n = 23$) produce appreciably less gastroscopically observed mucosal injury than 20 mg piroxicam ($n = 20$) daily over a four-week treatment period (Bianchi-Porro et al, 1989). There were no statistically significant differences in the therapeutic responses to either of these drugs. These results were confirmed in patients with rheumatoid arthritis (Montrone et al, 1989). Thus it is shown consistently that salsalate is among the least irritant or ulcerogenic NSAIDs in the gastrointestinal tract under controlled conditions.

Studies in animal models; comparative studies of mechanisms

Almost without exception it can now be said with hindsight that the animal model studies accurately predicted the lower gastric toxicity of salicylate as the acid or salts and salsalate compared with that of aspirin and other NSAIDs (Whitehouse et al, 1977; Rainsford, 1977, 1978b, 1981; Rainsford and Whitehouse, 1976, 1980a; Whitehouse and Rainsford, 1982). With the current criticisms of the use of laboratory species for investigations of drug toxicities, this outcome is both gratifying and reassuring for the patient. As noted, however, by Grossman et al (1961), these non-acetylated salicylates are not without their potential for toxic actions in the gastrointestinal mucosa, and this aspect is confirmed in the laboratory animal models (Rainsford, 1977, 1978b, 1981, 1984; Rainsford and Whitehouse, 1980; Whitehouse et al, 1977; Whitehouse and Rainsford, 1982). Our interest should also extend to the reasons for the differences in gastrointestinal ulcerogenicity of the non-acetylated salicylates compared with aspirin and other NSAIDs.

Hurley and Crandall (1963) performed quantitative endoscopic observations on the effects of oral or intravenous sodium salicylate (0.6 g daily) and various aspirin preparations (0.6 g daily) given to dogs for 21–34 days. The observations were performed five times over this time period. They showed that intravenous sodium salicylate failed to produce mucosal damage. Oral administration of the drug produced minimal damage, which was much less severe than that produced by plain aspirin tablets. In most of the animals the gastric erosions developed within the first few days.

In contrast to these observations, Davenport and colleagues showed that 20 μM salicylic acid in 0.1 M HCl produced equivalent damage to the gastric mucosal barrier (as evidenced by loss of physiologic ions into the gastric lumen) to that of an equimolar solution of aspirin in vagally denervated dogs (Davenport et al, 1965; Davenport, 1966). The gastric absorption of salicylic acid was slightly greater than that of aspirin under these conditions. Similar results have been observed on the gastric absorption of these drugs in both 0.1 M HCl and saline in pyloric ligated rats (Schanker et al, 1957). The slightly greater absorption of salicylic acid and the strongly acidic conditions may be a major factor in the irritancy of this drug. Accumulation of salicylic acid into parietal as well as mucous cells (Brune et al, 1977a, b) would appear to account for the selective toxicity of this drug as well as aspirin and other NSAIDs in these cells (Rainsford, 1975; Rainsford et al, 1980, 1981).

The unique distribution of the acetyl moiety compared with that of salicylate also has profound consequences for the more pronounced gastrointestinal ulcerogenicity of aspirin, e.g. acetylation of biomolecules (Rainsford et al, 1983).

The role of luminal acid in salicylic acid-induced mucosal damage has been shown in pyloric ligated rats (Rowe et al, 1987), dogs (Davenport et al, 1965; Davenport, 1966) and from electropotential difference measurements and K^+ loss from gastric mucosal damage in rats (Bruggeman et al, 1979; Morris et al, 1984) provided direct evidence of the back diffusion of hydrogen ions into the mucosa. This would appear to explain some of the irritant and barrier-breaking effects of salicylic acid on the mucosa. These authors also showed that a rapid drop in vascular resistance occurs when 20–30 μM salicylic acid is infused intragastrically to dogs with 100–160 μM HCl; the effect was evident within a minute and was not produced by the acid alone. The authors suggested that the back diffusion of acid was a cause of the drop in vascular resistance. They also showed that treatment with both histamine H_1 and H_2 blocking agents prevented the drop in vascular resistance. Johnson and Overholt (1967) showed that histamine is released into the stomach circulation of anaesthetized dogs within 10 minutes of perfusing the gastric lumen with 20 μM salicylic acid in 0.1 M HCl. Thus histamine release by salicylic acid would appear to be a major factor accounting for the reduction in vascular resistance induced by this drug. It also appears that salicylate (2.5–10 μM) has direct effects in enhancing release of intracellular hydrogen ions in exchange for extracellular sodium ions in rabbit gastric mucosal cells in vitro, a process that is sensitive to the inhibitory effects of the Na^+ channel blocker, amiloride (Olender et al, 1986). Thus, salicylic acid may stimulate exchange by ion trapping of H^+ but does not appear to influence HCO_3 movement (Olender et al, 1986), and these effects may account for the observed permeability changes which this drug induces.

Inhibition of the biosynthesis of gastroprotective prostaglandins (PGs) is thought to be one of a number of major factors accounting for the ulcerogenicity of NSAIDs (Rainsford, 1988, 1989). However, sodium salicylate does not appear to reduce gastric mucosal PG concentrations in the rat (Whittle et al, 1980) so that other mechanisms should be invoked to explain the irritancy of salicylate. Certainly the added effects of inhibiting PGs by other NSAIDs that are potent PG synthesis inhibitors (e.g. aspirin) would appear to account in part for their more profound ulcerogenicity (Rainsford, 1988, 1989). Salsalate has been reported to be without the inhibitory effects on PG synthesis exhibited by other NSAIDs (Morris et al, 1985).

Direct sloughing of gastric mucosal cells upon instillation of salicylic acid in acid, at pH 2, to guinea-pigs has been shown to be comparable with that produced by aspirin (Garner, 1977), suggesting that this exfoliation process is probably independent of drug-induced changes of PG synthesis.

A range of biochemical studies has been reported on the effects of salicylate and aspirin on mucosal metabolic processes. Thus, inhibition of the production of high-energy phosphate intermediates (ATP) and un-coupling of oxidative phosphorylation in pig gastric mucosal mitochondria has been shown (Glarborg Jorgensen et al, 1976; Rainsford and Whitehouse, 1980b). These effects may have importance in the long-term synthesis of biomolecules, especially gastric mucus synthesis. Inhibition of gastric mucosal cyclic AMP production by salicylate and aspirin has been observed (Mitznegg et al, 1977), and this could have consequences for the control of AMP-dependent intracellular reactions. Variations in the mucosal metabolism of salicylate to its glucuronides may also be important in the cyclical production of gastric lesions (Heitanen, 1975). Enterohepatic recirculation of salicylate may occur from the biliary excretion of salicylate, which has been shown in laboratory species (Pugh and Rutishauser, 1978; Cooper et al, 1980). This may be important for damage in the intestinal tract thought to be associated with aspirin in humans (Bjarnason et al, 1986; Jenkins et al, 1987).

The studies in laboratory animal models shows that oral salicylate or salicylic acid can be irritant to the upper gastrointestinal tract, but that it is probably less so than aspirin or other NSAIDs (Rainsford, 1977, 1978b, 1981, 1984; Whitehouse and Rainsford, 1982). Multiple mechanisms account for the actions of salicylate on the cellular and vascular integrity, biochemical and metabolic detoxification processes. The additional inhibitory actions of aspirin on PG synthesis probably account for the more pronounced ulcerogenicity of this drug compared with salicylate. It is probable that salsalate is even less ulcerogenic than salicylic acid (Rainsford, 1977) because of its pro-drug properties, i.e. as exemplified by effects of esterification of salicylates and other NSAIDs (Rainsford and Whitehouse, 1976; White-house and Rainsford, 1980). However, in comparison with the extensive studies that have been performed on the reactions of the gastric mucosa to NSAIDs, really very little is known about the effects of salsalate. Diflunisal is also of low ulcerogenicity (Torchiana et al, 1979) compared with other NSAIDs on the basis of relative anti-inflammatory actions (Rainsford, 1981).

CONCLUSION

A strong case can be made for the use of salicylate or salsalate in place of aspirin and probably even of other NSAIDs in the therapy of rheumatic conditions. The ultimate success of these non-acetylated salicylates will depend on patient preferences, toxicity and relative efficacy in the long term. Thus estimates of the drop-out rates of non-acetylated salicylates versus aspirin and other NSAIDs after one to five years of therapy will provide a good guide as to the acceptability of these drugs. We must await more detailed investigations on these points, together with further studies on the mode of action of salsalate and sodium salicylate, and development of formulations of the latter with improved safety and tolerability.

The reasons why aspirin was overlooked as effective therapy for rheumatoid arthritis for over half a century have been ably reviewed (Goodwin and Goodwin, 1981). The question arises: why did it take so long for clinicians and pharmacologists to appreciate that non-acetylated salicylates were just as effective as anti-inflammatory analgesics? The reason may well be that aspirin was known to acetylate albumin and other proteins (Hawkins et al, 1968; Pinckard et al, 1968; Samter, 1969), to inhibit adherence of platelets (O'Brien, 1968) and leucocytes (MacGregor et al, 1974), and to enhance platelet aggregation (Pinckard et al, 1968; Rosenkranz et al, 1986), whereas non-acetylated salicylates did not. Did this not prove that aspirin was a more powerful drug? The German proverb cited at the beginning of this chapter, that good medicines always have a bitter taste, may well hold for physicians as for patients. Max et al (1988) in a recent study of analgesics in herpetic neuralgia pain clearly showed that pain relief was potentiated by drug side-effects, whether mild or severe. The colour of the tablet, especially red, has been shown to potentiate the analgesic effects of placebo (Huskisson, 1974), and Schapira et al (1970) have shown that tablet colour is also important in the treatment of anxiety states. So that not only have we learnt that the acetyl moiety confers no added anti-inflammatory analgesia, but perhaps also about some of the factors that influence physicians' and patients' beliefs about medication.

In pragmatic terms we conclude that non-acetylated salicylates should be preferred to aspirin in rheumatology because:

1.   They are clinically equipotent.
2.   There is less gastrointestinal ulceration from non-acetylated salicylates (Leonards, 1969; Cohen, 1979; Mielants et al, 1981; Roth et al, 1990).
3.   There is a lower incidence of bronchial asthma from non-acetylated salicylates (Samter, 1973; Nizankowska et al, 1987; Morassut et al, 1989).
4.   Acetylated forms of salicylates are clearly more damaging to the kidneys than non-acetylated forms (Antillon et al, 1989; Bergamo et al, 1989); though it should be noted that salicylates themselves can cause some renal injury (Rainsford, 1984).

While non-acetylated salicylates may not be without their problems from side-effects it is apparent that the acetylated analogues, especially aspirin, are clearly more likely to produce these side-effects. Further work is clearly indicated to redefine the safety profile and efficacy of non-acetylated salicylates in rheumatologic practice and to develop more effective and safe formulations thereof.

REFERENCES

Abramson SB & Weissmann G (1989) The mechanisms of action of non-steroidal anti-inflammatory drugs. *Arthritis and Rheumatism* **32:** 1–9.

Anonymous (1983) Clinical pharmacology of the anti-rheumatic drugs. In Rodnan GP, Schumacher HR & Zvaifler NJ (eds) *Primer on the Rheumatic Diseases*, 8th edn, p 189. Atlanta: Arthritis Foundation.

Antillon M, Comimelli F, Reynolds TD & Zipser RD (1989) Comparative acute effects of diflunisal and indomethacin on renal function in patients with cirrhosis and ascites. *American Journal of Gastroenterology* **84**: 153–155.

April P, Abeles M, Baraf H et al (1990) Does the acetyl group of aspirin contribute to the anti-inflammatory efficacy of salicylic acid in the treatment of rheumatoid arthritis? *Seminars in Arthritis and Rheumatism* **19 (supplement 2)**: 20–28.

Arrigoni-Martelli E (1985) Pharmacology of free radical scavenging in inflammation. *International Journal of Tissue Reactions* **7**: 513–519.

Bergamo RR, Cominelli F, Kopple JD & Zipser RD (1989) Comparative acute effects of aspirin, diflunisal, ibuprofen and indomethacin on renal function in healthy man. *American Journal of Nephrology* **9**: 460–463.

Betts W & Cleland G (1982) Effect of metal chelators and anti-inflammatory drugs on the degradation of hyaluronic acid. *Arthritis and Rheumatism* **25**: 1469–1476.

Bianchi-Porro G, Petrillo M & Ardizzone S (1989) Salsalate in the treatment of rheumatoid arthritis: a double-blind clinical and gastroscopic trial versus piroxicam. II. Endoscopic evaluation. *Journal of International Medical Research* **17**: 320–323.

Biemond P, Swaak AJG, Penders JMA, Beindorff CM & Koster JF (1986) Superoxide production by polymorphonuclear leucocytes in rheumatoid arthritis and osteoarthritis: *in vivo* inhibition by the anti-rheumatic drug piroxicam due to interference with the activation of the NADPH-oxidase. *Annals of the Rheumatic Diseases* **45**: 249–255.

Biemond P, Swaak AJG, van Eijk HG & Koster JF (1988) Superoxide dependent iron release from ferritin in inflammatory diseases. *Free Radical Biology and Medicine* **4**: 185–198.

Bjarnason I, Zanelli G, Prouse P et al (1986) Effect of non-steroidal anti-inflammatory drugs on the human small intestine. *Drugs* **32 (supplement 1)**: 35–41.

Blechman WJ & Lechner BL (1979) Clinical comparative evaluation of choline magnesium trisalicylate and acetylsalicylic acid in rheumatoid arthritis. *Rheumatology and Rehabilitation* **18**: 119–124.

Bloomfield SS, Barden TP & Hille R (1970) Clinical evaluation of flufenisal, a long-acting analgesic. *Clinical Pharmacology and Therapeutics* **11**: 747–754.

Bruggeman TM, Wood JG & Davenport HW (1979) Local control of blood flow in the dog's stomach: vasodilatation caused by acid back-diffusion following topical application of salicylic acid. *Gastroenterology* **77**: 736–744.

Brune K, Graf P & Rainsford K (1977a) A pharmacokinetic approach to the understanding of therapeutic and side effects of salicylates. In Rainsford KD, Brune K & Whitehouse MW (eds) *Aspirin and Related Drugs: Their Actions and Uses*. Agents and Actions Supplement 1, pp 9–26. Basel: Birkhaeuser.

Brune K, Schweitzer A & Eckert H (1977b) Parietal cells of the stomach trap salicylates during absorption. *Biochemical Pharmacology* **26**: 1735–1740.

Caillier I, Bannwarth B, Monot C et al (1990) Differences in sodium salicylate protein binding in serum and synovial fluid from patients with a knee effusion. *International Journal of Clinical Pharmacology, Therapy and Toxicology* **28**: 7–13.

Capell HA, Rennie JAN, Rooney PJ et al (1979) Patient compliance: a novel method of testing non-steroidal anti-inflammatory analgesics in rheumatoid arthritis. *Journal of Rheumatology* **6**: 586–593.

Carlin G, Djursater R, Smedegard G & Gerdin B (1985) Effect of anti-inflammatory drugs on xanthine oxidase and xanthine oxidase-induced depolymerization of hyaluronic acid. *Agents and Actions* **16**: 377–384.

Chistoni A & Lapresa F (1909) Richerche farmacologiche sull' aspirina. *Archivo di Farmacologia Sperimentale e Scienze* **8**: 63–80.

Cohen A (1979) Fecal blood loss and plasma salicylate study of salicylsalicylic acid and aspirin. *Journal of Clinical Pharmacology* **19**: 242–247.

Cooper MJ, Baker AL & Moossa AR (1980) Sodium salicylate effects on determinants of bile flow and cholesterol solubility in rhesus monkeys. *Digestive Diseases and Sciences* **25**: 427–432.

Cowan RA, Hartnell GG, Lowdell CP, Baird IM & Leak AM (1984) Metabolic acidosis induced by carbonic anhydrase inhibitors and salicylates in patients with normal renal function. *British Medical Journal* **289**: 347–348.

Cox NL & Doherty SM (1987) Non-steroidal anti-inflammatories: outpatient audit of patient preferences and side-effects in different diseases. In Rainsford KD & Velo GP (eds) *Side Effects of Anti-Inflammatory Drugs. I. Clinical and Epidemiological Aspects*, pp 137–148. Lancaster: MTP Press.

Csuka ME & McCarty DJ (1989) Aspirin and the treatment of rheumatoid arthritis. *Rheumatic Disease Clinics of North America* **15:** 439–454.

Davenport HW (1966) Fluid produced by the gastric mucosa during damage by acetic salicylic acids. *Gastroenterology* **50:** 487–499.

Davenport HW, Cohen BJ, Bree M & Davenport VD (1965) Damage to the gastric mucosa: effects of salicylates and stimulation. *Gastroenterology* **49:** 189–196.

Deodhar SD, Dick WC, Hodgkinson R & Buchanan WW (1973) Measurement of clinical response to anti-inflammatory drug therapy in rheumatoid arthritis. *Quarterly Journal of Medicine* **42:** 387–401.

Deodhar SD, McLeod MM, Dick WC & Buchanan WW (1977) A short-term comparative trial of salsalate and indomethacin in rheumatoid arthritis. *Current Medical Research and Opinion* **5:** 185–188.

Dick C, Dick PH, Nuki G et al (1969) Effect of anti-inflammatory drug therapy on clearance of 133-Xe from knee joints of patients with rheumatoid arthritis. *British Medical Journal* **3:** 278–280.

Dick WC, Grayson MF, Woodburn A, Nuki G & Buchanan WW (1970) Indices of inflammatory activity. Relationship between isotope studies and clinical methods. *Annals of the Rheumatic Diseases* **29:** 643–648.

Droomgoole SH, Cassell S, Furst DE & Paulus HE (1983) Availability of salicylate from salsalate and aspirin. *Clinical Pharmacology and Therapeutics* **34:** 539–545.

Empire Rheumatism Council (1950) Multicentre controlled trial comparing cortisone acetate and acetylsalicylic acid in long-term treatment of rheumatoid arthritis. *Annals of the Rheumatic Diseases* **14:** 353–370.

Empire Rheumatism Council (1955) Multicentre controlled trial comparing cortisone acetate and acetylsalicylic acid in the long-term treatment of rheumatoid arthritis. Results up to one year. *Annals of the Rheumatic Diseases* **14:** 353–370.

Empire Rheumatism Council (1957) Multicentre controlled trial comparing cortisone acetate and acetylsalicylic acid in long-term treatment of rheumatoid arthritis. Results of three years' treatment. *Annals of the Rheumatic Diseases* **16:** 277–289.

Empire Rheumatism Council (1960) Gold therapy in rheumatoid arthritis: report of a multi-centre controlled trial. *Annals of the Rheumatic Diseases* **19:** 95–119.

Empire Rheumatism Council (1961) Gold therapy in rheumatoid arthritis: final report of a multicentre controlled trial. *Annals of the Rheumatic Diseases* **20:** 315–334.

Erhlich GE, Miller SB & Zeiders RS (1980) Choline magnesium trisalicylate versus ibuprofen in rheumatoid arthritis. *Rheumatology and Rehabilitation* **19:** 30–38.

Essigman WK, Chamberlain MA & Wright V (1979) Diflunisal in osteoarthrosis of the hip and knee. *Annals of the Rheumatic Diseases* **38:** 148–151.

Estes D & Kaplan K (1986) Lack of platelet effect with the aspirin analog, salsalate. *Arthritis and Rheumatism* **23:** 1303–1307.

Fazarinc F & Steen SN (1980) Long-term management of rheumatoid arthritis with disalcid. *Journal of International Medical Research* **8:** 339–342.

Forbes A, Foor M, Bowser MW, Calderazzo P, Shackleford W & Beaver WT (1982) A 12-hour evaluation of the analgesic efficacy of diflunisal, propoxyphene, a propoxyphene-acetaminophen combination, and placebo in postoperative oral surgery pain. *Pharmacotherapy* **2:** 43–49.

Forbes JA, Calderazzo JP, Bowser MW et al (1982b) A 12-hour evaluation of the analgesic efficacy of diflunisal, aspirin, and placebo in postoperative dental pain. *Journal of Clinical Pharmacology* **22:** 89–96.

Fremont-Smith K & Bayles TB (1965) Salicylate therapy in rheumatoid arthritis. *Journal of the American Medical Association* **192:** 1133–1136.

Furst DE, Blocka K, Cassell S et al (1987) A controlled study of concurrent therapy with a nonacetylated salicylate and naproxen in rheumatoid arthritis. *Arthritis and Rheumatism* **30:** 146–154.

Garner A (1977) Influence of salicylates on the rate of accumulation of deoxyribonucleic acid in gastric washings from the guinea pig. *Toxicology and Applied Pharmacology* **42:** 119–128.

Gay JC, Lukens JN & English DK (1984) Differential inhibition of neutrophil superoxide generation by non-steroidal anti-inflammatory drugs. *Inflammation* **8**: 209–222.

Ginsburg I, Sela MN, Morag A et al (1981) The role of leukocyte factors and cationic polyelectrolytes in the phagocytosis of group A streptococci and *Candida albicans* by neutrophils, macrophages, fibroblasts and epithelial cells. Modulation by anionic polyelectrolytes in relation to the pathogenesis of chronic inflammation. *Inflammation* **5**: 289–312.

Ginsburg I, Borinski R, Malamud D, Struckmayer F & Klimetzek V (1985) Chemiluminescence and superoxide generation by leukocytes stimulated by polyelectrolyte-opsonized bacteria. Role of polyarginine, polylysine, polyhistidine, cytochalasins and inflammatory exudates as modulators of the oxygen burst. *Inflammation* **5**: 245–271.

Ginsburg I, Borinski R, Sadovnic M, Eilam Y & Rainsford K (1987) Poly L-histidine. A potent stimulator of superoxide generation in human blood leukocytes. *Inflammation* **11**: 253–277.

Glarborg Jorgensen T, Weis-Fogh US, Nielsen HH & Olesen HP (1976) Salicylate and aspirin-induced uncoupling of oxidative phosphorylation in mitochondria isolated from the mucosal membrane of the stomach. *Scandinavian Journal of Clinical and Laboratory Investigation* **36**: 649–654.

Goldenberg A, Rudnicki RD & Koonce ML (1978) Clinical comparison of the safety of choline magnesium trisalicylate and indomethacin in treating osteoarthritis. *Current Therapeutic Research* **24**: 245–254.

Goodwin JS & Goodwin JM (1981) Failure to recognise efficacious treatments: a history of salicylate therapy in rheumatoid arthritis. *Perspectives in Biology and Medicine* **25**: 78–92.

Graham GG, Champion GD, Day RO et al (1977) Salicylates in rheumatoid arthritis: pharmacokinetics and analgesic response. In Rainsford KD, Brune K & Whitehouse MW (eds) *Aspirin and Related Drugs: Their Actions and Uses*, pp 37–42. Basel: Birkhauser.

Grootveld M & Halliwell B (1988) 2,3-Dihydroxybenzoic acid is a product of human aspirin metabolism. *Biochemical Pharmacology* **37**: 271–280.

Grossman MI, Matsumoto KK & Lichter RJ (1961) Fecal blood loss produced by oral and intravenous administration of various salicylates. *Gastroenterology* **40**: 383–388.

Hawkins D, Pinckard RN & Farr RS (1968) Acetylation of human serum albumin by acetylsalicylic acid. *Science* **160**: 780–781.

Hicklin JA (1978) Relationship of plasma salicylate levels to pain relief with two different salicylates. *Current Medical Research and Opinion* **5**: 572–579.

Hietanen E (1975) Mucosal and hepatic metabolism during spontaneous disappearance of salicylate-induced gastric lesions. *American Journal of Digestive Diseases* **20**: 31–41.

Higgs GA, Salmon JA, Henderson B & Vane JR (1987) Pharmacokinetics of aspirin and salicylate in relation to inhibition of arachidonate cyclo-oxygenase and anti-inflammatory activity. *Proceedings of the National Academy of Sciences of the USA* **84**: 1417–1420.

Higuchi S, Tanaka N, Shioiri Y, Otomo S & Aihara H (1986) Two modes of analgesic action of aspirin, and the site of analgesic action of salicylic acid. *International Journal of Tissue Reactions* **8**: 327–331.

Hurley JW & Crandall A (1963) The effect of various salicylates upon the dog's stomach: a gastroscopic photographic evaluation. In Dixon A St J, Martin BK, Smith MJH & Wood PHN (eds) *Salicylates: An International Symposium*, pp 213–216. London: Churchill.

Hurst NP (1987) Review. Molecular basis of activation and regulation of the phagocyte respiratory burst. *Annals of the Rheumatic Diseases* **46**: 265–272.

Hurst A & Lintott GAM (1939) Aspirin as a cause of haematemesis: a clinical and gastroscopic study. *Guy's Hospital Reports* **89**: 173–176.

Huskisson EC (1974) Simple analgesics for arthritis. *British Medical Journal* **4**: 196–200.

Jenkins RT, Rooney PJ, Jones DB, Bienenstock J & Goodacre RL (1987) Increased intestinal permeability in patients with rheumatoid arthritis: a side-effect of oral non-steroidal anti-inflammatory drug therapy? *British Journal of Rheumatology* **26**: 103–107.

Johnson LR & Overholt BF (1967) Release of histamine into gastric venous blood following injury by acetic and salicylic acid. *Gastroenterology* **52**: 505–509.

Kleinveld HA, Swaak AJG, Hack CE & Koster JF (1989) Interactions between oxygen free radicals and proteins: implications for rheumatoid arthritis. An overview. *Scandinavian Journal of Rheumatology* **18**: 334–352.

Lanza F, Rack MF, Doucette M et al (1989) An endoscopic comparison of the gastroduodenal injury seen with salsalate and naproxen. *Journal of Rheumatology* **16:** 1570–1574.

Larkai EN, Smith JL, Lidsky MD & Graham DY (1987) Gastroduodenal mucosa and dyspeptic symptoms in arthritic patients during chronic non-steroidal anti-inflammatory drug use. *American Journal of Gastroenterology* **82:** 1153–1158.

Lasagna L (1960) Analgesic drugs. *American Journal of Medical Sciences* **242:** 620–627.

Lecher BJ & Blechman WJ (1978) Double-blind comparison—trilisate tablets vs aspirin. *Florida Family Physicians* **28:** 50–56.

Lee P, Ahola SJ, Grennan D, Brooks P & Buchanan WW (1974) Observations on drug prescribing in rheumatoid arthritis. *British Medical Journal* **1:** 424–426.

Leonards JR (1969) Absence of gastrointestinal bleeding following administration of salicysalicylic acid. *Journal of Laboratory and Clinical Medicine* **74:** 911–914.

Levy G (1965) Aspirin: absorption rate and analgesic effect. *Anesthesiology and Analgesics* **44:** 837–841.

Liyanage SP & Tambar PK (1978) Comparative study of salsalate and aspirin in osteoarthrosis of the hip or knee. *Current Medical Research and Opinion* **5:** 450–453.

Luggan ME, Gartside PS & Hess EV (1989) Non-steroidal anti-inflammatory drugs in rheumatoid arthritis: duration of use as a measure of relative value. *Journal of Rheumatology* **16:** 1565–1569.

Lunec J, Halloran P, White AG & Dormandy TL (1981) Free-radical oxidation (peroxidation) products in serum and synovial fluid in rheumatoid arthritis. *Journal of Rheumatology* **8:** 233–245.

MacGregor RR, Spangnuolo PJ & Lentnek AL (1974) Inhibition of granulocyte adherence by ethanol, prednisone and aspirin measured by an assay system. *New England Journal of Medicine* **291:** 642–646.

McLaughlin G (1982) Choline magnesium trisalicylate versus naproxen in rheumatoid arthritis. *Current Therapeutic Research* **32:** 579–590.

McPherson TC (1984) Salsalate for arthritis: a clinical evaluation. *Clinical Therapeutics* **6:** 388–403.

Martin BK (1971) The formulation of aspirin. *Advances in Pharmaceutical Sciences* **3:** 107–171.

Max MB, Schafer SC, Culnane M, Dubner R & Gracely RH (1988) Association of pain relief with drug side-effects in post herpetic neuralgia: a single-dose study of clonidine, codeine, ibuprofen and placebo. *Clinical Pharmacology and Therapeutics* **43:** 363–371.

Medical Research Council (1954) A comparison of cortisone and aspirin in the treatment of early cases of rheumatoid arthritis. *British Medical Journal* **1:** 1223–1227.

Medical Research Council (1957) A comparison of cortisone and aspirin in the treatment of early cases of rheumatoid arthritis. *British Medical Journal* **1:** 847–850.

Medical Research Council & Nuffield Foundation (1954) A report by the Joint Committee of the Medical Research Council and Nuffield Foundation on clinical trials of cortisone, ACTH and other therapeutic measures in chronic rheumatic diseases. A comparison of cortisone and aspirin in the treatment of early cases of rheumatoid arthritis. *British Medical Journal* **1:** 1223–1227.

Medical Research Council & Nuffield Foundation (1955) A second report by the Joint Committee of the Medical Research Council and Nuffield Foundation on clinical trials of cortisone ACTH and other therapeutic measures in chronic rheumatic diseases. A comparison of cortisone and aspirin in the treatment of early cases of rheumatoid arthritis. *British Medical Journal* **2:** 695–700.

Medical Research Council & Nuffield Foundation (1957a) A report by the Joint Committee of the Medical Research Council and Nuffield Foundation on clinical trials of cortisone, ACTH and other therapeutic measures in chronic rheumatic diseases. A comparison of cortisone and prednisone in the treatment of rheumatoid arthritis. *British Medical Journal* **2:** 199–202.

Medical Research Council & Nuffield Foundation (1957b) A third report by the Joint Committee of the Medical Research Council and Nuffield Foundation on clinical trials of cortisone, ACTH and other therapeutic measures in chronic rheumatic diseases. Long-term results in early cases of rheumatoid arthritis treated with either cortisone or aspirin. *British Medical Journal* **1:** 847–850.

Medical Research Council & Nuffield Foundation (1959) Report by the Joint Committee of the Medical Research Council and Nuffield Foundation on clinical trials of cortisone, ACTH and other therapeutic measures in chronic rheumatic diseases. A comparison of prednisolone with aspirin or other analgesics in the treatment of rheumatoid arthritis. *Annals of the Rheumatic Diseases* **18**: 173–176.

Medical Research Council & Nuffield Foundation (1960) A second report by the Joint Committee of the Medical Research Council and Nuffield Foundation on clinical trials of cortisone, ACTH and other therapeutic measures in chronic rheumatic diseases. A comparison of prednisolone with aspirin or other analgesics in the treatment of rheumatoid arthritis. *Annals of the Rheumatic Diseases* **19**: 331–337.

Melzack R, Jeans ME, Kinch RA & Katz J (1983) Diflunisal (1000 mg single dose) versus acetaminophen (650 mg) and placebo for the relief of post-episiotomy pain. *Current Therapeutic Research* **34**: 929–939.

Mielants H, Veys EM, Verbruggen G & Schelstrete K (1981) Comparison of serum salicylate levels and gastrointestinal blood loss between salsalate and other forms of salicylates. *Scandinavian Journal of Rheumatology* **10**: 169–173.

Mitznegg P, Estler C-J, Loew FW & van Seil J (1977) Effect of salicylates on cyclic AMP in isolated rat gastric mucosa. *Acta Hepato-Gastroenterologica* **24**: 372–376.

Montrone F, Caruso I & Cazzola M (1989) Salsalate in the treatment of rheumatoid arthritis: a double-blind clinical and gastroscopic trial versus piroxicam. I. Clinical trial. *Journal of International Medical Research* **17**: 316–319.

Morassut P, Yang W & Karsh J (1989) Aspirin intolerance. *Seminars in Arthritis and Rheumatism* **18**: 22–30.

Morris GP, Wallace JL & Harding PL (1984) Effects of prostaglandin E2 on salicylate-induced damage to the rat gastric mucosa. Cytoprotection is not associated with preservation of the gastric mucosa. *Canadian Journal of Physiology and Pharmacology* **62**: 1065–1069.

Morris GH, Sherman NA, McQuain C et al (1985) Effects of salsalate (non-acetylated salicylate) and aspirin on serum prostaglandins in humans. *Therapeutic Drug Monitoring* **7**: 435–438.

Multicentre Salsalate/Aspirin Comparison Study Group (1989) Does the acetyl group of aspirin contribute to the antiinflammatory efficacy of salicylic acid in the treatment of rheumatoid arthritis? *Journal of Rheumatology* **16**: 321–327.

Nizankowska E, Czerniawska-Mysik G & Szczeklik A (1987) The effect of prostacyclin on asthma precipitated by aspirin. *Allergie et Immunologie* **19**: 22–24.

O'Brien JR (1968) Effect of anti-inflammatory agents on platelets. *Lancet* **i**: 894–895.

Olender EJ, Woods D, Kozol R & Fromm D (1986) Salicylate effects on proton gradient dissipation by isolated gastric mucosal surface cells. *Proceedings of the Society for Experimental Biology and Medicine* **183**: 177–185.

Oyanagui Y (1978) Inhibition of superoxide anion production in non-stimulated guinea pig peritoneal exudate cells by anti-inflammatory drugs. *Biochemical Pharmacology* **27**: 777–782.

Paulus HE (1989) Aspirin versus non-acetylated salicylate (editorial). *Journal of Rheumatology* **16**: 264–265.

Pelletier JP, Cloutier JM & Martel-Pelletier J (1989) *In vitro* effects of tiaprofenic acid, sodium salicylate and hydrocortisone on the proteoglycan metabolism of human osteoarthritis cartilage. *Journal of Rheumatology* **16**: 646–655.

Pinckard RN, Hawkins D & Farr RS (1968) *In vitro* acetylation of plasma proteins, enzymes and DNA by aspirin. *Nature* **219**: 68–69.

Pincus T & Callahan LF (1989) Clinical use of multiple non-steroidal anti-inflammatory preparations within individual rheumatology practices. *Journal of Rheumatology* **16**: 1253–1258.

Preston SJ, Arnold MH, Beller EM, Brooks PM & Buchanan WW (1989) Comparative analgesic and anti-inflammatory properties of sodium salicylate and acetylsalicylic acid (aspirin) in rheumatoid arthritis. *British Journal of Clinical Pharmacology* **27**: 607–611.

Pugh PM & Rutishauser SCB (1978) Comparative effects of 2,4-dinitrophenol and sodium salicylate on bile secretion in the dog, cat, rabbit and guinea pig. *Biochemical Pharmacology* **9**: 119–121.

Radeke HH, Meier B, Topley N, Floge J, Habermehl GG & Resch K (1990) Interleukin 1-α and tumor necrosis factor-α induce oxygen radical production in mesangial cells. *Kidney International* **37**: 767–775.

Rainsford KD (1975) Electronmicroscopic observations on the effects of orally administered

662666666

aspirin and aspirin bicarbonate mixtures on the development of gastric mucosal damage in the rat. *Gut* **16:** 514–527.

Rainsford KD (1977) Gastrointestinal damage from aspirin and non-steroidal anti-inflammatory drugs: thoughts for safer therapy from biochemical studies. *Drugs under Experimental and Clinical Research* **2:** 121–132.

Rainsford KD (1978a) The effects of aspirin and other non-steroidal anti-inflammatory drugs on the gastrointestinal mucus glycoprotein biosynthesis *in vivo*. Relationship to ulcerogenic actions. *Biochemical Pharmacology* **27:** 877–885.

Rainsford KD (1978b) Structure–activity relationships of non-steroidal anti-inflammatory drugs. I. Gastric ulcerogenic activity. *Agents and Actions* **8:** 587–605.

Rainsford KD (1981) Comparison of the gastric ulcerogenic activity of new non-steroidal anti-inflammatory drugs in stressed rats. *British Journal of Pharmacology* **73:** 79c–80c.

Rainsford KD (1984) *Aspirin and the Salicylates*. London: Butterworths.

Rainsford KD (1988) Mechanisms of gastrointestinal toxicity of non-steroidal anti-inflammatory drugs. *Scandinavian Journal of Gastroenterology* **24** (supplement 163): 9–16.

Rainsford KD (1989) Mechanisms of gastrointestinal damage by non-steroidal anti-inflammatory drugs. In Szabo S & Pfeiffer CJ (eds) *Ulcer Disease: New Aspects of Pathogenesis and Pharmacology*, pp 3–13. Boca Raton: CRC Press.

Rainsford KD & Velo GP (1987) *Side Effects of Anti-Inflammatory Drugs. I. Clinical and Epidemiological Aspects*. Lancaster: MTP Press.

Rainsford KD & Whitehouse MW (1976) Gastric irritancy of aspirin and its congeners: anti-inflammatory activity without this side-effect. *Journal of Pharmacy and Pharmacology* **8:** 599–601.

Rainsford KD & Whitehouse MW (1980a) Are all aspirins alike? A comparison of gastric ulcerogenicity with bioefficacy in rats. *Pharmacological Research Communications* **12:** 85–95.

Rainsford KD & Whitehouse MW (1980b) Biochemical gastro-protection from acute ulceration induced by aspirin and related drugs. *Biochemical Pharmacology* **29:** 1281–1289.

Rainsford KD, Schweitzer A, Green P, Whitehouse MW & Brune K (1980) Biodistribution in rats of some salicylates with low gastric ulcerogenicity. *Agents and Actions* **10:** 457–464.

Rainsford KD, Schweitzer A & Brune K (1981) Autoradiographic and biochemical observations on the distribution of non-steroidal anti-inflammatory drugs. *Archives Internationales Pharmacodynamie et de Thérapie* **250:** 180–194.

Rainsford KD, Schweitzer A & Brune K (1983) Distribution of the acetyl compared with the salicyl moiety of acetylsalicylic acid. Acetylation of biomolecules in organs wherein side effects are manifest. *Biochemical Pharmacology* **32:** 1301–1308.

Rainsford KD, Davies A, Mundy L & Ginsburg I (1989) Comparative effects of azapropazone on cellular events at inflamed sites. Influence on joint pathology, leucocyte superoxide and eicosanoid production, platelet aggregation, synthesis of cartilage proteoglycans, synovial production and actions of interleukin-1 induced cartilage resorption correlated with drug uptake into cartilage *in vitro*. *Journal of Pharmacy and Pharmacology* **41:** 322–330.

Re ON (1979) Salicylsalicylic acid revisited: a multicentre study. *Journal of International Medical Research* **7:** 90–95.

Regalado RG (1978) The use of salsalate for control of long-term musculoskeletal pain: an open non-comparative assessment. *Current Medical Research and Opinion* **5:** 454–460.

Reynolds JEF (ed.) (1989) *Martindale: The Extra Pharmacopoeia*, 29th edn. London: Pharmaceutical Press.

Roch M (1912) 1. Acide acetyl-salicylique et salicylate de soude. *Bulletin Générale de Thérapeutique Médicale de Paris* **163:** 218–223.

Rosenbloom D, Brooks PM, Bellamy N & Buchanan WW (1985) *Clinical Trials in the Rheumatic Diseases: a Selected Critical Review*. New York: Praeger.

Rosenkranz B, Rischer C, Meese CO & Frolich JC (1986) Effects of salicylic and acetylsalicylic acid alone and in combination on platelet aggregation and prostanoid synthesis in man. *British Journal of Clinical Pharmacology* **21:** 309–317.

Roth SH, Mitchell CS, Bennett RE et al (1989) Gastrointestinal effects of salsalate vs. naproxen in patients with rheumatoid arthritis (abstract). *Arthritis and Rheumatism* **32** (supplement): R46.

Roth S, Bennett R, Caldron P et al (1990) Reduced risk of NSAID gastropathy (GI mucosal toxicity) with nonacetylated salicylate (salsalate): an endoscopic study. *Seminars in Arthritis and Rheumatism* **19:** 11–19.

Rothwell KG (1983) Efficacy and safety of a non-acetylated salicylate, choline magnesium trisalicylate, in the treatment of rheumatoid arthritis. *Journal of International Medical Research* **11:** 343–348.

Rowe PH, Starlinger MJ, Kasdon E, Hollands MJ & Silen W (1987) Parenteral aspirin and sodium salicylate are equally injurious to the rat gastric mucosa. *Gastroenterology* **93:** 863–871.

Sagone AL & Husney RM (1987) Oxidation of salicylates by stimulated granulocytes: evidence that these drugs act as free radical scavengers in biological systems. *Journal of Immunology* **138:** 2177–2183.

Samter M (1969) The acetyl in aspirin. *Annals of Internal Medicine* **71:** 208–209.

Samter M (1973) Intolerance to aspirin. *Hospital Practice* **8:** 85–90.

Schanker LS, Shore A, Brodie B & Hogben CM (1957) Absorption of drugs from the stomach of the rat. *Journal of Pharmacology and Experimental Therapeutics* **120:** 528–539.

Schapira K, McClelland HA, Griffiths NR & Newell DJ (1970) Study on the effects of tablet colour on the treatment of anxiety states. *British Medical Journal* **2:** 446–449.

Scheiman JM, Behler EM, Berardi RR & Elta GH (1989) Salicylic acid causes less gastroduodenal mucosal damage than enteric-coated aspirin. An endoscopic comparison. *Digestive Diseases and Sciences* **34:** 229–232.

Scott DL, Roden S, Marshall T & Kendall MJ (1982) Variations in responses to non-steroidal anti-inflammatory drugs. *British Journal of Clinical Pharmacology* **14:** 691–694.

Seed JC (1965) A clinical comparison of the antipyretic potency of aspirin and sodium salicylate. *Clinical Pharmacology and Therapeutics* **6:** 353–358.

Singleton PT (1980) Salsalate: its role in the management of rheumatic diseases. *Clinical Therapeutics* **3:** 80–101.

Smith MJH (1978) Aspirin and prostaglandins. Some recent developments. *Agents and Actions* **8:** 427–429.

Smith MJH, Ford-Hutchinson AW, Walker JR & Slack JA (1979) Aspirin, salicylate and prostaglandins. *Agents and Actions* **9:** 483–487.

Soren A (1975) Transport time for salicylates from blood to joint fluid—a test of histopathology of the synovial membrane. *Zeitschrift für Rheumatologie* **34:** 213–220.

Soren A (1977) Dissociation of acetylsalicylic acid in blood and joint fluid. *Scandinavian Journal of Rheumatology* **6:** 17–22.

Spisani S, Marangoni C, Dovigo L & Traniello S (1984) Effect of antiinflammatory agents on neutrophil superoxide production in rheumatoid arthritis. *Inflammation* **8:** 45–53.

Steven MM, Small M, Pinkerton L, Madhok R, Sturrock RD & Forbes CD (1985) Non-steroidal anti-inflammatory drugs in haemophilic arthritis. A clinical and laboratory study. *Haemostasis* **15:** 204–209.

Strauss MB (ed.) (1968) *Familiar Medical Quotations*, p 127. Boston: Little, Brown.

Stone CA, Van Arman CG, Lotti VJ et al (1977) Pharmacology and toxicology of diflunisal. *British Journal of Clinical Pharmacology* **4:** 19S–29S.

Suzuki M, Inauen W, Kvietys PR et al (1989) Superoxide mediates reperfusion-induced leukocyte–endothelial cell interactions. *American Journal of Physiology* **257:** H1740–H1745.

Torchiana ML, Wiese SR & Westrick BL (1979) Comparison of the effects of diflunisal and other salicylates on the intragastric electropotential. *Journal of Pharmacy and Pharmacology* **31:** 112–114.

Van Dyke K, Peden D, Van Dyke C et al (1982) Inhibition by non-steroidal anti-inflammatory drugs of luminol-dependent human-granulocyte chemiluminescence and [3-H]FMLP binding. Effect of sulindac sulfide, indomethacin metabolites, and optical enantiomers (+) and (−) MK830. *Inflammation* **6:** 113–125.

Walker JR, Smith MJH & Ford-Hutchinson AW (1976) Anti-inflammatory drugs, prostaglandins and leucocyte migration. *Agents and Actions* **6:** 602–606.

Weitz Z, Moak SA & Greenwald RA (1988) Degradation of hyaluronic acid by neutrophil derived oxygen radicals is stimulus dependent. *Journal of Rheumatology* **15:** 1250–1253.

Whitehouse MW, Rainsford KD, Young IG, Ardlie NG & Brune K (1977) Alternatives to aspirin, derived from biological sources. *Agents and Actions* **7** (supplement 1): 43–57.

Whitehouse MW & Rainsford KD (1980) Esterification of acidic anti-inflammatory drugs suppresses their gastrotoxicity without adversely affecting their anti-inflammatory activity in rats. *Journal of Pharmacy and Pharmacology* **32:** 795–796.

Whitehouse MW & Rainsford KD (1982) Comparison of the gastric ulcerogenic activities of different salicylates. In Pfeiffer CJ (ed.) *Drugs and Peptic Ulcer Disease*, vol. 2, pp 127–141. Boca Raton: CRC Press.

Whittle BJ, Higgs GA, Eakins KE, Moncada S & Vane JR (1980) Selective inhibition of prostaglandin production in inflammatory exudates and gastric mucosa. *Nature* **234:** 271–272.

Zoschke DC & Kaja J (1989) Suboptimal levels of hydrogen peroxide scavengers in synovial fluid: *in vitro* augmentation with slow acting antirheumatic drugs. *Journal of Rheumatology* **16:** 1233–1240.

6

The management of NSAID gastropathy

JOHN M. HOWARD
NICOLE G. H. LE RICHE

Pain is a feature of most rheumatic diseases. Inflammation is the key pathological feature in many rheumatic diseases. Non-steroidal anti-inflammatory drugs (NSAIDs), which possess both analgesic and anti-inflammatory components, would appear to be ideal drugs to manage many of these diseases. In fact, in a survey of the patterns of NSAID use, NSAIDs were prescribed in 55% of visits for the broad diagnosis of arthritis (Baum et al, 1985). While NSAIDs can relieve pain and inflammation they can also cause gastrointestinal upset, ulceration, perforation, gastrointestinal bleeding and rarely death. Although the benefits of NSAIDs are fairly clear, the magnitude of the risks of using them and the way in which to avoid these risks are less clear. This chapter reviews the risks of NSAIDs to the upper gastrointestinal tract, treatment of the gastrointestinal effects of NSAIDs and ways in which to prevent or minimize these effects.

NSAIDs can cause significant injury to many areas of the luminal gastrointestinal tract, including the oesophagus, stomach, duodenum and small bowel. NSAID gastropathy refers to injury to the stomach caused by NSAIDs. It is sometimes difficult to separate out the specific effects of NSAIDs on the stomach alone, since many trials report both duodenal and gastric injury. Injury to the stomach and duodenum is responsible for most significant gastrointestinal complications. The emphasis of this chapter is on injury to the stomach, but where appropriate, injury to the duodenum is also discussed.

MECHANISMS OF NSAID INJURY

There are two distinct aspects of NSAID-induced injury: first, the acute injury to the gastric and duodenal mucosa which occurs within 24 hours of ingestion of the NSAID; and second, the development of chronic gastric or duodenal ulceration which may occur, if it does, over several weeks. In order to understand the way in which NSAIDs can cause injury to the upper gastrointestinal tract it is necessary to consider the constituents of the mucosal barrier.

Baillière's Clinical Rheumatology—
Vol. 4, No. 2, August 1990
ISBN 0–7020–1480–X

Defence mechanisms—the gastric mucosal barrier

The constituents of the gastric mucosal barrier have recently been reviewed (Schoen and Vender, 1989); they include the mucus layer, the phenomenon of surface hydrophobicity, the presence of bicarbonate secretion, a rich mucosal blood supply, the availability of neutralizing sulfhydryl compounds and the ability of the mucosal cells to cover rapidly any injured areas. Which component is most important to mucosal defence remains controversial. The gastric mucus is directly in contact with gastric acid in the lumen; the mucus is a high-viscosity gel which impedes hydrogen ion diffusion (Allen and Garner, 1980), resulting in a pH gradient across the mucus (Bahari et al, 1982). Hills et al (1983) showed that the gastric mucosa was very hydrophobic leading to repulsion of the aqueous acid solution within the stomach lumen. Bicarbonate, which can neutralize the back diffusion of acid, is actively secreted from the surface of the gastric mucosa but probably neutralizes less than 10% of the total acid secretion of the stomach (Allen and Garner, 1980). The gastric mucosal blood flow appears to play a defensive role in that blood flow increases if there is back diffusion of acid into the mucosa (Guth, 1984). Sulfhydryl compounds in the form of reduced glutathione are found in high concentration in the gastric mucosa; these are then available to bind free radicals which are generated following mucosal injury (Boyd et al, 1979). Very rapid mucosal re-epithelialization appears to occur following mucosal injury (Rutten and Ito, 1983).

The role of prostaglandins

Prostaglandins are a family of unsaturated fatty acids which are made in most kinds of cells. There is ample evidence to confirm the importance of prostaglandins in the maintenance of the gastric mucosal barrier. Prostaglandins are found in high concentration throughout the gut. Active immunization of rabbits with prostaglandins results in gastrointestinal mucosal ulceration, as does the passive immunization of rabbits with prostaglandin antibodies—strongly suggesting the role of prostaglandins in the maintenance of mucosal integrity (Redfern and Feldman, 1989). A major stimulus for their formation is mild injury, including acid damage (Robert et al, 1983). Administration of selected prostaglandins prior to injury by such diverse agents as hot liquids, alcohol, and acidic, alkaline and hypertonic solutions can significantly reduce subsequent mucosal injury (Robert et al, 1979). These findings lead to the concept of 'cytoprotection', perhaps more accurately termed 'mucosal protection', and form the basis for the use of exogenously administered prostaglandins for the prevention of mucosal injury.

    Exogenously administered prostaglandins have been found to have a number of actions that can be interpreted as improving the gastric mucosal barrier. These include production of mucus gel with increased thickness (McQueen et al, 1983), increased mucosal bicarbonate secretion (Domschke et al, 1978), induction of increased mucosal surface hydrophobicity (Lichtenberger et al, 1985) and increased mucosal blood flow

(Kauffman et al, 1979). These findings provide the basis for the use of prostaglandins for the prevention of NSAID-induced gastrointestinal damage in patients.

The process of mucosal injury by NSAIDs

Mucosal damage occurs very soon after aspirin administration. Ultrastructural damage is seen as early as one minute following exposure of the gastric mucosa to aspirin (Hingson and Ito, 1971). Damage is maximal by eight minutes following exposure. Cellular disruption occurs with the subsequent development of intramucosal haemorrhages which can be detected at endoscopy (Graham and Smith, 1986). Within several hours, erosions develop in areas where haemorrhages were most concentrated. Healing of haemorrhages occurs within several days of a single dose of NSAID but erosions take longer to resolve, often taking more than a week to resolve totally.

There are many acute cellular effects of aspirin on the gastric mucosa. Other NSAIDs, including indomethacin and phenylbutazone, produce similar changes in the gastric mucosa (Schoen and Vender, 1989) but the effects of asprin are discussed here. Aspirin is a weak organic acid that becomes unionized in an acid environment which encourages its absorption into the mucosal cells. Upon absorption it enters a neutral environment where it becomes ionized and is trapped in the cell. The absorption of aspirin has several effects on cell function. The mucus layer shows decreased thickness, increased permeability to acid and increased breakdown by proteases (Sarosiek et al, 1986). Tight junctions are disrupted (Meyer et al, 1986). Rapid back-diffusion of acid into the mucosa occurs with subsequent loss of the transmucosal potential difference (Murray et al, 1974). Bicarbonate secretion is reduced (Garner, 1978) as is the surface hydrophobicity (Lichtenberger et al, 1985). The two mechanisms mainly responsible for this injury are the inhibition of cyclo-oxygenase and the toxic effects of salicylate on the cell itself (Kauffman, 1989). Cyclo-oxygenase inhibition appears to be responsible for the inhibition of mucus secretion, the alteration of the physicochemical properties of the mucus, the inhibition of bicarbonate secretion and the reduction of hydrophobicity of the epithelial cell surface. Acetylsalicylate is rapidly deacetylated to salicylate which is directly toxic to cells.

Tissue repair occurs through a process called restitution, which is the migration of cells from the surrounding gastric glands. The initial stages of repair appear to occur without a significant increase in cell division or an increase in protein synthesis and are not significantly influenced by prostaglandins (Silen and Ito, 1985).

The continued administration of an injurious agent appears to result in an adaptive response by the mucosa which results in less severe signs of injury (Graham et al, 1983). Almost all subjects given a single dose or a short course of aspirin will demonstrate endoscopic signs of injury. However, 32% of patients receiving chronic doses of various NSAIDs had no endoscopic evidence of damage (Larkai et al, 1987). This phenomenon is referred to as 'adaptive cytoprotection'. It is interesting that pre-treatment of the mucosa with a variety of irritants significantly reduces the degree of injury caused by subsequent application of an irritant (Robert et al, 1983). This phenomenon may help us to explain the lack of correlation between the presence of acute injury to the mucosa and the infrequent occurrence of mucosal ulceration after chronic administration of NSAIDs.

Lack of correlation between acute injury and chronic injury

Despite much information describing the acute effects of NSAIDs on the mucosa, the mechanisms that determine why some patients develop ulcers following chronic administration of NSAIDs while others do not are unknown. The assumption that acute gastric injury is a precursor for chronic ulceration may not be correct. In fact there is good evidence to refute this assumption. Pro-drugs—drugs that are activated following absorption—have at least the same propensity to cause chronic ulceration as do drugs that are inherently active and cause immediate injury to the stomach and duodenum. Sulindac, which requires activation in the liver and has no local irritant effects, was the leading cause of bleeding associated with NSAIDs in the first month of treatment in one study (Carson et al, 1987a). It is critically important to realize that *all* of the prospective prevention trials deal with acute damage or acute ulceration rather than chronic ulceration. All reported treatment trials may turn out to have little or no relevance to clinical practice, since the most important life-threatening process which we try to prevent with the use of concomitant medication is the chronic deep ulcer, rather than erosions or acute ulceration.

THE UPPER GASTROINTESTINAL RISKS OF NSAIDS

Before attempting to prevent the gastrointestinal complications of the use of NSAIDs, it is important to understand the scope of the problem. NSAIDs frequently cause gastrointestinal side-effects, which are usually of symptomatic importance only; however, NSAIDs can occasionally cause peptic ulceration, which can become life-threatening as a result of bleeding or perforation. The physician must try to reduce the symptoms of gastrointestinal intolerance caused by NSAIDs without compromising their anti-inflammatory and analgesic effects. However, if a patient has an ulcer, the physician's overriding aim is to heal the ulcer, thereby preventing possible life-threatening complications of the ulcer.

NSAID-induced upper gastrointestinal symptoms

Symptoms referable to the upper gastrointestinal tract are common in patients receiving NSAIDs. Studies of large numbers of patients treated with a variety of NSAIDs indicate that the risk of gastrointestinal side-effects is between 16% (Cox and Doherty, 1987) and 35% (Husby et al,

1986). A recent study by Larkai et al (1989) reported on 245 arthritic patients on continuous treatment with various NSAIDs. Heartburn, indigestion and sour stomach occurred in 37% of patients at least once in the two months prior to questioning. Twenty-nine per cent had experienced these symptoms in the previous week. Sixteen per cent reported at least daily dyspepsia and 4% reported episodes of dyspepsia more than five times daily. Twenty-three per cent of patients gave a history of peptic ulcers. There was no correlation between reports of dyspepsia and the history of previous ulcer disease.

Risk of ulcer perforation or haemorrhage

It is commonly believed that the use of NSAIDs is associated with the development of gastrointestinal ulceration. The risk of developing mucosal damage immediately following NSAID administration is high, whereas the risk of developing a life-threatening gastrointestinal complication is fortunately low. The reported risk of a life-threatening complication depends on the type of study performed. In order to assess accurately the risk of complication in any one patient, one must be aware of the data on which the ulceration association is based.

Case-control studies provide the most direct evidence that NSAIDs play a significant role in ulcer causation. When patients with gastric ulcers or duodenal ulcers and hospital controls are asked about NSAID use, more patients with gastric ulcers are found to have been taking NSAIDs than either duodenal ulcer patients or controls (McIntosh et al, 1985; Duggan et al, 1986). In studies of patients presenting with perforated ulcers, there is a highly significant association between perforation and NSAID use compared to a hospital control population (Collier and Pain, 1985). In a case-control study of patients admitted for bleeding duodenal or gastric ulcers, 35% were taking NSAIDs as compared to only 15% of controls (Somerville et al, 1986). Non-aspirin NSAIDs were taken more than twice as often by patients presenting with bleeding, compared with community or hospital controls. Clearly, ingestion of NSAIDs is associated with an increased risk of ulcer complication.

Pincus and Callahan (1986) performed a meta-analysis of all studies of patients with rheumatoid arthritis in which mortality was considered. This analysis gives some idea as to the relative risk of taking NSAIDs in any one patient. Of 11 studies analysed, 5% of all deaths were secondary to gastrointestinal causes. The control frequency was 2.4%, giving a doubled risk of death due to gastrointestinal causes in patients with rheumatoid arthritis. A more recent study (Fries et al, 1989) of hospitalizations in 1949 patients with rheumatoid arthritis demonstrated a sixfold increase in hospitalization in patients who had been NSAID users compared with rheumatoid arthritis patients who had never been NSAID users. Death from gastrointestinal causes were twice those in patients who received NSAIDs compared to non-NSAID users. Increasing disability, use of prednisone and increasing age were also factors associated with increased admissions for gastrointestinal problems.

Given that NSAID use is associated with gastrointestinal ulceration, other studies have attempted to look at the actual risk for any one patient developing a gastrointestinal complication. The risks reported in surveillance studies indicate a relatively low, sometimes undetectable occurrence of significant gastrointestinal side-effects. Inman (1985) reported that no serious side-effects were detectable in patients on courses of NSAIDs, compared with times when the patients were not on NSAIDs. His estimate of the rate of ulcer perforation associated with upper gastrointestinal bleeding was one occurrence every 200 patient years of NSAID use. Carson (1987b) reported a relative risk of significant upper gastrointestinal bleeding of 1.5 in patients receiving NSAIDs compared with unexposed patients. The occurrence of bleeding was 1.27 per 10 000 patient months of treatment in patients receiving NSAIDs, compared with 0.83 per 10 000 patient months in non-exposed patients. Most comparative trials of NSAIDs are too small and have a number of exclusion criteria so that results are not applicable to the general rheumatologic population. However, in the largest trial (Husby, 1986), which compared piroxicam and naproxen, 2035 patients were randomized. Over 30% of each treatment group suffered from at least one gastrointestinal event, of which approximately 1% of the total were considered severe (Husby, 1986). Chalmers et al (1988) performed a meta-analysis of the side-effects of 44 aspirin and 123 non-aspirin placebo-controlled NSAID trials. Three times as many ulcers were documented in the aspirin group compared with the placebo group, with one proven ulcer occurring per 70 patients on aspirin. No difference was seen in the non-aspirin NSAID groups, but the rate of ulcer diagnosis was extremely small in both the placebo group (none of 6355 patients) and the treated group (2 of 6460 patients). More patients treated with aspirin suffered from a gross haemorrhage than did patients treated with placebo. These studies indicate the rare occurrence of ulcer complication in patients treated with NSAIDs. The risk of occurrence has critical importance when considering risk prevention trials. For example misoprostol has been reported to prevent NSAID-induced ulceration, but not a single patient had a complicated ulcer in either the active or placebo arm of the study. From their extensive analysis, Chalmers et al (1988) concluded that the detection of a 50% reduction in the aspirin-induced ulceration would require 3346 subjects on chronic aspirin therapy, if clinically significant ulceration was the end-point.

What is the absolute risk of a significant gastrointestinal complication in any one patient receiving NSAIDs? Langman (1989) recently reviewed the studies evaluating the epidemiologic evidence of the association between peptic ulceration and anti-inflammatory drug use. He states that 'a reasonable synthesis suggests that the risk is perceptibly increased by a factor between 2 and 4 for gastric ulcer occurrence, for ulcer complications (particularly bleeding), and for ulcer death'. It appears that the incidence of a significant complication is in the order of a single case per 10 000 courses of treatment.

Identification of patients at risk for NSAID-induced ulceration

The problem would be simple if gastrointestinal intolerance could predict the patients at risk of developing gastrointestinal ulceration. However, this is not the case. Acute administration of aspirin produces acute damage in almost all subjects (Jiranek et al, 1989). On the other hand, the risk of a significant complication of ulceration is about 1 per 10 000 treatment months (Langman, 1989). The correlation between gastrointestinal symptoms and endoscopic findings is poor (Doube and Morris, 1988), with some patients experiencing significant gastrointestinal side-effects with little or no change in the gastric or duodenal mucosa or endoscopy. On the other hand, some subjects have no symptoms but have significant mucosal injury on endoscopy. This lack of correlation between symptoms and gastric or duodenal damage is particularly important, because patients with ulcers frequently have no symptoms but can present with a life-threatening complication. It is a cause for concern that the first sign of gastrointestinal intolerance of NSAIDs is frequently a catastrophe. One-third of patients presenting with ulcers were asymptomatic in one study (Silvoso et al, 1979), whereas in another (Armstrong and Blower, 1987) 58% of patients presenting with complications of ulceration leading to death or surgery had had no previous gastrointestinal symptoms. Finally, drugs that cause little or no acute gastric damage can have at least the same potential for causing chronic ulcers as drugs that induce significant acute damage following their administration (Carson et al, 1987b). The lack of correlation between gastrointestinal symptoms and complications makes it difficult for the clinician concerned about the serious side-effects of NSAIDs. The patient with excellent symptomatic tolerance of NSAIDs may be as likely—or more likely—to develop life-threatening complications.

The elderly are at particular risk of developing gastrointestinal ulceration on NSAID treatment (Collier and Pain, 1985; CSM, 1986; Somerville et al, 1986; Armstrong and Blower, 1987; Griffin et al, 1988). In a study by Jick et al (1987) the adjusted rate ratio for a patient 60–79 years old taking NSAIDs was 20 times the risk of a similar patient 10–39 years old. The risk for a patient over 80 years old was more than twice that of a patient 60–79 years old. This increased risk is of particular importance given the increased occurrence of certain kinds of arthritis and resultant NSAID use with increasing age.

No other risk factors for the development of NSAID-induced gastrointestinal damage have been clearly established. Whether the patient has rheumatoid arthritis or osteoarthritis, and which NSAIDs are used, does not seem to be important in determining the risk of complications. Perhaps the most important question is whether any one NSAID causes a lower incidence of ulceration or bleeding. Somerville et al (1986) found a possible increase in bleeding with all NSAIDs except ibuprofen. Carson et al (1987b) found an increased risk of bleeding with sulindac as compared to ibuprofen.

Gastrointestinal ulceration is clearly a complication that can occur with the use of NSAIDs. The data to support this association are conclusive. However, NSAIDs have a definite role in the management of rheumatic diseases and in general have lower side-effect profiles than the remittive agents used in the treatment of certain kinds of inflammatory arthritis. Improvement of the risk–benefit ratios of NSAIDs includes consideration of the optimal treatment of ulcers should they occur and the use of agents that protect against the injurious effects of NSAIDs.

TREATMENT OF ESTABLISHED NSAID-INDUCED ULCERATION

Efficacy of available drugs

How should NSAID ulcers be treated? Many effective drugs exist. These include the histamine H_2-receptor antagonists, sucralfate, misoprostol and omeprazole. Any of these agents heal both gastric and duodenal ulcers as compared with placebo in clinical trials. The choice of which agent to use should be based on cost, possible side-effects and, perhaps to a lesser extent, differences in efficacy.

Histamine H_2-receptor antagonists

The available histamine H_2-receptor antagonists include cimetidine, ranitidine, famotidine and nizatidine. All of these drugs heal both gastric and duodenal ulceration well with minimal side-effects. All act on the parietal cell by competing with histamine—a powerful acid secretagogue—for the histamine H_2-receptor. The drugs do differ in potency and side-effects. Many trials have shown superiority of one agent over another, but equipotent doses of these agents were not used in these trials. Famotidine appears to be approximately nine times more potent than ranitidine which is approximately four times more potent than cimetidine (Howard et al, 1985). Therefore, given the administration of equipotent doses, there are likely to be no real differences in efficacy. Cimetidine does produce side-effects in selected indivuduals; it has antiandrogenic side-effects and can cause impotence, particularly in the older male. It interferes with hepatic metabolism of a number of drugs. Confusion has been reported in the elderly using this drug particularly if they also have renal insufficiency. The incidence of these side-effects is less or absent with ranitidine, famotidine and nizatidine. On the other hand, depending on the availability of the generically manufactured drugs, cimetidine is usually the cheapest of the H_2-receptor antagonists and is well tolerated in most subjects.

Sucralfate

Sucralfate is an effective drug in the treatment and long-term prevention of gastric and duodenal ulcers. It is an analogue of sucrose with eight aluminium and eight sulphate radicals attached to the sucrose core. It does not suppress gastric acid secretion, yet treatment of ulcers with sucralfate is as successful as treatment with histamine H_2-receptor antagonists. The drug probably acts by forming a protective barrier by attaching to the exudate over the ulcer, protecting it from further damage by acid and pepsin. Sucralfate has also been shown to have bile and pepsin binding properties, to increase bicarbonate secretion by the gastric mucosa and to have some properties suggestive of cytoprotection (Szabo and Hollander, 1989). No consistent significant side-effects have been reported. The local action of sucralfate and its excellent side-effect profile have made it an attractive choice of drug in the treatment of NSAID-induced injury.

Prostaglandins

Prostaglandins have received significant attention for the treatment of NSAID-induced gastric and duodenal injury. Aspirin and other NSAIDs inhibit the formation of prostaglandins. Prostaglandins appear to play a major role in maintaining the integrity of the gastric mucosal barrier (as discussed earlier). Therefore, it is attractive to consider that replacement of the depleted prostaglandins may heal or lessen the injury caused by NSAIDs. Several synthetic prostaglandins have been tested, with misoprostol, a commercially available drug, having received the most attention.

Although not as extensively investigated as the histamine H_2-receptor antagonists and sucralfate, prostaglandins do heal gastric and duodenal ulcers better than placebo therapy. For gastric ulcer, misoprostol 100 μg four times daily had an eight-week healing rate of 62%, compared with the 45% healing rate of placebo (Agrawal et al, 1985). Misoprostol (Brand et al, 1985), enprostil (Thomson et al, 1986) and arbaprostil (Vantrappen et al, 1982) were superior to placebo in the treatment of duodenal ulcers. Diarrhoea was a frequently reported side-effect in these studies. Despite their efficacy in acute ulceration, these agents are not commonly prescribed to patients who are not taking NSAIDs, since fewer side-effects are seen with the use of H_2-receptor antagonists. For the primary treatment of ulcers, prostaglandins are no better and may be less efficacious than the H_2-receptor antagonists (Hawkey and Walt, 1986).

Omeprazole

Omeprazole is a benzimadazole derivative which inhibits the gastric mucosal hydrogen-potassium ATPase. This enzyme is responsible for the secretion of acid from the parietal cell. Omeprazole, which is ionized in an acid environment, is sequestered in the parietal cell. Ionization results in activation of the drug which acts by covalently binding to proteins with sulfhydryl groups. Binding of omeprazole to the hydrogen-potassium ATPase inactivates the enzyme. New enzyme needs to be formed before there is resumption of acid secretion. This drug has proved to be a most powerful suppressor of gastric acid secretion (Lind et al, 1983). Healing rates for duodenal ulcers (Bardhan et al, 1986), gastric ulcers (Walan et al, 1989) and particularly erosive oesphagitis (Sandmark et al, 1988) are greater than with conventional doses of histamine H_2-receptor antagonists. Omeprazole appears to provide the greatest potential for rapid healing in patients with peptic ulceration.

Use of any of these drugs will lead to healing of gastric or duodenal ulceration in most patients and thus prevent future complications. The studies that assessed the efficacy of all these drugs did not specifically consider the patient on NSAIDs. The choice of ulcer therapy is probably not as important as the decision whether to continue NSAIDs in a patient who has demonstrated clear benefit from NSAIDs. Therefore, it is important to consider the efficacy of the act of discontinuing the NSAID, a known cause of ulcers, as well as to consider the need for stopping the NSAID to allow healing of the ulcer.

The effect of NSAID discontinuation on ulcer healing

Is the discontinuation of the NSAID an active form of therapy for gastric ulcer? The need for the anti-inflammatory component of NSAIDs varies from patient to patient. NSAIDs might be discontinued in patients where arthritis is predominantly degenerative rather than inflammatory. Prior to the era of histamine H_2-receptor antagonists, Gerber et al (1981) reported on 35 evaluable cases of patients with rheumatoid arthritis and peptic ulcer. Complete healing in a six-month period as assessed radiologically occurred in all 8 cases treated with antacids alone in whom NSAIDs were stopped. It is interesting that in 27 patients in whom NSAIDs were continued, 21 (78%) also healed, indicating the usually benign course for peptic ulceration in patients receiving NSAIDs. Manniche et al (1987) performed a nine-week trial of sucralfate and ranitidine in 67 patients with duodenal or gastric ulcers who were on NSAIDs. In half of the patients, the NSAIDs were stopped. For all types of ulceration, 91% healed when the NSAIDs were stopped as opposed to 77% when the NSAIDs were continued. Despite the limitations of this evidence, it would seem reasonable that in patients in whom peptic ulceration is identified discontinuation of the NSAIDs leads to improved ulcer healing.

The necessity of discontinuing NSAIDs in the patient with an ulcer

Does the presence of a gastric ulcer necessitate stopping NSAIDs? Discontinuation of NSAIDs in a patient with arthritis may result in significant worsening of the arthritis and increased disability. In patients with a life-threatening complication such as perforation or bleeding, maximal therapy would include stopping the NSAIDs. The same imperative does not apply to the patient without a complication. Most comparative trials have either excluded patients on NSAIDs or have had too few patients continuing on NSAIDs to determine the effects of these drugs. Looking at trials that examined the effects of NSAIDs, Croker et al (1980) found that 11 of 14 gastric ulcers and 7 of 7 duodenal ulcers were healed with continued NSAID use after 12 weeks of cimetidine in a dose of 1 g per day. In 18 patients on NSAIDs with gastric ulceration, O'Laughlin (1982) found eight-week healing rates of 55% in patients treated with cimetidine 300 mg four times daily, compared with 40% in patients treated with placebo. They stated that all but one ulcer did eventually heal with up to 26 months of treatment. In the trial by Manniche (1987), 77% of all ulcers and 50% (3 of 6) of gastric ulcers were healed with either sucralfate 1 g four times daily or ranitidine 150 mg twice daily after nine weeks of treatment despite continued NSAID treatment. On the other hand, in a study by Jaszewski et al (1989), none of 7 patients with gastric ulcers who had been on NSAIDs and were continued on enteric coated aspirin healed on cimetidine, compared with 15 of 16 patients in whom no aspirin was given. In a study comparing ranitidine with omeprazole—the most powerful acid suppressant—for the treatment of gastric ulceration, over 80% healed with eight weeks of omeprazole as compared to 53% healing after eight weeks of ranitidine (Walan et al, 1989). Analysing the data, it appears that duodenal ulceration, and to a lesser extent gastric ulceration, will heal with medical treatment in a significant number of patients in whom NSAIDs are continued. It should be stated that there are no data as to whether or not continued NSAID administration leads to increased complications.

Conclusions regarding treatment of an established NSAID-induced ulcer

Recognizing the limitations of the available data, the following recommendations are suggested. Since NSAIDs are a major cause of ulceration, NSAIDs should be discontinued if at all possible. Therefore, in all patients presenting with a complication and in patients in whom the anti-inflammatory benefits of NSAIDs are small, the NSAID should be stopped to ensure maximum opportunity for healing. However, in patients with either duodenal or gastric ulcer in whom there is a clear benefit from the anti-inflammatory effects of NSAIDs, an argument can be made for the continuation of the NSAIDs in the uncomplicated patient. These patients could be treated with any of the standard ulcer therapies while receiving NSAIDs. Omeprazole may well be the most efficacious drug for healing the NSAID-induced ulcer. These patients, particularly those with gastric ulcers, should be followed until complete healing has occurred as assessed by X-ray or preferably by endoscopy. If no healing has been documented over a period of four to eight weeks, and in the case of gastric ulcer, gastroscopic biopsies have been negative for malignancy, the NSAIDs should be discontinued.

THE PREVENTION OF NSAID INJURY

Problems with trials evaluating NSAID injury prevention

Controversies over the definition of mucosal protection

Before one reads the literature regarding the prevention and treatment of NSAID-induced gastrointestinal injury, it is important to recognize the limitations of available studies. Initially there appears to be a wide choice of 'effective drugs' available to provide 'protection' against the damaging effects of NSAIDs. However, the 'protection' provided by the 'effective drug' may be of little (if any) clinical significance. Most studies have used elaborate endoscopic scoring systems to describe grades of injury—erythema, haemorrhages, erosions and acute ulcers. A reported improvement based on the reduction of the degree of erythema or the number of haemorrhages is of questionable significance since these injuries are thought to be quickly reversible. For example, sucralfate was found to be 'effective' in relieving symptoms and reducing gastric mucosal damage in patients receiving concomitant NSAID therapy (Caldwell et al, 1987). The frequency and severity of dyspeptic symptoms were reduced to a greater extent in the sucralfate group than in the placebo group. Closer evaluation, however, reveals no significant difference in the mean score between placebo or sucralfate-treated groups at the end of treatment (patients treated with sucralfate had slightly higher mean symptom scores prior to treatment). Sucralfate-treated patients had a mean symptom intensity score of 0.65 compared to a score of 0.72 for placebo-treated patients at the end of six weeks (symptom scoring method was not described, but on entry the mean score was in the order of 1.4). Similarly, a difference in the endoscopic score between the groups at the end of six weeks was reported, with patients on sucralfate experiencing a reduction in score from 3.5 to 2.5 and patients on placebo a reduction in score from 2.9 to 2.5. A score of 2.0 in this study denoted presence of mucosal oedema, friability, one to three erosions and possibly more than one haemorrhage. The clinical significance of the 'statistically significant' differences found in this study is dubious.

Similar comments can be made about trials involving histamine H_2-receptor antagonists. Ranitidine did reduce the numbers of erosions and haemorrhages in the stomachs of normal men given aspirin for four weeks (Berkowitz et al, 1987). The authors concluded that ranitidine was effective in preventing gastroduodenal damage. However, only 21% of patients given ranitidine were free of gastric erosions at the end of the study (11% with placebo). A smaller percentage (25%) of subjects had submucosal haemorrhages on ranitidine treatment as compared to placebo (89%), but the significance of this is not known. The practising clinician must seriously consider the clinical usefulness of differences frequently reported in therapeutic studies evaluating the protective properties of various drugs against NSAID damage.

Lack of correlation between acute injury and chronic complications

Acute mucosal injury, gastrointestinal intolerance and chronic ulceration appear to affect different subgroups of patients receiving NSAIDs. This has made the problem of assessment of NSAID intolerance and NSAID-induced ulceration most difficult. Figure 1 summarizes the patient subgroups having side-effects caused by NSAIDs as typified by aspirin. Most patients who ingest aspirin develop acute mucosal injury. Many also experience gastrointestinal intolerance—a different subgroup of the patients receiving aspirin (some with acute injury, others with no injury). A smaller number will develop ulcers—again a different subgroup (some who demonstrate acute injury, perhaps some who did not, some with symptoms, some without symptoms). A very small number of the patients with ulcers develop complications, some of whom will have had gastrointestinal symptoms, others who will not. The physician's aim is to minimize symptoms of

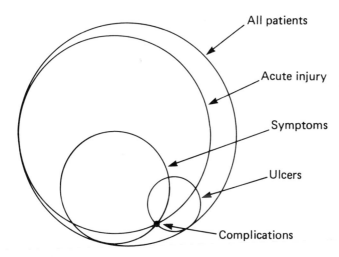

Figure 1. Venn diagram of side-effects in patients taking NSAIDs, using aspirin as an example. This figure illustrates the lack of predictive value of acute mucosal NSAID-induced injury for the development of gastrointestinal intolerance and the development of chronic ulceration, and the lack of predictive value of gastrointestinal intolerance for ulceration and its complications.

gastrointestinal intolerance and minimize complications. As Figure 1 illustrates, symptoms are not predictive of the presence of an ulcer. In addition, the presence of acute mucosal injury does not appear to predict the development of chronic ulceration. Most studies have studied ways in which to prevent acute gastric or duodenal injury following single or short-term doses of NSAIDs. These studies assume that acute gastric injury is the precursor of chronic ulceration. This assumption may well be false. Prevention of acute damage due to NSAIDs does not necessarily predict prevention of chronic ulceration and its risks of bleeding or perforation.

Low incidence of significant ulcer complications

Since the incidence of catastrophic complications due to NSAID use is so low—approximately one case per 10 000 patient months of NSAID use—a trial designed to study the prevention of complications of NSAIDs would require enormous numbers of subjects to provide meaningful data. The presence of an ulcer could be a logical alternative end-point, because ulcers occur with much greater frequency than do their complications. Unfortunately, not all ulcers are the same. While erosions are technically ulcers, they are superficial lesions which typically occur very soon after NSAID administration, heal rapidly on discontinuation of the NSAID and pose little if any risk. However, a chronic ulcer has the potential to perforate or erode a blood vessel. The problem is that there is a continuum of pathologic change from erosions to ulcers. Studies using less stringent criteria which would include smaller acute ulcers would require fewer subjects, but are less likely to address the question of risks of bleeding and perforation associated with

NSAID use. If the criteria were more stringent, requiring that ulcers be defined as larger, deeper lesions, the studies done would be more useful in answering questions about prevention of clinically important ulcers but would result in fewer lesions being defined as ulcers, requiring enrolment of more subjects.

Unfortunately, no studies have looked at the prevention of complications of ulceration. Very few studies have looked at the prevention of NSAID-induced ulcers. Knowing that NSAID use does carry significant risk of ulceration and its complications, the physician must use this incomplete information to make decisions about patients on NSAIDs.

Primary prevention—the necessity for and the choice of NSAIDs

The best therapy is prevention. Not all patients with arthritis need to be treated with NSAIDs. The analgesic rather than the anti-inflammatory properties of NSAIDs may be the desired effect in some patients. These patients may be better managed with paracetamol (acetaminophen), a drug not associated with increased gastrointestinal ulceration. Unfortunately, the short half-life of paracetamol requires frequent dosing to maintain analgesia, a factor that may lead to apparent failure of this drug in relieving pain. Establishing the need for an NSAID is particularly pertinent in the elderly. There is an increased risk associated with NSAIDs in the older patient. Osteoarthritis is more common in the elderly and the anti-inflammatory effects of NSAIDs may be less important than the analgesic ones.

Pharmaceutical companies have spent enormous amounts of money developing NSAIDs that do not possess the mucosal damaging properties of aspirin. These efforts include enteric coating of tablets, formation of slow-release preparations and administration of the inactive pro-drug. These efforts do reduce the acute damage as assessed endoscopically, but may have little effect on the development of chronic ulcerations (Carson et al, 1987a).

The use of drugs to prevent NSAID-induced ulceration

Given the lack of success in developing an NSAID with good anti-inflammatory effects and low risk to the mucosa, the next alternative is to give the NSAID in combination with a drug that could protect the gastric mucosa. All of the drugs used for the acute treatment of ulcer disease have been used in clinical trials to determine their protective effects against NSAID damage.

Histamine H_2-receptor antagonists

There is little doubt that the histamine H_2-receptor antagonists reduce the mucosal damage caused by acute administration of aspirin and other NSAIDs (Rachmilewitz et al, 1986; Kimmey and Silverstein, 1988; Lanza et al, 1988b; Berkowitz et al, 1987). The effect of the histamine H_2-receptor antagonists on the prevention of gastric ulceration is less evident. Roth et al (1987) evaluated the use of cimetidine 300 mg four times daily in 94 patients with endoscopically proven NSAID gastropathy. No reduction in the percentage of patients with gastric mucosal damage was seen with cimetidine after eight weeks of treatment. Berkowitz et al (1987) showed that in 43 healthy individuals given aspirin or placebo for four weeks there was a reduction in the number of mucosal haemorrhages when ranitidine 150 mg twice daily was given, as compared with placebo-treated patients, but there was no reduction in the incidence of erosions. In a trial by Ehsanullah et al (1988) on 263 patients receiving NSAIDs with a normal pre-treatment endoscopy, there was a reduction in the number of duodenal ulcers but not gastric ulcers occurring during the eight weeks when ranitidine 150 mg twice daily was given, compared with placebo-treated patients. Lanza et al (1988b) found a reduction in the amount of duodenal injury with ranitidine given 150 mg twice daily compared with placebo in 119 patients being treated with a variety of NSAIDs. No difference was seen between the placebo and ranitidine groups with regard to the degree of gastric injury. These trials indicate a reduction in the amount of duodenal injury but, more importantly, no significant benefit from the H_2-receptor antagonists in the prevention of NSAID-induced gastric ulceration. Once again we emphasize that these studies were looking at relatively short-term and probably innocuous ulceration. Whether histamine H_2-receptor antagonists prevent the development of life-threatening haemorrhage or perforation remains to be determined.

Sucralfate

Studies looking at the prevention of acute NSAID-induced gastric ulceration with sucralfate have been even less encouraging. Sucralfate has been reported to have cytoprotective properties. (Tarnawski et al, 1987) suggesting a potential for its use in prevention of NSAID-induced gastric injury. Studies by Stiel et al (1986) and Stern et al (1987) demonstrated protective effects on gastric mucosa in normal volunteers against the acute administration of aspirin. However, Wu and Castell (1984) showed protection of the duodenum but not the stomach with sucralfate, and Graham et al (1983) showed no significant effect of sucralfate versus placebo. Although a trial by Caldwell et al (1987) concluded that there was no protection against injury (as judged by endoscopy), there was precisely the same degree of injury after six weeks of NSAIDs with sucralfate as with placebo. In a trial of 26 patients with rheumatoid arthritis and gastric or duodenal lesions taking NSAIDs, 11 of 14 patients given sucralfate 1 g four times daily and 8 of 12 patients taking cimetidine had improved endoscopic scores after six weeks of treatment (Shepherd et al, 1989). Given the paucity of positive data, it is difficult to recommend sucralfate for the treatment or prevention of NSAID-induced gastrointestinal damage.

Prostaglandins

Synthetic prostaglandins administered orally prevent the acute damage seen with NSAID administration and do so better than histamine H_2-receptor antagonists given at doses with greater antisecretory effects. In an acute study of 130 healthy individuals given 975 mg of aspirin four times daily, misoprostol in doses of 100 µg or 200 µg given concurrently with aspirin reduced the percentage of subjects exhibiting erosions from 90% to about 20% (Jiranek et al, 1989). Misoprostol 200 µg four times daily was superior to cimetidine 300 mg four times daily in the reduction of tolmetin-induced injury (400 mg four times daily) in a study of 900 normal volunteers taking both drugs for six days (Lanza et al, 1988a). Both drugs were equally effective in preventing duodenal injury.

Prostaglandins have shown the most promise in the prevention of NSAID-induced gastric ulceration. A large, multicentre trial of misoprostol performed by Graham et al (1988) requires special consideration. In this double-blind, placebo-controlled study, two dosage regimens of miso-prostol (100 µg or 200 µg four times daily) were compared to placebo in the prevention of NSAID-induced ulcers. Only patients with osteoarthritis receiving ibuprofen, piroxicam or naproxen and who had NSAID-induced abdominal pain were studied. Four hundred and twenty patients without ulcers at entry were studied. Ulcers, defined as circumscribed breaks in the gastric mucosa of 3 mm or greater, occurred in 21% of placebo-treated patients, compared with 5.6% of patients treated with misoprostol 100 µg four times daily and 1.4% of patients treated with 200 µg of misoprostol four times daily. For ulcers defined as breaks larger than 5 mm, ulcers occurred in 12.3%, 4.2% and 0.7% of patients respectively. It was interesting that in these patients who had NSAID-induced abdominal pain at entry, 57% of patients treated with placebo were pain-free after three months indicating a major spontaneous or placebo-induced response. The 70% pain relief with misoprostol was not significantly different from the placebo group. Thirty-nine per cent of patients treated with misoprostol 200 µg four times daily, 25% treated with misoprostol 100 µg four times daily and 12% treated with placebo experienced diarrhoea. About 6% of patients treated with miso-prostol 200 µg four times daily had to be withdrawn from treatment because of diarrhoea. This study is important in that it is the only study that has shown prevention of gastric ulceration by concomitantly administered medi-cation.

Administration of oral prostaglandins to patients with documented NSAID injury results in improvement of the gastric mucosal appearance. A summary report on the three trials of arbaprostil versus placebo given for four weeks in 658 patients with rheumatoid arthritis or osteoarthritis receiv-ing NSAIDs in whom endoscopic damage was seen prior to entry has recently been published (Euler et al, 1990). The endoscopic score improved in more patients treated with arbaprostil than in placebo-treated patients. Healing of gastric ulcers (defined as lesions greater than 4 mm in diameter) was also seen with increased frequency in the arbaprostil-treated patients compared with placebo-treated patients. Significant improvement in the endoscopic score in healing of ulcers was seen in doses as low as 10 µg given four times daily.

Before instituting a policy of administering prostaglandins to all patients at risk of NSAID ulceration, one needs to understand some of the shortcomings of the data on which this policy would be based. Any study that will show a significant difference has to be large, since gastric ulceration occurs in only one of five placebo-treated patients. The studies outlined above were large studies, each with over 400 patients. They are large enough to detect a significant reduction in gastric ulcer occurrence. No other similarly designed study with other agents has included such a large number of patients and, therefore, real differences can be missed. Before agents other than prosta-glandins are dismissed as ineffective, they should be evaluated in similar placebo-controlled trials. Perhaps more important is the fact that the pre-vention of ulcers defined as circumscribed lesions of more than 3 mm or even 5 mm in depth does not necessarily translate into the prevention of chronic ulceration with the potential for bleeding or perforation. None of the 1080 patients on placebo or active drug in the above prostaglandin trials developed significant bleeding or perforation. Although these trials suggest significant benefit from prostaglandins in the short term, we cannot assume that misoprostol will prevent the occurrence of ulcer complications. This is particularly important, given that a misoprostol regimen is not without significant occurrence of diarrhoea.

Omeprazole

The available literature is insufficient to allow comment on the efficacy of omeprazole in preventing NSAID-induced damage. A single study using an endoscopic scoring system in healthy volunteers given aspirin did not show any benefit with omeprazole in doses lower than are given for treatment of ulcer disease (Muller et al, 1986). Omeprazole 20 mg once daily reduced the gastrointestinal blood loss caused by aspirin (given 900 mg twice daily for one week) by 80% (Daneshmend et al, 1990). The profound acid-lowering effect of omeprazole and its ability to heal gastric ulcers rapidly with conti-nuation of NSAIDs (Walan et al, 1989) suggest that given appropriate trials omeprazole may play a role in the prevention of NSAID ulceration.

The use of drugs to prevent NSAID-induced gastrointestinal symptoms

The discussion to this point has dealt with the prevention of gastric injury. Although ulceration is the main risk of NSAID use, the rheumatologist is much more concerned about improving the gastrointestinal symptomatic tolerance of NSAIDs. Unfortunately, the literature does not provide much information in this regard. In a trial of patients on NSAIDs with gastroin-testinal symptoms and normal endoscopy, complete resolution of symptoms occurred in 72% of patients treated with a low dose of cimetidine, compared with 49% treated with placebo (Bijlsma, 1988). Sucralfate was also reported to improve symptoms of gastric intolerance better than placebo (Caldwell et al, 1987) but as discussed in depth above, the beneficial effect was minimal if at all clinically significant. In the large prostaglandin trials by Graham et al (1988) and Euler et al (1990) there was no significant improvement in the symptoms of gastrointestinal intolerance despite the entry criteria of the former trial requiring abdominal pain as an inclusion criterion. It is not that the patients on active treatment did not experience improvement of symptoms, but that there was an equally impressive improvement in symptoms in patients given placebo (Caldwell et al, 1987; Graham et al, 1988; Euler et al, 1990). Therefore, there is no firm evidence as yet that prostaglandins should be prescribed to prevent symptoms, minimal evidence that prescription of histamine H_2-receptor antagonists is indicated and debatable evidence as to whether sucralfate improves gastrointestinal tolerance of NSAIDs.

Recommendations for the prevention of NSAID-induced upper gastrointestinal symptoms and injury

Table 1 summarizes the available data for the therapeutic efficacy of the drugs used for the prevention and treatment of NSAID-induced gastric and duodenal injury. Histamine H_2-receptor antagonists, sucralfate, prostaglandins and omeprazole heal gastric and duodenal ulcers caused by NSAIDs, with omeprazole being slightly more efficacious than the rest. The prostaglandins have been shown to prevent the acute damage caused by NSAIDs to the gastric and duodenal mucosa. The histamine H_2-receptor

Table 1. Efficacy of drugs shown to have mucosal protective properties for the prevention of upper gastrointestinal side-effects.

Drug	Ulcer healing	Acute injury prevention	Symptom relief	Ulcer prevention	Complication prevention
H_2-Antagonists	+ +	+ +	+	?	?
Sucralfate	+ +	+	±	?	?
Prostaglandins	+	+ + +	—	+ +	?
Omeprazole	+ + +	?	?	?	?

? indicates no data to make judgement of efficacy, ± indicates conflicting data, + indicates minimal efficacy, + + indicates good efficacy, + + + indicates best efficacy compared to other agents.

antagonists afford some protection. The few data available on relief of gastrointestinal intolerance caused by NSAIDs indicate some effect from the histamine H_2-receptor antagonists, a questionable effect from sucralfate and no demonstrable effect from the prostaglandins. Prostaglandins have been the only drugs shown to prevent gastric ulcers. The table is incomplete because nothing has been reported about the ability of omeprazole—the most powerful ulcer-healing drug available—to prevent acute injury, improve tolerance of NSAIDs or prevent development of ulcers in patients on NSAIDs. Similarly there are no equivalent trials of sucralfate and the histamine H_2-receptor antagonists examining the ability of these agents to prevent ulceration in patients receiving NSAIDs. Finally, there are no trials showing prevention of ulcer complications by any drug.

Given the many uncertainties regarding NSAID-induced gastrointestinal injury, it is extremely difficult to make recommendations with respect to improving the gastrointestinal tolerances of NSAIDs based on existing data. In the patient with purely symptomatic intolerance, a trial of a histamine H_2-receptor antagonist is warranted. If there is a strong indication for the prevention of chronic ulcer, and if one believes that the aforementioned acute studies predict the prevention of the chronic ulcer, the best evidence supports the use of a prostaglandin. However, if the criteria were more stringent, requiring that ulcers be defined as larger, deeper lesions, the studies done would be more useful in answering questions about prevention of clinically important ulcers but would result in fewer lesions being defined as ulcers, requiring enrolment of more subjects.

Unfortunately, no studies have looked at the prevention of complications of ulceration. Very few studies have looked at the prevention of NSAID-induced ulcers. Knowing that NSAID use does carry significant risk of ulceration and its complications, physicians must use this incomplete information to make decisions about their patients on NSAIDs.

CONCLUSION

It is clear that non-steroidal anti-inflammatory drugs play a major role in the causation of both acute and chronic gastrointestinal injury. Acute injury and symptomatic intolerance are common but the life-threatening complications of ulceration are fortunately rare. Neither the presence of symptomatic gastrointestinal intolerance nor the development of acute gastric injury are predictive of the development of chronic ulceration and its complications. Although some NSAIDs cause less acute gastric and duodenal injury, it appears that all drugs have a similar propensity for causing chronic gastric ulceration. There are several effective drugs that will heal gastric and duodenal ulcers in patients who have received NSAIDs. Stopping the NSAIDs, although not always necessary, does appear to improve the chances of healing. The best method for the prevention of NSAID-induced ulceration and its complications has not been established. Orally administered prostaglandins have shown the most promise for protecting the gastric mucosa, but it must be pointed out that these are the only class of antiulcer drugs that have been adequately studied.

Many important questions remain. Is there a relationship between the acute gastric mucosal injury and the development of chronic gastric ulceration? Do any of the available agents prevent the development of chronic gastric ulceration with its attendant risks of perforation or bleeding? What is the most appropriate drug for prevention of gastrointestinal ulceration with NSAIDs? Should all patients, or a subgroup of patients, receiving NSAIDs also receive an agent that reduces gastrointestinal ulceration? Particularly applicable to the young person with inflammatory arthritis, what is the long-term effect of the mucosal protecting drugs given with or without the NSAIDs? Much more information needs to be available before one can recommend the routine use of drugs that have been reported to be protective against the injury caused by NSAIDs.

Given the rarity of complications and the incompleteness of knowledge with regard to the prevention of ulcer complications, there is little indication for widespread use of any of the available drugs for prophylaxis against NSAID injury.

REFERENCES

Agrawal NM, Saffouri, B, Kruss DM et al (1985) Healing of benign gastric ulcer. A placebo-controlled comparison of two dosage regimens of misoprostol, a synthetic analog of prostaglandin E1. *Digestive Diseases and Sciences* **30:** 164S–170S.

Allen A & Garner A (1980) Mucus and bicarbonate secretion in the stomach and their possible role in mucosal protection. *Gut* **21:** 249–262.

Armstrong CP & Blower AL (1987) Non-steroidal anti-inflammatory drugs and life threatening complications of peptic ulceration. *Gut* **28:** 527–532.

Bahari HMM, Ross IN & Turnberg LA (1982) Demonstration of a pH gradient across the mucus layer on the surface of human gastric mucosa in vitro. *Gut* **23:** 513–516.

Bardhan KD, Bianchi Porro G, Bose K et al (1986) A comparison of two different doses of omeprazole versus ranitidine in treatment of duodenal ulcers. *Journal of Clinical Gastroenterology* **8:** 408–413.

Baum C, Kennedy DL & Forbes MB (1985) Utilization of nonsteroidal antiinflammatory drugs. *Arthritis and Rheumatism* **28:** 686–692.

Berkowitz JM, Rogenes PR, Sharp JT & Warner CW (1987) Ranitidine protects against gastroduodenal mucosal damage associated with chronic aspirin therapy. *Archives of Internal Medicine* **147:** 2137–2139.

Bijlsma JWJ (1988) Treatment of endoscopy-negative NSAID-induced upper gastrointestinal symptoms with cimetidine: an international multicenter collaborative study. *Alimentary Pharmacology and Therapeutics* **2S:** 75–83.

Boyd SC, Sasame HA & Boyd MR (1979) High concentrations of glutathione in glandular stomach—possible implications for carcinogenesis. *Science* **205:** 1010–1012.

Brand DL, Roufail WM, Thomson ABR & Tapper EJ (1985) Misoprostol, a synthetic PGE1 analog, in the treatment of duodenal ulcers. A multicenter double-blind study. *Digestive Diseases and Sciences* **30:** 147S–158S.

Caldwell JR, Roth SH, Wu WC et al (1987) Sucralfate treatment of nonsteroidal anti-inflammatory drug-induced gastrointestinal symptoms and mucosal damage. *American Journal of Medicine* **83** (supplement 3B): 74–82.

Carson JL, Strom BL, Morse LM et al (1987a) The relative gastrointestinal toxicity of the non-steroidal anti-inflammatory drugs. *Archives of Internal Medicine* **147:** 1054–1059.

Carson JL, Strom BL, Soper KA et al (1987b) The association of non-steroidal anti-inflammatory drugs with upper gastrointestinal bleeding. *Archives of Internal Medicine* **147:** 85–88.

Chalmers TC, Berrier J, Hewitt P et al (1988) Meta-analysis of randomized controlled trials as a method of estimating rare complications of non-steroidal anti-inflammatory drug therapy. *Alimentary Pharmacology and Therapeutics* **2** (supplement): 9–26.

Collier DS & Pain JA (1985) Non-steroidal anti-inflammatory drugs and peptic ulcer perforation. *Gut* **26:** 359–363.

Cox NL & Doherty SM (1987) Non-steroidal anti-inflammatories: outpatient audit of patient preferences and side-effects in different diseases. In Rainsford KD & Velo GL (eds) *Side Effects of Anti-inflammatory Drugs. 1. Clinical and Epidemiological Aspects*, pp 137–150. Lancaster: MTP Press.

Croker J, Cotton PB, Boyle AC & Kinsella P (1980) Cimetidine for peptic ulcer in patients with arthritis. *Annals of Rheumatic Disease* **39:** 275–278.

CSM (1986) Committee on Safety of Medicines Update: Non-steroidal anti-inflammatory drugs and serious gastrointestinal adverse reactions—2. *British Medical Journal* **292:** 1190–1191.

Daneshmend TK, Stein AG, Bhaskar NK & Hawkey CJ (1990) Abolition by omeprazole of aspirin induced gastric mucosal injury in man. *Gut* **31:** 514–517.

Domschke W, Domschke S, Hornig D & Demling L (1978) Prostaglandin-stimulated gastric mucus secretion in man. *Acta Hepatogastroenterology* **25:** 292–294.

Doube A & Morris A (1988) Non-steroidal anti-inflammatory drug-induced dyspepsia—is *Campylobacter pyloridis* implicated? *British Journal of Rheumatology* **27:** 110–112.

Duggan JM, Dobson AJ, Johnson H & Fahey P (1986) Peptic ulcer and non-steroidal anti-inflammatory agents. *Gut* **27:** 929–933.

Ehsanullah RSB, Page MC, Tildesley G & Wood JR (1988) NSAID-induced gastroduodenal damage: effect of ranitidine prophylaxis (abstract). *Gastroenterology* **94:** A111.

Euler AR, Safdi M, Rao J et al (1990) A report of three multiclinic trials evaluating arboprostil in arthritic patients with ASA/NSAID gastric mucosal damage. *Gastroenterology* **98:** 1549–1557.

Fries JF, Miller SR, Spitz PW, Williams CA, Hubert HB & Bloch DA (1989) Toward an epidemiology of gastropathy associated with nonsteroidal antiinflammatory drug use. *Gastroenterology* **96:** 674–655.

Garner A (1978) Mechanisms of action of aspirin on the gastric mucosa of the guinea pig. *Acta Physiologica Scandinavica* (special supplement): 101–110.

Gerber LH, Rooney PJ & McCarthy DM (1981) Healing of peptic ulcers during continuing anti-inflammatory drug therapy in rheumatoid arthritis. *Journal of Clinical Gastroenterology* **3:** 7–11.

Graham DY & Smith JL (1986) Aspirin and the stomach. *Annals of Internal Medicine* **104:** 390–398.

Graham DY, Smith JL & Dobbs SM (1983) Gastric adaptation with aspirin administration in man. *Digestive Diseases and Sciences* **28:** 1–6.

Graham DY, Agrawal NM & Roth SH (1988) Prevention of NSAID-induced gastric ulcer with misoprostol: multicentre, double-blind, placebo-controlled trial. *Lancet* **ii:** 1277–1280.

Griffin MR, Ray WA & Schaffner W (1988) Nonsteroidal anti-inflammatory drug use and death from peptic ulcer in elderly persons. *Archives of Internal Medicine* **109:** 359–363.

Guth PH (1984) Local metabolism and circulation in mucosal defense. In Allen A, Flemstrom G & Garner A (eds) *Mechanisms of Mucosal Protection in the Upper Gastrointestinal Tract*, pp 235–258. New York: Raven Press.

Hawkey CJ & Walt RP (1986) Prostaglandins for peptic ulcer: a promise unfulfilled. *Lancet* **ii:** 1084–1086.

Hills BA, Butler BD & Lichtenberger LM (1983) Gastric mucosal barrier: hydrophobic lining to the lumen of the stomach. *American Journal of Physiology (Gastrointestinal and Liver Physiology)* **244:** G561–568.

Hingson DJ & Ito S (1971) Effect of aspirin and related compounds on the fine structure of mouse gastric mucosa. *Gastroenterology* **61:** 156–177.

Howard JM, Chremos AA, Collen MJ et al (1985) Famotidine, a new, potent, long-acting histamine H_2-receptor antagonist: comparison with cimetidine and Ranitidine in the Zollinger-Ellison syndrome. *Gastroenterology* **88:** 1026–1033.

Husby G, Holme I, Rugstad HG, Herland OB & Giercksky K-E (1986) A double-blind multi-centre trial of piroxicam and naproxen in osteoarthritis. *Clinical Rheumatology* **5:** 84–91.

Inman WhW (1985) Comparative study of five NSAIDs. *PEM News* **3:** 3–13.

Jaszweski RJ, Cal-zada R & Dhar R (1989) Persistence of gastric ulcers caused by plain aspirin or nonsteroidal anti-inflammatory agents in patients treated with a combination of cimetidine, antacids and enteric-coated aspirin. *Digestive Diseases and Sciences* **34:** 1361–1364.

Jick SS, Perera DR, Walker AM & Jick H (1987) Non-steroidal anti-inflammatory drugs and hospital admission for perforated peptic ulcer. *Lancet* **ii:** 380–382.

Jiranek GC, Kimmey MB, Saunders DR, Willson RA, Shanahan W & Silverstein FE (1989) Misoprostol reduces gastroduodenal injury from one week of aspirin: an endoscopic study. *Gastroenterology* **96:** 656–661.

Kauffman G (1989) Aspirin-induced gastric mucosal injury: lessons learned from animal models. *Gastroenterology* **96:** 606–614.

Kauffman GL, Whittle BJR, Aures D, Vane JR & Grossman MI (1979) Effects of prostacyclin and a stable analogue, 6 beta-PGI$_1$ on gastric acid secretion, mucosal blood flow, and blood pressure in conscious dogs. *Gastroenterology* **77:** 1301–1306.

Kimmey MB & Silverstein FE (1988) Role of H_2-receptor blockers in the prevention of gastric injury resulting from nonsteroidal anti-inflammatory agents. *American Journal of Medicine* **84** (supplement 2A): 49–52.

Langman MJS (1989) Epidemiologic evidence on the association between peptic ulceration and antiinflammatory drug use. *Gastroenterology* **96:** 640–644.

Lanza FL, Aspinall RL, Swabb EA et al (1988a) Double-blind, placebo-controlled endoscopic comparison of the mucosal protective effects of misoprostol versus cimetidine on tolmetin-induced mucosl injury to the stomach and duodenum. *Gastroenterology* **95:** 289–294.

Lanza F, Robinson M, Bowers J et al (1988b) A multi-center double-blind comparison of ranitidine vs placebo in the prophylaxis of nonsteroidal antiinflammatory drug (NSAID) induced lesions in gastric and duodenal mucosae (abstract). *Gastroenterology* **94**: A250.

Larkai EN, Smith JL, Lidsky MD & Graham DY (1987) Gastroduodenal mucosa and dyspeptic symptoms in arthritic patients during chronic nonsteroidal anti-inflammatory drug use. *American Journal of Gastroenterology* **82**: 1152–1158.

Larkai EN, Smith JL, Lidsky MD, Sessoms SL & Graham DY (1989) Dyspepsia in NSAID users: the size of the problem. *Journal of Clinical Gastroenterology* **11**: 158–162.

Lichtenberger LM, Richards JE & Hills BA (1985) Effect of 16,16-dimethyl prostaglandin E_2 on the surface hydrophobicity of aspirin-treated canine gastric mucosa. *Gastroenterology* **88**: 308–314.

Lind T, Cederberg C, Ekenved G, Haglund U & Olbe L (1983) Effects of omeprazole—a gastric proton pump inhibitor—on pentagastrin stimulated acid secretion in man. *Gut* **24**: 270–276.

Manniche C, Malchow-Moller A, Anderson JR et al (1987) Randomized study of the influence of non-steroidal anti-inflammatory drugs on the treatment of peptic ulcer in patients with rheumatic disease. *Gut* **28**: 226–229.

McIntosh JH, Byth K & Piper DW (1985) Environmental factors in aetiology of chronic gastric ulcer: a case control study of exposure variables before the first symptoms. *Gut.* **26**: 789–798.

McQueen S, Hutton D, Allen A & Garner A (1983) Gastric and duodenal surface mucus gel thickness in rat: effects of prostaglandins and damaging agents. *American Journal of Physiology (Gastrointestinal and Liver Physiology)* **245**: G388–G393.

Meyer RA, McGinley D & Posalaky Z (1986) Effects of aspirin on tight junction structure of the canine gastric mucosa. *Gastroenterology* **91**: 351–359.

Muller VP, Dammann HG & Simon B (1986) Akute schadigung der magen schleinhaut durch acetylsalicylsaure. Eine endoskopische vergleichsstudie am menschen mit oral virksamen prostaglandin-analoga, omeprazol und ranitidine. *Arzneimittelforsch* **36**: 265–268.

Murray HS, Strottman MP & Cooke AR (1974) Effect of several drugs on gastric potential difference in man. *British Medical Journal* **1**: 19–21.

O'Laughlin JC, Silvoso GK & Ivey KJ (1982) Resistance to medical therapy of gastric ulcers in rheumatic disease patients taking aspirin. *Digestive Diseases and Sciences* **27**: 976–980.

Pincus T & Callahan LF (1986) Taking mortality in rheumatoid arthritis seriously—predictive markers, socioeconomic status and comorbidity. *Journal of Rheumatology* **13**: 841–845.

Rachmilewitz D, Polak D, Eliakim R et al (1986) Cimetidine significantly decreases indomethacin induced gastroduodenal mucosal damage (abstract). *Gastroenterology* **90**: 1596.

Redfern JS & Feldman M (1989) Role of endogenous prostaglandins in preventing gastrointestinal ulceration: induction of ulcers by antibodies to prostaglandins. *Gastroenterology* **96**: 596–605.

Robert A, Nezamis JE, Lancaster C & Hanchar AJ (1979) Cytoprotection by prostaglandins in rats: prevention of gastric necrosis produced by alcohol, HCl, NaOH, hypertonic NaCl and thermal injury.

Robert A, Nezamis JE, Lancaster C et al (1983) Mild irritants prevent gastric necrosis through 'adaptive cytoprotection' mediated by prostaglandins. *American Journal of Physiology (Gastrointestinal and Liver Physiology)* **245**: G113–G121.

Roth SH, Bennett RE, Mitchell CS & Hartman RJ (1987) Cimetidine therapy in nonsteroidal anti-inflammatory drug gastropathy. Double-blind long-term evaluation. *Archives of Internal Medicine* **147**: 1798–1801.

Rutten MJ & Ito S (1983) Morphology and electrophysiology of guinea pig gastric mucosal repair in vitro. *American Journal of Physiology (Gastrointestinal and Liver Physiology)* **244**: G171–G182.

Sandmark S, Carlsson R, Fausa O & Lundell L (1988) Omeprazole or ranitidine in the treatment of reflux esophagitis: results of a double-blind, randomized, Scandinavian multicenter study. *Scandinavian Journal of Gastroenterology* **23**: 625–632.

Sarosiek J, Mizuta K, Slomiany A & Slomiany BL (1986) Effect of acetylsalicylic acid on gastric mucin viscosity, permeability to hydrogen ion, and susceptibility to pepsin. *Biochemical Pharmacology* **35**: 4281–4295.

Schoen RT & Vender RJ (1989) Mechanisms of non-steroidal anti-inflammatory drug-induced gastric damage. *American Journal of Medicine* **86**: 449–458.

Shepherd HA, Fine D, Hillier K, Jewell R & Cox N (1989) Effect of sucralfate and cimetidine on rheumatoid patients with active gastroduodenal lesions who are taking nonsteroidal anti-inflammatory drugs. *American Journal of Medicine* **86:** 49–54.

Silen W & Ito S (1985) Mechanisms for rapid re-epithelialization of the gastric mucosal surface. *Annual Review of Physiology* **47:** 217–229.

Silvoso GR, Ivey KJ, Butt JH et al (1979) Incidence of gastric lesions in patients with rheumatic disease on chronic aspirin therapy. *Annals of Internal Medicine* **91:** 517–520.

Somerville K, Faulkner G & Langman M (1986) Non-steroidal anti-inflammatory drugs and bleeding peptic ulcer. *Lancet* **i:** 462–464.

Stern AI, Ward F & Hartley G (1987) Protective effect of sucralfate against aspirin-induced damage to the human gastric mucosa. *American Journal of Medicine* **83** (supplement 38): 83–85.

Stiel D, Ellard KT, Hills LJ & Brooks PM (1986) Protective effect of enprostil against aspirin-induced gastroduodenal mucosal injury in man. *American Journal of Medicine* **81** (supplement 2A): 54–58.

Szabo S & Hollander D (1989) Pathways of gastrointestinal protection and repair: mechanisms of action of sucralfate. *American Journal of Medicine* **86:** 23–31.

Tarnawski A, Hollander D & Cergely H (1987) Cytoprotective drugs. Focus on essential fatty acids and sucralfate. *Scandinavian Journal of Medicine* **22** (supplement 127): 39–43.

Thomson ABR, Navert H, Halvorsen L et al (1986) *American Journal of Medicine* **81** (supplement 2a): 59–63.

Vantrappen G, Janssens J, Popiela T et al (1982) Effect of 15(R)-15-methylprostaglandin E_2 (arbaprostil) on the healing of duodenal ulcer. A double-blind multicenter study. *Gastroenterology* **83:** 357–363.

Walan A, Bader J-P, Classen M et al (1989) Effect of omeprazole and ranitidine on ulcer healing and relapse rates in patients with benign gastric ulcer. *New England Journal of Medicine* **320:** 69–75.

Wu WC & Castell DO (1984) Does sucralfate protect against aspirin induced mucosal lesions? Yes and no! (abstract). *Gastroenterology* **86:** 1303.

7

Chondroprotection: myth or reality?

PETER M. BROOKS
PETER GHOSH

Osteoarthritis is the most prevalent rheumatic disorder affecting man. It has been estimated to affect approximately 15% of the world's population, making it one of the most common causes of chronic disability (Kellgren and Lawrence, 1957; Kellgren, 1961; Rejholec, 1987). With our aging population, the economic and social costs of osteoarthritis are considerable (Andrews and Ward, 1985). Within recent years research has focused on the changes that take place in cartilage in normal and pathological states and the influence that non-steroidal anti-inflammatory drugs (NSAIDs) may have on the synthesis and degradation of matrix components. The optimal function of diarthroidal joints is dependent on the integrity of articular cartilage, synovial fluid and the synovial membrane. Activated synovial cells as seen in the inflammatory forms of arthritis, such as rheumatoid arthritis or seronegative arthropathies, produce a variety of mediators which can induce cartilage cells to absorb their extracellular matrix in vitro and in vivo. These soluble factors include the interleukin family of proteins (Dingle et al, 1979; Saklatvala, 1981; Wood et al, 1983; van de Loo and van den Berg, 1990) and prostaglandins (Dayer et al, 1976; Mitrovic et al, 1984; Carroll, 1985). Although these and similar factors obviously play a major role in cartilage destruction in inflammatory joint diseases there is still only limited evidence that they are implicated in the pathogenesis of cartilage failure in osteo-arthritis (Pelletier and Martel-Pelletier, 1988). While the integrity of cartilage is maintained by the chondrocytes, a major function of the synovial lining type B cells is to synthesize hyaluronic acid, which is the principal non-proteinaceous component of synovial fluid and is essential for the nourishment, protection and lubrication of synovial tissues (Fraser, 1989; Ghosh et al, 1990). The constituents of synovial fluid, as well as the extra-cellular matrix of cartilage, undergo continuous turnover which may increase during normal physical activity (Engström-Laurent and Hallgren, 1987). In normal joints the biosynthetic capacities of the chondrocytes and the synovial lining cells are sufficient to replenish the levels of proteoglycans and hyaluronic acid which are lost from the tissues by the catabolic pro-cesses. However, in the arthritic joint there is a net depletion of proteo-glycans from articular cartilage even though chondrocytes are actively engaged in biosynthesis (Mankin et al, 1971; Carney et al, 1984) and

Baillière's Clinical Rheumatology—
Vol. 4, No. 2, August 1990
ISBN 0–7020–1480–X

replication (Fassbender, 1983). This occurs because the rate at which proteoglycans are catabolized exceeds their rate of synthesis.

In order to assess whether NSAIDS contribute to the progression of cartilage damage in osteoarthritis, it is necessary to review the clinical evidence available and examine this in conjunction with laboratory studies on the effects of these drugs on cartilage metabolism.

Following the introduction of indomethacin as an NSAID in 1965, case reports began appearing which described instances where the osteoarthritis worsened following administration of this drug (Coke, 1967; Arora and Maudsley, 1968; Allen and Murray, 1971; Milner, 1973; Solomon, 1973; Rönningen and Langeland, 1979; Newman and Ling, 1985). However, in many of these cases other factors such as inflammatory joint disease (rheumatoid arthritis) or steroid therapy might also have contributed to joint destruction (Allen and Murray, 1971; Milner, 1973; Isdale, 1962; Storey, 1968; Bossingham et al, 1978). The finding that rapid joint deterioration also occurred in patients not receiving NSAIDs led some workers to doubt the association of NSAID therapy with the exacerbation of osteoarthritis (Watson, 1976; Doherty et al, 1986). In a study of 19 patients with rapid destructive atrophic arthropathy involving both femoral and acetabular components. Doherty et al (1986) found that only 10 of the 19 patients had received NSAIDs and 4 had taken no medication at all. They also noted that a number of the patients had complained of severe and persistent pain (even when on NSAID therapy) and this was considered to discount suggestions that the so-called 'analgesic hip' might be due to 'overuse' of a diseased joint rendered relatively pain-free by drug treatment. These workers likened the condition to the destructive joint disease seen in association with calcium pyrophosphate dihydrate crystal deposition (Richards and Hamilton, 1974; Menkes et al, 1985).

Recently Rashad et al (1989) described 105 patients with osteoarthritis awaiting hip arthroplasty who were treated prospectively with either indomethacin (a strong prostaglandin synthetase inhibitor) or azapropazone (a weak prostaglandin synthetase inhibitor). Pain and radiological joint space changes were monitored from the time of entry into the trial to the time when arthroplasty was performed. The authors state that the timing of arthroplasty was determined by 'failure to control pain, severe restriction of joint movement or inability to perform normal tasks'. The study showed that there was a significant difference in the time to arthroplasty between the group treated with indomethacin (10.4 months) and the group receiving azapropazone (15.7 months). Using serial x-rays, the overall reduction in joint space was less in both hips of patients treated with azapropazone compared with patients treated with indomethacin, though the differences were not statistically significant. Analysis of the resected hip cartilage and synovium demonstrated that the proteoglycan content was higher in the cartilage of those patients receiving azapropazone (13.42 µg/mg) than in those receiving indomethacin (7.8 µg/mg). The synovium of the azapropazone-treated patients also contained significantly more prosta-glandin E_2, thromboxane B_2 and 5-hydroxy-eicosatetraenoic acid. The problem with this study was that the initial pain scores for the azapropazone group tended to be higher than in the indomethacin group, and there was a statistically significantly higher final day pain score for the azapropazone group than the indomethacin group. Since pain was a determinant of arthroplasty, these data would suggest that for some reason different criteria were used either by the investigators or by the patients in determining when an operation was to be performed. Although this was a carefully conducted study presenting interesting data, because of the methodological problems outlined it failed to resolve the question whether NSAIDs alter the course of osteoarthritis.

ANIMAL MODELS

Salicylates, phenylbutazone and flufenamic acid uncouple oxidative phosphorylation and have been shown to reduce the incorporation of radioactive inorganic sulphate ($^{35}SO_4^{2-}$) into rat rib cartilage in vitro and in vivo (Whitehouse and Bostrom, 1962; Bostrom et al, 1964). However, the drug concentrations used in these studies were far in excess of those achieved in blood during normal treatment with these agents. Watson (1976) reported a reduction of $^{35}SO_4^{2-}$ incorporation into the articular cartilage of rabbits treated with pharmacological doses of indomethacin, but interestingly this did not greatly influence the progression of the degenerative arthritis induced.

A number of researchers have consistently shown that aspirin and (to a lesser extent) indomethacin can depress proteoglycan synthesis in different animal species at therapeutic concentrations (Videman et al, 1981; Maier and Wilhelmi, 1983; Palmoski and Brandt, 1980, 1982, 1983a,b). Using histological techniques including stereo-electron microscopy, Kalbhen and co-workers (Kalbhen, 1982, 1984, 1989; Kalbhen et al, 1986) have demonstrated that while some NSAIDs (including salicylates, indomethacin and phenylbutazone) when injected into rat or chicken knee joints caused rapid loss of joint space due to cartilage destruction, weekly intra-articular injections of 2 mg diclofenac for four months did not. In other studies using intra-articular iodoacetate to produce chondrocyte degeneration, the progression of cartilage damage (as determined by joint space measurements and radiologically determined criteria) was found to be attenuated by thrice weekly intramuscular injections of diclofenac. This effect was shown to be dose dependent and statistically significant when 3 mg/kg of the drug was used, which is a dose not dissimilar to that used in humans (Kalbhen et al, 1986). In contrast to Kalbhen's studies, Eronen and Videman (1985) using a rabbit atrophy model of osteoarthritis reported that diclofenac resulted in increased loss of chondroitin sulphate from joint articular cartilage.

Experiments employing the spontaneous osteoarthritis model in C57 black mice have shown that several NSAIDs administered systemically over a period of four to five months would significantly accelerate the progression of the osteoarthritic lesion. Diclofenac and piroxicam appeared to be the exception (Maier and Wilhelmi, 1982, 1983). In the same model, oral administration of 1 mg or 3 mg of diclofenac for four months reduced the frequency and severity of spontaneous osteoarthritis which normally developed in this strain of mice. In these studies it was reported that lower doses (0.5 and 1.5 mg/kg orally) of diclofenac given intermittently for nine months reduced the severity of the osteoarthritic lesions. Mohr et al (1984) investigated whether piroxicam was harmful to articular cartilage of normal canine joints. Adults beagles were given daily 0.3 mg/kg piroxicam orally during an eight-week period; light microscopy and $^{35}SO_4^{2-}$ autoradiographic evaluation of sections of femoral condyles, tibial plateaux and patellae showed no evidence of deleterious changes to cartilage. In an osteoarthritis model induced in dogs by severance of the anterior cruciate ligament, degenerative changes in articular cartilage were increased in animals receiving postoperative aspirin treatment (120 mg/kg daily). The proteoglycan content as well as its synthesis in joint cartilage were both reduced, whereas the cartilage of animals not receiving drugs showed some recovery of these parameters after surgery (Palmoski and Brandt, 1982). Brandt's group also established a positive correlation between the suppression of proteoglycan synthesis by indomethacin and salicylate in unloaded areas of articular cartilage derived from canine joints and the proteoglycan content of the tissue (Brandt and Palmoski, 1983; Palmoski and Brandt, 1983a,b). Depletion of glycosaminoglycans (by digestion with testicular hyaluronidase) from the loaded cartilage regions confirmed that drugs were more inhibitory when the cartilage levels of these components were reduced. Taken together these data suggest that the response of osteoarthritic cartilage to NSAIDs may be more rapid than that of normal cartilage.

Using a rabbit model of joint atrophy induced by immobilization, Ghosh and co-workers (Ghosh, 1990) have demonstrated that tiaprofenic acid when administered subcutaneously for four weeks at 5.0 mg/kg exhibited a chondroprotective effect on cartilage, but at 10.0 mg/kg the same drug exacerbated cartilage destruction. These studies indicate that the dosage of NSAIDs used can be critical to their effects on cartilage. Tiaprofenic acid has also been shown by others to exhibit positive effects on osteoarthritic cartilage metabolism in vitro (Pelletier et al, 1989; Pelletier and Martel-Pelletier, 1988a) and in vivo (Martel-Pelletier et al, 1988; de Vries et al, 1988a,b; Vignon et al, 1989, 1990).

Recently Pettipher et al studied the effects of indomethacin on antigen-induced arthritis in rabbits (Pettipher et al, 1989). Arthritis was induced in the knee joints of sensitized rabbits by intra-articular injection of ovalbumin. The joint swelling was measured over the 14 days after antigen challenge and groups of animals were killed on days 1, 7 or 14, with collection of synovial fluid, cartilage and synovium. Indomethacin, at oral doses of 1 mg/kg three times daily over the experimental period, significantly reduced joint swelling and prostaglandin E_2 concentrations in synovial fluid, but in addition increased the loss of proteoglycan from joint articular cartilage. This study thus demonstrated experimentally that the symptomatic benefits of indomethacin on inflammation may occur at the expense of joint cartilage integrity.

IN VITRO STUDIES

Several groups have demonstrated that NSAIDs can inhibit some of the proteinases capable of degrading matrix proteoglycans and collagens (Kruze et al, 1976a,b; Stephens et al, 1980; Shinmei et al, 1985; Pelletier and Martel-Pelletier, 1988b; Ghosh, 1989). Studies by Perper and Oronsky (1974), using ^{35}S-labelled rabbit articular cartilage and IgG-stimulated polymorphonuclear leucocytes (PMNs), found that aspirin, phenylbutazone, oxyphenylbutazone and indomethacin partially inhibited the non-phagocytic release of neutral proteinases from cells at concentrations between 10^{-4} and 10^6 mol. At these concentrations, however, there was little or no direct inhibitory effect on the enzymes. Kruze et al (1976a,b) also showed that diclofenac at 2×10^{-4} mol inhibited leucocyte neutral proteinase degradation of cartilage by approximately 25%. The latter study confirmed that phenylbutazone, sulindac and piroxicam were only moderate inhibitors of elastase while sulindac and diflunisal exhibited significant inhibition. It was also shown that the metabolites derived from some of the NSAIDs were more potent inhibitors of these enzymes than the parent molecule (Lentini et al, 1987). For example, sulindac sulphide was twenty times more potent as an elastase inhibitor than sulindac, and salicyluric acid was twenty times more potent than salicylic acid as a cathepsin G inhibitor (Lentini et al, 1987). These findings highlight the need to include drug metabolites during in vitro evaluations of NSAIDs.

Oxygen-derived free radicals (particularly superoxide) are thought to play an important role in matrix degradation in the inflammatory arthropathies, particularly when leucocyte and monocyte infiltration of the synovium is significant. Hyaluronic acid, proteoglycans and collagen are substrates for these high-energy species, and the suppression of these radicals by drugs must be considered to be of some benefit in preserving cartilage both directly and indirectly. Salicylic acid and some of its derivatives have been shown to be scavengers of the superoxide radical in vitro (Haggag et al, 1986). Minta and Williams (1985) examined the effects of NSAIDs on the generation of superoxide anions by activated PMNs. Diclofenac was the most potent of the drugs studied in suppressing superoxide anion production, having an ID_{50} of 7.7×10^{-5} mol. Piroxicam has been reported to be particularly effective in preventing the production of superoxide by PMNs when these cells were collected from patients with osteoarthritis and rheumatoid arthritis who had been given the drug for several weeks beforehand (Biemond et al, 1986; van Epps et al, 1987). The influence of anti-inflammatory drugs on the depolymerization of hyaluronic acid by xanthine oxidase-derived free radicals has been reported by Betts and Cleland (1982) and Carlin et al (1985). In these studies, salicylic acid, aspirin, gentisic acid, azodisalicylic acid and sulphasalazine were effective scavengers of free radicals at concentrations of 0.5 mmol, but paracetamol, ibuprofen and benoxaprofen were less effective.

The interleukin-I (IL-I) induced resorption of cartilage has, in general, shown a disappointing response to currently prescribed anti-inflammatory drugs. Sheppeard et al (1982) showed that indomethacin, aspirin, clozic and flubiprofen produced no effect either on the release of IL-I from synovial cells or on the resorption of cartilage by IL-1 stimulated chondrocytes. Isoxicam, however, appeared to be the exception in this assay since at concentrations between 5 µg/l and 30 µg/l it consistently reduced cartilage resorption by about 12% (Sheppeard and Couchman, 1986). Tiaprofenic acid was reported to reduce the levels of IL-I as well as phospholipase A_2, prostaglandins and proteinases in synovial fluids of patients receiving the drug (Vignon et al, 1989). Neutral proteinase activities were also demonstrated to be suppressed in human osteoarthritic cartilage (Shinmei et al, 1985, 1988; Martel-Pelletier and Pelletier, 1989; Vignon et al, 1990).

In a recent study, Herman et al (1987) showed that piroxicam, in contrast to indomethacin and sodium salicylate, generally suppressed the synthesis of IL-I in cultures of synovial tissues obtained from rheumatoid arthritis joints. In contrast to this, none of the NSAIDs studied consistently blocked the catabolism inducing activity in osteoarthritis tissue. This study again indicates that there might be differences between osteoarthritic and rheumatoid synovial tissue regarding the response to cytokines and other mediators.

Palmoski and Brandt (1980) have demonstrated that fenoprofen and ibuprofen—but not indomethacin or sulindac sulphide—inhibited proteoglycan synthesis in normal canine cartilage articular slices in vitro in a concentration-dependent manner. Earlier studies by McKenzie et al (1976), using aged normal and osteoarthritic human femoral head articular cartilage obtained at the time of surgery, showed suppression of glycosaminoglycan synthesis by sodium salicylate, phenylbutazone, hydrocortisone, indomethacin and ibuprofen at concentrations within the usual therapeutic range achieved in humans. Herman and Hess (1984) reported that piroxicam at therapeutic concentrations (5–10 mg/l) did not suppress proteoglycan synthesis in porcine cartilage explant cultures. These findings were compatible with those of Kirkpatrick et al (1983), Mohr et al (1983), Mohr and Kirkpatrick (1984) and—more recently—Verbruggen et al (1989). Franchimont et al (1983) studied the effect of tiaprofenic acid, salicylate and acetylsalicylic acid on the incorporation of $^{35}SO_4$ into chicken embryo cartilage in vitro. They showed that while salicylates resulted in a significant decrease in sulphate incorporation into cartilage proteoglycans, there were no significant changes in synthesis observed when the same tissues were incubated with tiaprofenic acid at concentrations between 5 mg/l and 200 mg/l. More recently Muir et al (1988) demonstrated that indomethacin, aspirin and naproxen decreased the in vitro biosynthesis of proteoglycan in canine cartilages while tiaprofenic acid did not.

Kato et al studied the effects of NSAIDs on soft agar growth of rabbit articular chondrocytes. They showed that while acetyl salicylic acid, naproxen and tiaprofenic acid did not significantly affect colony formation, indomethacin at concentrations of 10^{-5} to 10^{-4} mol significantly depressed chondrocyte colony formation in both the presence and absence of fibroblast growth factor (Kato et al, 1989). Using rabbit chondrocyte monolayer cultures maintained over eight days, Collier and Ghosh (1989) showed that while the sulphated polysaccharide glycosaminoglycan polysulphate ester and pentosan polysulphate stimulated the secretion of ^{35}S-labelled proteoglycans into media at therapeutic concentrations, indomethacin, diclofenac, ketoprofen and tiaprofenic acid did not. However, at supranormal concentration (50 and 100 mg/l) indomethacin and diclofenac strongly inhibited secretion, whereas ketoprofen and tiaprofenic acid were less severe. In a study of collagen biosynthesis by cultured chick embryo sternal chondrocytes, Fujii et al (1989) showed that while indomethacin and acetylsalicylic acid depressed the biosynthesis of type II collagen by 70–80%, tiaprofenic acid has no significant effect. Aspirin is reported to stimulate dedifferentiation of chondrocytes in vitro (Gay et al, 1983).

It seems clear from these laboratory studies that NSAIDs can have significant effects on several aspects of cartilage metabolism both in vitro and in vivo. However, the relevance of these studies to humans can be questioned from several standpoints, including species differences (Annefeld, 1985a,b) and the high concentrations of drugs employed by some workers to produce an effect. Nevertheless, the experimental studies can be useful in identifying drugs that might endanger the patient during chronic high-dose administration. Furthermore, at present the laboratory-based studies are all that is available to enable decision-making to be placed on a scientific footing; for patients still require treatment, and existing clinical methods of assessing cartilage changes in response to drug therapy are far from satisfactory.

The recently described innovations in imaging techniques (Sabiston et al, 1987; Dacre et al, 1989) as well as biochemical markers of cartilage breakdown (Saxne et al, 1986, 1987; Lohmander et al, 1989) in conjunction with long-term clinical assessment of function may resolve this dilemma (Doherty, 1989; Ghosh, 1990).

REFERENCES

Allen EH & Murray O (1971) Iatrogenic arthropathies. *European Association of Radiology Proceedings* **249**: 204–210.

Andrews RNL & Ward C (1985) Arthritis and public policy. In Napier NM & Gillings DB (eds) *Arthritis and Society*, pp 269–289. London: Butterworth.

Annefeld M (1985a) Ultrastructural and morphometrical studies on the articular cartilage of rats: the destructive effect of dexamethasone and the chondroprotective effect of Rumalon. *Agents and Actions* **17**: 320–321.

Annefeld M (1985b) The influence of steroidal and non-steroidal anti-inflammatory drugs on rat articular cartilage. In Nilsen OG (ed.) *Tiaprofenic Acid*, pp 47–52. International Congress of Rheumatology. Amsterdam: Excerpta Medica.

Arora JS & Maudsley RH (1968) Indocid arthropathy of hips. *Proceedings of the Royal Society of Medicine* **61**: 669.

Betts WH & Cleland LG (1982) Effects of metal chelators and antiinflammatory drugs on the degradation of hyaluronic acid. *Arthritis and Rheumatism* **25**: 1469–1476.

Biemond P, Swaak AJG, Penders JMA, Beindorff CM & Koster JF (1986) Superoxide production by polymorphonuclear leucocytes in rheumatoid arthritis and osteoarthritis: in vivo inhibition by the antirheumatic drug piroxicam due to interference with the activation of the NADPH-oxidase. *Annals of the Rheumatic Diseases* **45**: 249–255.

Bossingham DH, Schorn D, Morgan GW & Mowat AG (1978) Progression of hip disease in rheumatoid arthritis. *Rheumatology and Rehabilitation* **17**: 170–178.

Bostrom H, Berntsen K & Whitehouse MW (1964) Biochemical properties of anti-inflammatory drugs. II. Some effects on sulphate-^{35}S-metabolism in vivo. *Biochemical Pharmacology* **13**: 413–420.

Brandt KD & Palmoski MJ (1983) Proteoglycan content determines the susceptibility of articular cartilage to salicylate-induced suppression of proteoglycan synthesis. *Journal of Rheumatology* **10 (supplement 9):** 78–80.

Carlin G, Djursater R, Smedegard G & Gerdin B (1985) Effect of anti-inflammatory drugs on xanthine oxidase and xanthine oxidase induced depolymerization of hyaluronic acid. *Agents and Actions* **16:** 377–384.

Carney SL, Billingham MEJ, Muir H & Sandy JD (1984) Demonstration of increased proteoglycan turnover in cartilage explants from dogs with experimental osteoarthritis. *Journal of Orthopaedic Research* **2(3):** 201–206.

Carroll GJ (1985) Porcine catabolin stimulates prostaglandin E_2 secretion but does not affect intracellular cyclic AMP production in pig synovial fibroblasts. *Annals of the Rheumatic Diseases* **44:** 631–636.

Coke H (1967) Long term indomethacin therapy of coxarthrosis. *Annals of the Rheumatic Diseases* **26:** 364–367.

Collier S & Ghosh P (1989) Evaluation of the effects of antiarthritic drugs on the secretion of proteoglycans by lapine chondrocytes using a novel assay procedure. *Annals of the Rheumatic Diseases* **48:** 372–381.

Dacre JE, Coppock JS, Herbert KE, Perrett D & Huskisson EC (1989) Development of a new radiographic scoring system using digital image analysis. *Annals of the Rheumatic Diseases* **48:** 194–200.

Dayer J-M, Krane SM, Russell RGG & Robinson DR (1976) Production of collagenase and prostaglandins by isolated adherent rheumatoid synovial cells. *Proceedings of the National Academy of Sciences of the USA* **73:** 945–949.

De Vries BJ, Vandenbe WB, Vitters E & Vandeput LB (1988a) The influence of antirheumatic drugs on basal and accelerated breakdown of articular proteoglycans. *Agents and Actions* **23:** 52–54.

De Vries BJ, Vandenberg WB, Vitters E & Vandeput LB (1988b) Effects of NSAIDs on the metabolism of sulfated glycosaminoglycans in healthy and (post) arthritic murine articular-cartilage. *Drugs* **35 (supplement 1):** 24–32.

Dingle JT, Saklatvala J, Hembry R, Tyler J, Fell HB & Jubb R (1979) A cartilage catabolic factor from synovium. *Biochemical Journal* **184:** 177–180.

Doherty M (1989) Chondroprotection by non-steroidal anti-inflammatory drugs. *Annals of the Rheumatic Diseases* **48:** 619–621.

Doherty M, Holt M, MacMillan P, Watt I & Dieppe P (1986) A reappraisal of 'analgesic hip'. *Annals of the Rheumatic Diseases* **45:** 272–276.

Engström-Laurent A & Hallgren R (1987) Circulating hyaluronic acid levels vary with physical activity in healthy subjects and in rheumatoid arthritis patients—relationship to synovitis mass and morning stiffness. *Arthritis and Rheumatism* **30:** 1333–1338.

Eronen I & Videman T (1985) Effects of sodium diclofenac on glycosaminoglycan metabolism in experimental osteoarthritis in rabbits. *Scandinavian Journal of Rheumatology* **14:** 37–42.

Fassbender HG (1983) Osteoarthrosis—not simply a degenerative process. In *Articular Cartilage and Osteoarthrosis*, pp 7–29. Bern: Huber.

Franchimont P, Gysen P, Lecomte-Yerna MJ & Gasper S (1983) Incorporation du soufre radioactif dans les proteoglycanes du cartilage in vitro. Effects de certains anti-inflammatoires non steroidiens. *Revue Rhumatologie* **50:** 249–253.

Fraser JRE (1989) Hyaluronan: sources, turnover and metabolism. In Lindh E & Thorell JI (eds) *Clinical Impact of Bone and Connective Tissue Markers*, pp 31. London: Academic Press.

Fujii K, Tajiri K, Sai S, Tanaka T & Murota K (1989) Effects of nonsteroidal antiinflammatory drugs on collagen biosynthesis of cultured chondrocytes. *Seminars in Arthritis and Rheumatism* **18 (supplement 1):** 16–18.

Gay RE, Palmoski MJ, Brandt KD & Gay S (1983) Aspirin causes in vivo synthesis of type I collagen by atrophic articular cartilage. *Arthritis and Rheumatism* **26:** 1231–1236.

Ghosh P (1989) Therapeutic modulation of cartilage catabolism by nonsteroidal anti-inflammatory drugs in arthritis. *Seminars in Arthritis and Rheumatism* **18:** 2–6.

Ghosh P (1990) Chondroprotective drugs and osteoarthritis. *Annals of the Rheumatic Diseases* **49:** 338–339.

Ghosh P, Wells C, Smith M & Hutadilok N (1990) Chondroprotection, myth or reality: an experimental approach. *Seminars in Arthritis and Rheumatism* **19 (supplement 1):** 3–9.

Haggag AA, Mohamed HF, Eldawy MA & Elbahrawy H (1986) Biochemical studies on the anti-inflammatory activity of salicylates as superoxide radical scavengers. *IRCS Medical Science—Biochemistry* **14:** 1104–1105.

Herman JH & Hess EV (1984) Nonsteroidal anti-inflammatory drugs and modulation of cartilageous change in osteoarthritis and rheumatoid arthritis—clinical implications. *American Journal of Medicine* **15:** 16–25.

Herman JH, Appel AM & Hess EV (1987) Modulation of cartilage destruction by select nonsteroidal antiinflammatory drugs—in vitro effect on the synthesis and activity of catabolism-inducing cytokines produced by osteoarthritic and rheumatoid synovial tissue. *Arthritis and Rheumatism* **30:** 257–265.

Isdale IC (1962) Femoral head destruction in rheumatoid arthritis and osteoarthritis. *Annals of the Rheumatic Diseases* **21:** 23–30.

Kalbhen DA (1982) Einflusse antirheumatischer Pharmaka auf den Gelenkknorpel. *Aktuelle Rheumatologie* **7:** 211–217.

Kalbhen DA (1984) Biochemically induced osteoarthritis in the chicken and rat. In Munthe E & Bjelle A (eds) *Effects of Drugs on Osteoarthritis*, pp 48–68. Bern: Huber.

Kalbhen DA (1989) Proteoglycan synthesis and cartilage protection in the hen model of osteoarthritis. In Moskowitz RW & Hirohata K (eds) *Diclofenac (Voltaren) and Cartilage in Osteoarthritis*, pp 22. Toronto: Hogrefe & Huber.

Kalbhen DA, Meiser SM, Buhl K et al (1986) Antidegenerative effect of diclofenac sodium on osteoarthrosis biochemically induced in animals. *Therapiewoche* **36:** 4945–4967.

Kato Y, Sato K, Koike T et al (1989) Effects of antiinflammatory drugs on soft agar growth of rabbit articular chondrocytes. *Seminars in Arthritis and Rheumatism* **18 (supplement 2):** 7–10.

Kellgren JH (1961) Osteoarthritis in patients and population. *British Medical Journal* **2:** 1–6.

Kellgren JH & Lawrence JS (1957) Radiological assessment of osteoarthrosis. *Annals of the Rheumatic Diseases* **16:** 494–501.

Kirkpatrick CJ, Mohr W, Wildfeuer A & Haferkamp O (1983) Influence of nonsteroidal anti-inflammatory agents on lapine articular chondrocyte growth in vitro. *Zeitschrift für Rheumatologie* **42:** 58–65.

Kruze D, Fehr K, Menninger H & Boni A (1976a) Effect of antirheumatic drugs on neutral protease from human leucocyte granules. *Zeitschrift für Rheumatologie* **35:** 337–346.

Kruze D, Fehr K & Boni A (1976b) Effect of antirheumatic drugs on cathepsin B1 from bovine spleen. *Zeitschrift für Rheumatologie* **35:** 95–102.

Lentini A, Ternai B & Ghosh P (1987) Synthetic inhibitors of human leucocyte elastase. 4. Inhibition of human granulocyte elastase and cathepsin G by non-steroidal anti-inflammatory drugs (NSAIDs). *Biochemistry International* **15:** 1069–1078.

Lohmander LS, Dahlberg L, Ryd L & Heinegard D (1989) Increased levels of proteoglycan fragments in knee joint fluid after injury. *Arthritis and Rheumatism* **32:** 1434–1442.

Maier R & Wilhelmi G (1982) Special pharmacological findings with diclofenac sodium. In Kass E (ed.) *Voltaren—New Findings*, pp 11–18. Bern: Huber.

Maier R & Wilhelmi G (1983) Evaluierung der Wirkung von Analgetika-Antiphlogistic auf die Progredienz der Spontanarthrose der C57-black-Maus. *Zeitschrift für Rheumalogie* **42:** 232–240.

Mankin HJ, Dorfman H, Lippiello L & Zarins A (1971) Biochemical and metabolic abnormalities in articular cartilage from osteoarthritic human hips. II. Correlation of morphology with biochemical and metabolic data. *Journal of Bone and Joint Surgery* **53A:** 523–537.

Martel-Pelletier J & Pelletier J-P (1989) Molecular basis for the action of tiaprofenic acid on human osteoarthritic cartilage degradation. *Seminars in Arthritis and Rheumatism* **18:** 19–26.

Martel-Pelletier J, Cloutier J-M, Pelletier J-P (1988) In vivo effects of antirheumatic drugs on neutral collagenolytic proteases in human rheumatoid arthritis cartilage and synovium. *Journal of Rheumatology* **15:** 1198–1204.

McKenzie LS, Horsburgh BA, Ghosh P & Taylor TKF (1976) Effect of anti-inflammatory drugs on sulphated glycosaminoglycan synthesis in aged human articular cartilage. *Annals of the Rheumatic Diseases* **35:** 487–497.

Menkes C-J, Decraemere W, Postel M & Forest M (1985) Chondrocalcinosis and rapid destruction of the hip. *Journal of Rheumatology* **12**: 130–133.

Milner JC (1973) Osteoarthritis of the hip and indomethacin. *Journal of Bone and Joint Surgery* **54B**: 752.

Minta JO & Williams MD (1985) Some nonsteroidal antiinflammatory drugs inhibit the generation of superoxide anions by activated polymorphs by blocking ligand–receptor interactions. *Journal of Rheumatology* **12**: 751–757.

Mitrovic D, McCall E, Front P, Aprile F, Darmon N & Dray F (1984) Antiinflammatory drugs, prostanoids and proteoglycan production by cultured bovine articular chondrocytes. *Prostaglandins* **28**: 417–434.

Mohr W & Kirkpatrick CJ (1984) In vitro experiments with chondrocytes. In Munthe E & Bjelle A (eds) *Effects of Drugs on Osteoarthritis*, pp 75–89. Bern: Huber.

Mohr W, Kirkpatrick CJ, Wildfeuer A & Leitold M (1983) Der Einfluss von Piroxicam auf Struktur und Funktionen des Gelenkknorpels. *Zeitschrift für Rheumatologie* **42**: 70–77.

Mohr W, Kirkpatrick CJ, Wildfeuer A & Leitold M (1984) Effect of piroxicam on structure and function of joint cartilage. *Inflammation* **8 (supplement):** 139–154.

Muir H, Carney SL & Hall LG (1988) Effect of tiaprofenic acid and other NSAIDs on proteoglycan metabolism in articular-cartilage explants. *Drugs* **35 (supplement 1):** 15–23.

Newman NM & Ling RSM (1985) Acetabular bone destruction related to non-steroidal anti-inflammatory drugs. *Lancet* **ii**: 11–14.

Palmoski MJ & Brandt KD (1980) Effects of some nonsteroidal antiinflammatory drugs on proteoglycan metabolism and organization in canine articular cartilage. *Arthritis and Rheumatism* **23**: 1010–1020.

Palmoski MJ & Brandt KJ (1982) Aspirin aggravates the degeneration of canine joint cartilage caused by immobilization. *Arthritis and Rheumatism* **25**: 1333–1342.

Palmoski MJ & Brandt KD (1983a) Relationship between matrix proteoglycan content and effects of salicylate and indomethacin on articular cartilage. *Arthritis and Rheumatism* **26**: 528–531.

Palmoski MJ & Brandt KD (1983b) In vivo effect of aspirin on canine osteoarthritic cartilage. *Arthritis and Rheumatism* **26**: 994–1001.

Pelletier J-P & Martel-Pelletier J (1988a) In vitro effects of tiaprofenic acid, sodium salicylate and hydrocorticone on human osteoarthritic cartilage degradation and synovial collagenase synthesis. *Drugs* **35 (supplement 1):** 42–45.

Pelletier J-P & Martel-Pelletier J (1988b) Evidence for the involvement of interleukin I in human osteoarthritic cartilage degradation: protective effect of NSAID. *Journal of Rheumatology* **16 (supplement 18):** 19–27.

Pelletier J-P, Cloutier JM & Martel-Pelletier J (1989) In vitro effects of tiaprofenic acid, sodium salicylate and hydrocortisone on the proteoglycan metabolism of human osteoarthritic cartilage. *Journal of Rheumatology* **16**: 646–655.

Perper RJ & Oronsky AL (1974) Enzyme release from human leukocyte and degradation of cartilage matrix. Effects of antirheumatic drugs. *Arthritis and Rheumatism* **17**: 47–55.

Pettipher ER, Henderson B, Edwards JCW & Higgs GA (1989) Effects of indomethacin on swelling, lymphocyte influx, and cartilage proteoglycan depletion in experimental arthritis. *Annals of the Rheumatic Diseases* **48**: 623–627.

Rashad S, Revell P, Hemingway A, Low F, Rainsford K & Walker F (1989) Effect of non-steroidal anti-inflammatory drugs on the course of osteoarthritis. *Lancet* **ii**: 519–522.

Rejholec V (1987) Therapeutic long-term studies with disease-modifying drugs in osteo-arthritis. *Seminars in Arthritis and Rheumatism* **17 (supplement 1):** 35–53.

Richards AJ & Hamilton EBD (1974) Destructive arthropathy in chondrocalcinosis articularis. *Annals of the Rheumatic Diseases* **33**: 196–203.

Rönningen H & Langeland N (1979) Indomethacin treatment in osteoarthritis of the hip joint. *Acta Orthopaedica Scandinavica* **50**: 169–174.

Sabiston CP, Adams ME & Li DKB (1987) Magnetic-resonance imaging of osteoarthritis—correlation with gross pathology using an experimental model. *Journal of Orthopaedic Research* **5**: 164–172.

Saklatvala J (1981) Characterisation of catabolin, the major product of pig synovial tissue that induces resorption of cartilage proteoglycans in vitro. *Biochemical Journal* **199**: 705–714.

Saxne T, Heinegard D & Wollheim FA (1986) Therapeutic effects on cartilage metabolism in arthritis as measured by release of proteoglycan structures into the synovial fluid. *Annals of the Rheumatic Diseases* **45**: 491–497.

Saxne T, Heinegard D & Wollheim FA (1987) Cartilage proteoglycans in synovial-fluid and serum in patients with inflammatory joint disease—relation to systemic treatment. *Arthritis and Rheumatism* **30**: 972–979.

Sheppeard H & Couchman KG (1986) Experience with isoxicam and catabolin. *British Journal of Clinical Pharmacology* **22**: 121S–124S.

Sheppeard H, Pilsworth L, Hazleman B & Dingle JT (1982) Effects of antirheumatoid drugs on the production and action of porcine catabolism. *Annals of the Rheumatic Diseases* **41**: 463–468.

Shinmei M, Shimada K, Shigeno Y, Kikuchi K & Miyazaki K (1985) Effects of anti-inflammatory drugs on proteoglycan synthesis and degradation in rabbit articular chondrocytes in vitro. In Nilsen OG (ed.) *Tiaprofenic Acid*, pp 59–68. International Congress of Rheumatology. Amsterdam: Excerpta Medica.

Shinmei M, Kikuchi T, Masuda K & Shimomura Y (1988) Effects of interleukin-1 and anti-inflammatory drugs on the degradation of human articular cartilage. *Drugs* **35 (supplement 1):** 33–41.

Solomon L (1973) Drug induced arthropathy and necrosis of the femoral head. *Journal of Bone and Joint Surgery* **55B:** 246–261.

Stephens RW, Walton EA, Ghosh P, Taylor TKF, Gramse M & Havemann K (1980) A radioassay for proteolytic cleavage of isolated cartilage proteoglycan. 2. Inhibition of human leukocyte elastase and cathepsin G by anti-inflammatory drugs. *Arzneimittelforschung* **30:** 2108–2112.

Storey GO (1968) Bone necrosis in joint disease. *Proceedings of the Royal Society of Medicine* **61:** 961–969.

van de Loo AAJ & van den Berg WB (1990) Effects of murine recombinant interleukin 1 on synovial joints in mice—measurement of patellar cartilage metabolism and joint inflammation. *Annals of the Rheumatic Diseases* **49:** 238–245.

van Epps DE, Greiwe S, Potter J & Goodwin J (1987) Alterations in neutrophil superoxide production following piroxicam therapy in patients with rheumatoid arthritis. *Inflammation* **11:** 59–72.

Verbruggen G, Veys EM, Malfait A-M et al (1989) Proteoglycan metabolism in tissue cultured human articular cartilage—influence of piroxicam. *Journal of Rheumatology* **16:** 355–362.

Videman T, Eronen I, Friman C, Ahtiala K & Mattila MJ (1981) Effects of indomethacin on glycosaminoglycan metabolism in the development of experimental osteoarthritis in rabbits. *Biochemical Pharmacology* **30:** 2135–2139.

Vignon E, Mathieu P, Couprie N et al (1989) Effects of tiaprofenic acid on interleukin-1, phospholipase A_2 activity, prostaglandins, neutral protease, and collagenase activity in rheumatoid synovial fluid. *Seminars in Arthritis and Rheumatism* **18 (supplement 1):** 11–15.

Vignon E, Mathieu P, Broquet P, Louisot P & Richard M (1990) Cartilage degradative enzymes in human osteoarthritis: effect of a nonsteroidal antiinflammatory drug administered orally. *Seminars in Arthritis and Rheumatism* **19 (supplement 1):** 26–29.

Watson M (1976) The suppressing effect of indomethacin on articular cartilage. *Rheumatology and Rehabilitation* **15:** 26–30.

Whitehouse MW & Bostrom H (1962) The effect of some anti-inflammatory (anti-rheumatism) drugs on the metabolism of connective tissues. *Biochemical Pharmacology* **11:** 1175–1201.

Wood DD, Ihrie EJ, Dinarello CA & Cohen PL (1983) Isolation of an interleukin-1-like factor from human joint effusions. *Arthritis and Rheumatism* **26:** 975–983.

8

The risks of local and systemic corticosteroid administration

CYRUS COOPER
JOHN R. KIRWAN

The pattern of use of corticosteroid therapy differs widely in rheumatology. The prevalence of steroid use in rheumatoid arthritis, for example, may vary markedly in different countries. Within Britain, beliefs about the uses of corticosteroid therapy are strongly held by rheumatologists, yet show wide variation (Byron and Mowat, 1985). Our knowledge about the efficacy and risk of corticosteroid administration remains in large part suboptimal. As might be expected with any group of drugs that exert a wide range of pharmacological actions and are routinely used in a variety of pathological conditions, reports of adverse effects of corticosteroids are frequent. However, much literature on the subject is derived from case reports and uncontrolled studies. In the case of several potential adverse effects, careful review of the evidence leads to the conclusion that the risk of their occurrence, if present at all, is small. The purpose of this review is to consider these adverse effects in relation to the three common routes of administration: oral, intravenous pulse and intrasynovial.

Corticosteroids are among the most effective agents currently available for the alleviation of symptoms attributable to inflammatory arthritis. The discovery of some of these effects by Hench at the Mayo Clinic over forty years ago (Hench, 1952) was rapidly followed by the widespread use of corticosteroids in rheumatoid arthritis. The optimism that cortisone might be a cure for the condition quickly evaporated as some of the toxic effects of systemic corticosteroid therapy came to light over the ensuing decades. There followed a backlash as the more serious of these effects, particularly at the high doses being used, were set against a failure of steroid therapy to alter longer term progression of rheumatoid arthritis. The tone of much subsequent debate on the balance of risks and benefits of corticosteroid therapy has been clouded by the emotional arguments of these earlier years.

ORAL CORTICOSTEROID THERAPY

The clinical complications which may occur during the use of corticosteroid therapy are protean (Table 1). Three putative sequelae of chronic steroid

Table 1. Adverse effects of systemic corticosteroid therapy.

1. Metabolic	Obesity
	Glucose/protein metabolism
	Electrolyte balance
	Enzyme induction
2. Predisposition to infection	
3. Musculoskeletal	Myopathy
	Osteoporosis
	Avascular necrosis
	Tendon rupture
	Steroid withdrawal syndrome
4. Gastrointestinal	Peptic ulcer disease
	Pancreatitis
5. Ophthalmic	Cataract
	Glaucoma
6. Central nervous system	Psychosis
	Depression
	Benign intracranial hypertension
7. Dermatological	Acne
	Striae
	Alopecia
	Bruising
	Skin atrophy
8. Growth retardation	
9. Hypothalamic–pituitary–adrenal axis suppression	

therapy have important clinical implications. For osteoporosis, the evidence implicating steroid therapy is unequivocal, for peptic ulceration it is discrepant, and in relation to atherosclerosis evidence is only now beginning to accrue. These examples highlight the difficulties faced by investigators in studying rare outcomes in patients with a heterogeneous group of inflammatory disorders, who are treated with varying doses of a single agent.

Cushingoid features, obesity and other metabolic effects

Glucocorticoids induce alterations of fat distribution that account for the classical cushingoid appearance. These include truncal obesity, 'buffalo hump' and moon facies, which occur in 13% of patients who receive steroids for two months and almost half of patients treated for five years or more (Shubin, 1965; Smyllie and Connolly, 1968; David et al, 1970). Other localized fat deposits may be found in the mediastinum (Bodman and Condemi, 1967) and temporal (Gottlieb, 1980) fat pads. Obesity and cushingoid features often resolve rapidly when patients are switched to alternate-day therapy (Ackerman and Nolan, 1968).

Exogenous glucocorticoids also influence glucose, protein and electrolyte metabolism, and hepatic enzyme function (David et al, 1970).

1. Glucose metabolism. It is well established that steroids produce a tendency towards hyperglycaemia, glycosuria, increased hepatic gluconeogenesis, increased hepatic glycogen deposition and insulin antagonism. Classically, steroid-induced diabetes mellitus is considered to be a mild, stable disorder, usually without ketoacidosis or hyperosmolarity (Blereau and Weingarten, 1964; Alavi et al, 1971; Dujovne and Azarnoff, 1975). Its severity is related to the dose and duration of steroid administration, and it is relatively resistant to insulin therapy. The diabetes appears to be reversible on discontinuation of steroid therapy but this reversal may take several months (Olefsky and Kimmerling, 1976; Bond, 1977).

2. Protein metabolism. Inhibition of protein synthesis, enhancement of protein catabolism and negative nitrogen balance are well-recognized consequences of steroid therapy (David et al, 1970). These consequences appear to be tissue-specific, however. Decreased protein content of muscle, bone and lymphoid tissue contrasts with increased nitrogen content in the liver, gastrointestinal and urinary tracts.

3. Electrolyte balance. Intravenous corticosteroid administration produces a transient (four-hour) increase in urinary sodium excretion. More prolonged use of steroids results in sodium retention with concomitant potassium loss, which corrects itself over a few weeks. This effect appears to be mediated by the weak mineralocorticoid properties of cortisone derivatives. Hypokalaemic alkalosis is an important (though rare) event in patients treated with large doses of steroids.

4. Hepatic enzymes. Pharmacological doses of glucocorticoids have been shown to increase the activities of various liver enzymes involved in transamination, gluconeogenesis and the urea cycle.

Predisposition to infection

Glucocorticoids have effects on several arms of the immune system (Figure 1). These may be conveniently divided into effects on the different leucocyte types and those on overall function of the system. Administration of steroids to healthy subjects produces a neutrophil leucocytosis within 4 to 6 hours (Fauci et al, 1976). However, this is accompanied by a suppression of neutrophil aggregation at any inflammatory site (Allison et al, 1955). Reduced granulocyte adherence to vascular epithelium after an inflammatory stimulus is one mechanism for this suppression (MacGregor et al, 1974). In addition, granulocytes in corticosteroid-treated patients demonstrate impairment of phagocytic capacity, although their bactericidal activity appears to be preserved (Hirsh and Church, 1961). This is in marked contrast to the blunted bactericidal activity of monocytes in these patients (Rinehart et al, 1975). Steroid therapy in animals and humans is also associated with lymphocytopenia (Claman, 1972). These changes lead to profound effects on several cell-mediated immunological processes, including delayed hypersensitivity, antigen processing, lymphocyte activation and

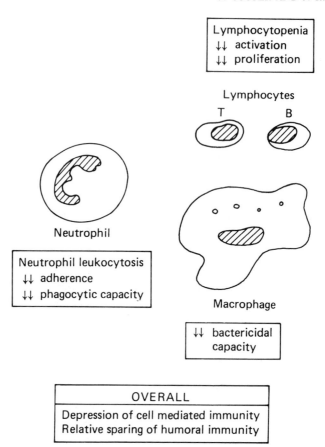

Figure 1. Effects of corticosteroid therapy on various arms of the immune response.

proliferation, and cell-mediated cytotoxicity (Fauci et al, 1976). In contrast, humoral immune function appears to be less compromised by steroid therapy.

The combined effects of these changes must be considered in trying to understand the relation between steroid therapy and infection. Soon after steroid therapy was introduced, it was recognized that these agents can dramatically alter the course of most infectious diseases. Fever was reduced, as were the malaise and toxicity from the illness, but the infection often worsened (Kass and Finland, 1958). Steroid therapy predisposes to a wide range of infections (Beisel and Rapoport, 1969). Among bacterial agents, staphylococcal, Gram-negative, tuberculous and *Listeria* infections appear most frequently associated. Certain viral, fungal and bacterial infections also occur often.

Clinical data to support a large increase in the risk of infection during steroid therapy are harder to obtain. In many published clinical trials, patients also have diseases that predispose to infection and are exposed to atypical organisms in a hospital environment (Staples et al, 1974; Grieco, 1984). The putative association between steroid therapy and reactivation of tuberculosis provides a good example. In large studies of patients receiving steroids in low doses over long periods of time for chest conditions, no increased risk of developing active tuberculosis has been observed (Smyllie and Connolly, 1968; Leiberman et al, 1972). Likewise cohorts of patients with positive tuberculin skin tests have been followed up for prolonged periods without development of active disease (Schatz et al, 1976). Those studies reporting an increased risk of tuberculosis in patients treated with steroids have often included patients on several immunosuppressive agents or with diseases predisposing to infection (Kaplan et al, 1974). These findings have led many authors to the view that the risk of developing active tuberculosis during steroid therapy is much lower than initially suspected (Haanaes and Bergman, 1983).

Musculoskeletal complications

The most important musculoskeletal complication of steroid therapy is osteoporosis; this condition is discussed in greater detail at the end of this section. Other effects of steroid therapy on bone and muscle include proximal myopathy, tendon rupture and avascular necrosis.

Chronic steroid treatment may produce muscle weakness which is typically proximal (Dujovne and Azarnoff, 1975). There is no relationship between the occurrence of steroid myopathy and age, sex, steroid dosage or duration of therapy (Afifi et al, 1968). It has been reported to be more frequent in patients receiving fluorinated compounds such as triamcinolone (Golding and Begg, 1960). The myopathy is usually associated with marked muscle wasting, and improvement usually begins as soon as steroids are withdrawn. No benefit has been found by administration of anabolic steroids or potassium supplements. Data have more recently become available on the ultrastructural changes of affected muscles (Horber et al, 1986). Chronic treatment (between 8 and 105 months) of renal transplant recipients with around 10 mg of prednisone resulted in atrophy of all three muscle fibre types, as well as features suggestive of compensatory hypertrophy. Thus subclinical myopathy may be a more frequent complication of steroid therapy than commonly appreciated, being obscured by an adaptive response equivalent to training.

Myalgia often occurs as part of a generalized syndrome in patients who are withdrawn from steroid treatment (Byyny, 1976; Dixon and Christy, 1980). This constellation of complaints (steroid withdrawal syndrome) includes fatigue, malaise, anorexia, nausea and weight loss. It has been reported in as many as 70% of patients treated with 30 mg of prednisone daily for longer than three months. There appears to be no correlation between symptoms and adrenal function. In certain clinical settings, however, such as polymyalgia rheumatica and polymyositis, it may be difficult to differentiate from poor control of the primary disease.

Tendon rupture, a complication usually associated with injected steroids,

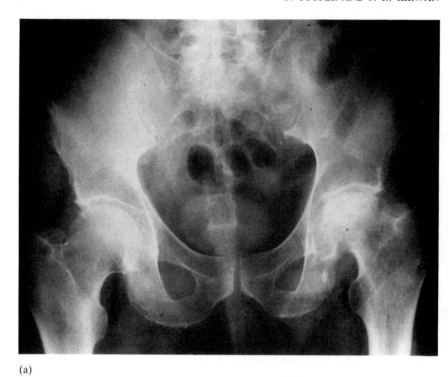

(a)

(b)

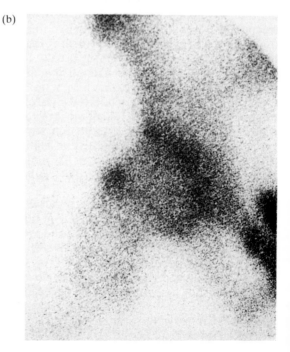

Figure 2. Avascular necrosis of the femoral head: (a) plain radiograph (b) isotope scintigram (reproduced with kind permission of Professor L. Solomon, Bristol). Note deformity of bony contour of femoral head on plain radiography, and band of increased isotope uptake on scintigram.

has also been reported with systemic therapy, although it must be extremely rare (Barnal, 1984).

Steroid therapy has also been implicated in the aetiology of aseptic necrosis (Figure 2). Over 150 cases of this association have been reported in the literature (Sutton et al, 1963), and it has been recorded in 1% of patients receiving steroids for pulmonary disease (Richards et al, 1980). However, aseptic necrosis does occur as part of the natural history of rheumatoid arthritis and other connective tissue diseases. In a review of 52 patients with aspetic necrosis (McConkey et al, 1962), around 10% gave a history of steroid use and 17% had a history of alcoholism. These two risk factors support the hypothesis that aseptic necrosis is caused by fat embolism arising from fatty degeneration of the liver or bone marrow (Richards et al, 1980).

Avascular necrosis may occur as early as six weeks after the start of glucocorticoid therapy (Sutton et al, 1963). It usually affects the femoral head and presents a major diagnostic challenge as the onset of pain may be insidious and without accompanying radiographic changes. Isotope bone scanning is twice as sensitive as conventional radiography in diagnosing avascular necrosis and may point to unsuspected contralateral disease (Conklin et al, 1983). The relationship between steroid dose and risk of avascular necrosis is not clear. Although an early study (Sutton et al, 1963) reported that the complication was not dose-related, a more recent analysis of 24 patient cohorts (Felson and Anderson, 1987), treated with oral or intravenous bolus corticosteroids and followed for at least three months, showed that oral steroid dose was highly correlated with the risk of avascular necrosis. Bolus steroids, in contrast, posed little risk. There was a preponderance of renal transplant patients in this series, however, and as this is the only situation in which data on bolus administration are widely available, generalization that bolus doses are safe in this regard may be unwarranted.

Gastrointestinal complications

The gastrointestinal complication of steroid therapy that has greatest clinical significance is peptic ulceration. The often conflicting evidence relating to the role of exogenously administered steroids in causing peptic ulceration is discussed in detail later in this review. Patients who develop peptic ulcer disease while on corticosteroids do not appear to be at increased risk of perforation or haemorrhage, but these complications tend to occur silently (Glenn and Grafe, 1967; Smyllie and Connolly, 1968; Conn and Blitzer, 1976). A recent series of 25 patients seen over a 25-year period who suffered a perforated peptic ulcer while taking steroids found that only 9 showed clinical evidence of peritoneal irritation (Dayton et al, 1987). A common sequence of events appeared to be an exacerbation of primary disease, followed by a significant increase in steroid dose and perforation. Overall mortality rose from 17% in those under 50 years old to 85% in those over 50 years old.

Almost every organ of the gastrointestinal tract has been reported to suffer adverse consequences of steroid therapy (Gallant and Kenny, 1986). Gastric upset, anorexia, nausea and vomiting have frequently been reported. Fatty liver, common in animals, has been documented in humans.

Adults receiving steroids appear to be at increased risk of acute pancreatitis. This is a rare condition, but fatal cases have been reported. A postmortem study of 54 patients who had received steroids for at least three days prior to death showed ectasia of the pancreatic ducts in 59% and acute focal pancreatitis in 28.5% of the cases. In contrast, changes of pancreatitis were detected in only 3.7% of a comparable group of control subjects who had not taken steroids (Carone and Liebon, 1957). A threefold increase in the risk of developing pancreatitis has also been reported in children who receive corticosteroids (Oppenheimer and Boitnott, 1960). No relationship can be detected, however, between the incidence of this complication and either dose or duration of therapy (Riemenschneider et al, 1968).

The mechanism whereby steroids induce pancreatitis is unknown. Pancreatic necrosis with hyperamylasaemia and hyperlipidaemia can be induced in rabbits by intravenous glucocorticoid administration (Stumpf et al, 1956). Steroid therapy increases the viscosity of pancreatic secretions and may result in inspissation and consequent obstruction of pancreatic excretory passages (Dujovne and Azarnoff, 1975).

There have been occasional reports of perforation of the caecum, colonic diverticula and rectum in association with corticosteroid administration (Cushman, 1970). Most patients with these disorders had underlying inflammatory bowel disease, so the role of therapy in producing these adverse effects is unclear. As with peptic ulceration, there is evidence to suggest that the features of colonic perforation might be masked by concomitant steroid administration (Sterioff et al, 1974).

Ophthalmic complications

Ocular reactions are among the better demonstrated complications of steroid therapy. Posterior subcapsular cataracts were initially recognized in over 30% of a group of 47 patients with rheumatoid arthritis who were treated with steroids (Black et al, 1960). Subsequent studies have shown children to be at greater risk than adults (Bihari and Grossman, 1968; Shiono et al, 1977). Steroid-related cataracts are almost always bilateral and often do not alter visual acuity (Furst et al, 1966). It is thought that they do not progress at steroid doses of around 10 mg daily, but are not precluded by alternate-day or intermittent therapy (Chai et al, 1975; Rooklin et al, 1978).

Increased intraocular pressure is the other major ophthalmic complication of steroid therapy (David and Berkowitz, 1969). It is found in as many as 40% of patients systemically treated with the drug (Burde and Becker, 1970). Although usually reversible by discontinuing treatment, irreversible glaucoma and blindness may occur, especially in patients who are diabetic or highly myopic.

Other less frequent ophthalmic effects of steroid therapy include scleral atrophy (Crews, 1965), exophthalmos (Cohen et al, 1981) and herpetic keratitis (Aaron, 1968).

Central nervous system complications

Corticosteroids are important determinants of behaviour pattern (Carpenter and Bunney, 1971). Administration of these agents has been reported to cause psychiatric reactions in 4% to 36% of patients (Ritchie, 1956; Hall et al, 1979). These reactions include psychosis, agitation, depression and suicidal tendency. Most reactions of this type are reversible and appear strongly related to steroid dose. The Boston Collaborative Drug Study (Boston Collaborative Drug Surveillance Group, 1972) noted a prevalence of reported psychotic events of less than 1% in patients receiving less than 30 mg prednisone daily, in contrast to 18% in those receiving more than 80 mg daily. It has been suggested that these adverse effects are more likely to occur in subjects with pre-existing personality disorders (Glaser, 1953). Management should include reduction in steroid dose and anti-psychotic drugs, especially lithium (Claman, 1983; Goggans et al, 1983).

Benign intracranial hypertension has also been reported with increased frequency in association with glucocorticoid therapy (Weisberg and Chutorian, 1977; Rimza, 1978; Fritz and Weston, 1984). The complication seems to occur particularly in children, in whom the condition is otherwise rare. Patients present with headaches, impaired vision or nausea, and are found on fundoscopy to have papilloedema. It usually responds to withdrawal of steroid therapy and therapeutic lumbar punctures. Failure to resolve, however, may prompt treatment with higher doses of a different steroid preparation.

Dermatological complications

A whole host of skin changes have been reported with the use of oral glucocorticoids (Gallant and Kenny, 1986). Most frequent among these are acne, striae, alopecia, purpura and skin atrophy with poor healing. Increased fragility and easy bruising appear more frequently in patients being treated for rheumatoid arthritis. Some patients have been noted to improve on oral ascorbic acid or vitamin A supplementation (Judge, 1960; Hunt et al, 1969).

Growth retardation

Physiological levels of glucocorticoids are required for normal growth in childhood (Loeb, 1976). Growth retardation may occur in children receiving corticosteroids as these agents inhibit linear bone growth and delay epiphyseal closure (Lucky, 1984). The mechanism of these influences on growth remains unknown, although suppression of growth hormone secretion and competition at insulin and somatomedin receptor sites are all candidates (Fritz and Weston, 1984).

Much information on steroid-induced growth retardation has come from studies of asthmatic children (Reimer et al, 1975; Murray et al, 1976; Godfrey et al, 1978; Balfour-Lynn, 1986; Elliot, 1987; Shohat et al, 1987). Regular daily steroid administration of 7.5 mg or above is associated with significant inhibition of linear growth (Lucky, 1984). At lower doses, the evidence for a growth effect is less convincing, and if it occurs, catch-up growth is possible prior to puberty on withdrawal of therapy. This catch-up phase cannot, however, extend beyond epiphyseal closure.

The growth-retarding effects of corticosteroids appear to be reduced by alternate-day administration (Reimer et al, 1975).

Suppression of the hypothalamic–pituitary–adrenal axis

Adrenal function is regulated through the hypothalamic–pituitary–adrenal axis. Two bodies of evidence relate to the suppression of this axis by exogenously administered corticosteroid therapy. First, postmortem studies of steroid-treated patients have shown pituitary and adrenal atrophy (Salassa et al, 1953; Axelrod, 1976). Second, studies measuring blood levels of adrenal steroids, their metabolites and precursors have confirmed the long-term suppressive effect of systemic steroids on the adrenal gland (Landon et al, 1976). Available data suggest that 10–12.5 mg of prednisone daily significantly blunts adrenal function in a third of patients, but that complete suppression only occurs in patients receiving 20 mg or more daily (Klinefelter et al, 1979). There is disagreement regarding the duration of suppression and how frequently this suppression leads to adrenal crisis under stress. In considering the vast number of patients who have received corticosteroids over the last three decades, the frequency of documented adrenal crisis is surprisingly low (Rees, 1981). It has been suggested that although prolonged corticosteroid therapy leads to relative suppression of the pituitary–adrenal axis, hypothalamic responsiveness might persist and be sufficient to prevent adrenal crisis under stress (Storrs, 1979). Thus, slow tapering of steroid dosage to allow recovery of the hypothalamic–pituitary–adrenal system may only serve to prolong exposure to unwanted effects of exogenous steroids. Tapering of dose, especially after relatively short periods of use (around one month) is more usefully tailored to disease control alone.

Steroid therapy and osteoporosis: a significant complication

Since Cushing first described his syndrome, it has been recognized that supraphysiological levels of endogenous corticosteroids are associated with excessive bone loss (Cushing, 1932). Soon after the introduction of cortisone as a therapeutic agent in 1949, it became apparent that exogeneous steroid excess also had skeletal consequences (Boland and Headley, 1950; Curtess et al, 1954; Rosenberg, 1958; Virkkunen and Lehtinen, 1958). Recent advances in the non-invasive assessment of bone density, in the histo-morphometric assessment of bone turnover and in the development of therapeutic strategies for osteoporosis have significant implications for our understanding of steroid-induced bone loss.

The bone loss associated with steroid therapy principally affects trabecular bone (Hahn, 1978; Baylink, 1983; Lukert and Raisz, 1990). Studies using photon absorptiometric measurement of bone mineral density have shown that bone loss is greater in the lumbar spine, less in the proximal femur and least in the forearm (Schaadt and Bohr, 1984). These observations are reflected in the pattern of fractures associated with steroid use. Vertebral wedge and crush fractures are a frequent complication of steroid-treated rheumatoid arthritis, with prevalence rates from 11% to 20% reported (Boland and Headley, 1950; Curtess et al, 1954; Adinoff and Hollister, 1983; Luengo et al, 1987). The increased risk of fractures at other skeletal sites in such patients, however, remains unclear (Hooyman et al, 1984; Verstraeten and Dequeker, 1986). In a recent case-control study of hip fracture in Britain (Cooper et al, 1988a), current use of corticosteroids was associated with a doubled hip fracture risk, which remained significantly elevated even after adjustment for confounding variables such as body mass index, smoking, alcohol consumption and physical inactivity (Figure 3). This observation supported the findings of a previous Californian epidemiological study (Paganini-Hill et al, 1981).

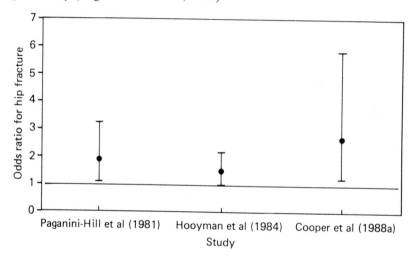

Figure 3. Relationship between steroid therapy and the risk of hip fracture: results of three epidemiological studies. Note consistent, statistically significant increase in hip fracture risk. (Bars show 95% confidence limits.)

The severity of bone loss associated with steroid use varies with the dosage used, the duration of therapy and perhaps the diseases for which steroids are prescribed (Reid, 1990a).

Malabsorption of calcium has been documented at prednisone doses of above 15 mg daily, but not at doses of 8–10 mg daily (Klein et al, 1977). There is, however, evidence that osteoblast function might be impaired by doses as low as 5 mg daily (Lund et al, 1985). Studies of bone loss in patients treated with steroids do not clearly suggest a threshold dose below which osteoporosis does not occur. In some cases, significant bone loss has been reported in groups on doses as low as 2.5–5 mg daily (Chesney et al, 1978; Als et al 1983, 1985). There appears to be a consistent relationship between doses above 7.5 mg daily and rate of bone loss.

It is now clear that the skeletal effects of corticosteroids begin almost immediately after commencement of therapy. Fractures often occur within the first year, and animal studies point to a rapid period of bone loss during a comparable period (Jee et al, 1970). Longitudinal histomorphometric data in humans suggested a rapid early phase of resorption, following which bone loss occurs more slowly (Duncan, 1972). It should be noted, however, that several studies have documented a relationship between bone mass and duration of steroid use. A synthesis of the available evidence suggests that the most rapid period of bone loss occurs within a few months of the introduction of steroid therapy, with a much more gradual loss thereafter (Reid et al, 1982, 1986).

The third determinant of bone loss in steroid-treated patients is the underlying disease. Many studies have been carried out in patients with rheumatoid arthritis, a condition characterized by marked juxta-articular osteoporosis, which itself manifests as a reduction in appendicular cortical bone mass (Cooper et al, 1988b). This cortical reduction is not found in patients who use corticosteroids for asthma (Reid et al, 1984).

The pathogenesis of steroid-induced osteoporosis probably involves

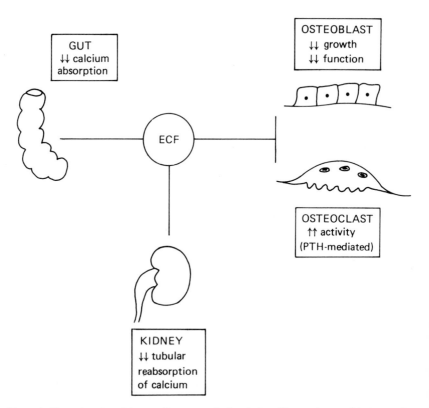

Figure 4. Alterations in calcium and bone metabolism induced by corticosteroids. Note effects on both major bone cell types, as well as gut and kidney. ECF: extracellular fluid.

direct inhibition of bone formation and indirect enhancement of bone resorption (Peck, 1984) (Figure 4). Glucocorticoids have an inhibitory effect on the growth and replication of cultured osteoblast cell lines (Rodan and Martin, 1981; Chyun and Raisz, 1982) and reduce formation of osteocalcin by human osteoblasts (Beresford et al, 1984). This effect may be achieved through interference with the surface receptor for 1,25-dihydroxy vitamin D. The indirect bone-resorptive effects of steroids are probably mediated through an impairment of vitamin D-induced calcium absorption (Beresford et al, 1986). Concomitant calcium malabsorption results in secondary hyperparathyroidism and a possible increase in 1,25-dihydroxy vitamin D, both of which serve as a stimulus to osteoclast-mediated bone resorption (Hahn et al, 1981).

The prevention and treatment of steroid-induced osteoporosis are subjects of much current research (Reid, 1990b). Potential preventive strategies include the use of different drug delivery systems, such as alternate-day therapy, pulse methylprednisolone, ACTH and inhaled corticosteroids. To date, none of these measures has produced encouraging results. Prevention with adjunctive therapy, most notably oestrogens in postmenopausal women and calcium, requires serious consideration. Finally, the results of using alternative steroid preparations such as deflazacort, which have decreased skeletal effects, are awaited (Gennari and Imbimbo, 1985). In terms of treatment of established disease, recent studies suggest a prominent role for orally administered diphosphonates (Reid et al, 1988).

Steroid therapy and peptic ulceration: a tenuous association

Peptic ulceration is not a common occurrence in endogenous Cushing's disease (Dujovne and Azarnoff, 1975) yet it is widely held that steroid therapy is frequently complicated by the appearance or reactivation of peptic ulcers. The basis for this view resides in a number of anecdotal reports of the development of peptic ulcer in patients receiving steroids, and several series of steroid-treated patients with a high incidence of ulcers (Lubin et al, 1951; Smyth, 1951; Bollett et al, 1955; Kern et al, 1957; Freiberger et al, 1958; Gedda and Moritz, 1958). Close scrutiny of the evidence from controlled studies of steroid therapy, however, suggests that the increased risk of peptic ulceration—if it exists at all—is considerably lower than is widely believed.

In the first synthesis of prospective, controlled investigations of steroid or ACTH therapy and peptic ulceration, Conn and Blitzer (1976) reviewed 42 studies of steroid therapy (26 of which were double-blind studies) with a total of 5331 patients. Steroid therapy was evaluated in a variety of clinical settings in these studies, including tuberculosis, chronic liver disease, multiple sclerosis, stroke and sarcoidosis. Steroid dosages varied from 10 mg to 60 mg of prednisone or equivalent, and exposures ranged from one week to over a year. The relative risk of peptic ulceration from steroid therapy in these studies is shown in Figure 5. Among the double-blind trials, ulcers occurred slightly more frequently in the steroid-treated patients (1.4%) compared with controls (1%) but the difference was not statistically

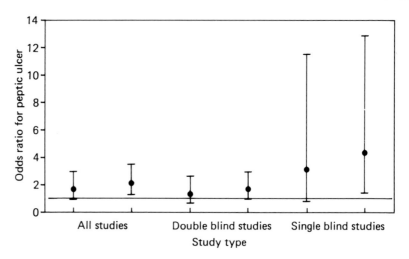

Figure 5. Results of controlled studies examining the relationship between steroid administration and peptic ulceration (after Conn and Poynard). Note lower odds ratios for peptic
ulceration in double blind studies compared to single blind studies. Risks on left of each pair
represent data of Conn et al (1976) and on right of each pair data of Messer et al (1983).

significant. There was a higher rate of ulcers, however, in subgroups of
patients who received steroids for more than 30 days or in total doses greater
than 1 g of prednisone.

Messer et al (1983), using a similar experimental design, re-examined the
issue in 71 studies and concluded that adrenal steroids significantly increased
the risk of peptic ulcer (Figure 5). In the 37 double-blind studies, ulcer
prevalence was 2.6% in steroid-treated patients compared with 1.5% in
controls, while in the non-double-blind investigations, ulcer prevalence was
almost six times greater in cases (1.1%) than in controls (0.2%).

In a subsequent critique of this study, Conn and Poynard (1985) highlighted
a number of methodological and statistical shortfalls. These included the
failure of several studies to report complications adequately, concomitant
use of antacids, inclusion of assymetric uncontrolled investigations and lack
of randomization. They reanalysed the data after correcting for some of
these deficiencies and found that more than four-fifths of the total number of
reported ulcers in the 37 double-blind studies reviewed by Messer et al arose
in a single study. Exclusion of this study (which may have been inappro-
priately included in any case) from the analysis resulted in the previously
significant association between steroids and ulcer becoming non-significant.

An overall synthesis of these data leads us to the conclusion that if an
association does exist between steroid therapy and peptic ulcer, it is likely to
be a small one. Theoretically, the issue could be resolved by a prospective,
randomized controlled trial. Such a trial is, however, unlikely ever to be
performed. It is difficult to conceive of a situation in which steroid treatment
could be randomly withheld from some patients, while current evaluations
of steroid therapy in disorders such as rheumatoid arthritis are unlikely ever

to have sufficient statistical power to detect with confidence an increased risk of this rare outcome. It is also worth mentioning that no pathogenetic mechanism has to date been suggested to explain the putative association between steroid treatment and peptic ulceration. Finally, it should be borne in mind that if rheumatologists see 15 new patients each week during 30 years of service, and treat around 4% of these with steroids, they will see at best one, and at worst two, steroid-induced peptic ulcers during their medical lifetime.

Steroid therapy and atherosclerosis: a potential complication of major significance

The only cardiovascular complications of steroids that have been consistently identified are hypertension and congestive cardiac failure. Information is beginning to accumulate, however, that prolonged steroid therapy may accelerate the development of atherosclerosis (Nashel, 1986). If true, even a small effect would have considerable clinical and public health significance. The evidence for this association may be broadly classified into two categories: (a) experiments on animals and *in vitro* human tissue suggesting that steroids enhance experimentally induced atherogenesis, and (b) epidemiological studies showing a link between steroid therapy and cardiovascular mortality.

In animal experiments, cortisone and ACTH have been shown to produce endothelial damage and alter vascular connective tissue (Rosenfeld et al, 1960; Lorenzen and Hansen, 1967). These changes, coupled with hyperlipidaemia, abnormal glucose tolerance and hypertension which are also recognised in some patients on steroid therapy, might easily lead to premature atherosclerosis.

A postmortem survey of 36 steroid-treated patients with systemic lupus erythematosus found that atherosclerotic plaques had caused coronary luminal occlusion greater than 50% in 8 of 19 subjects who received steroids for longer than a year (Bulkley and Roberts, 1975). This degree of narrowing was not found in any of the patients taking steroids for less than a year.

In a controlled study of this subject, Kalbak reported a prevalence of lower limb atherosclerosis of 60% in steroid-treated patients with rheumatoid arthritis, compared with only 20% in a non-steroid treated control group (Kalbak, 1972).

Finally, several studies of mortality in rheumatoid arthritis and other connective tissue diseases have detected an increased cardiovascular mortality among sufferers (Rasker and Cosh, 1981; Allebeck, 1982; Pincus et al, 1984; Prior et al, 1984; Vandenbroucke et al, 1984). These point to an approximate doubling in the death rate from ischaemic heart disease. Although data on steroid use in these studies are often incomplete, one study reported an excess of coronary artery deaths in a steroid-treated group when compared with a non-steroid treated control group (Million et al, 1984).

Clearly, the evidence linking steroid therapy with atherosclerosis falls far short of proof. Vasculitis is a prominent feature of many of the diseases for which steroid treatment is used, and controlled, comprehensive patho-logical studies of long-term treatment are not yet available. Nevertheless, the incidence of atherosclerotic disease in the general population and the frequency with which steroids are used in relatively young patients suggest that this putative association is worthy of consideration.

PULSED INTRAVENOUS CORTICOSTEROID THERAPY

Pulse therapy involves the intravenous infusion of a large dose of corti-costeroid (usually around 1 g of methylprednisolone) over a short time—around 30 minutes (Weiss, 1989). A variety of regimens are used currently, but most entail a course of three pulses on alternate days, followed by a resting phase of around six weeks. This form of treatment was initiated in renal transplant recipients, but gradually spread to the treatment of other renal disorders, most notably lupus nephritis. The observation was made in such patients that synovial inflammation responded rapidly, and for pro-longed periods, with intravenous therapy. Following anecdotal reports of benefit in rheumatoid arthritis, controlled studies were performed through the 1980s which suggested beneficial effects from this regimen, with rela-tively few side-effects (Leibling et al, 1981; Forster et al, 1982; Neumann et al, 1985; Radia and Furst, 1988). These trials are small, however, and therefore limited in statistical power.

Table 2. Adverse effects of pulse methylprednisolone therapy.

1. Sudden death/ventricular dysrhythmia
2. Severe infection
3. Transient arthralgia/synovitis
4. Hyperglycaemia
5. Pancreatitis
6. Gastrointestinal bleeding
7. Acute psychosis

Most reports of complications following pulse steroid therapy have arisen in renal transplant patients (Table 2). Most important among these is sudden death, most probably arising as a result of ventricular dysrhythmia and consequent myocardial infarction. In three such cases (Stubbs and Morrell, 1973), the intravenous bolus was administered rapidly (in one case over only 20 seconds) and all were taking frusemide, which may have induced hypo-kalaemia. It has been suggested that increasing infusion time to at least 30 minutes might prevent such events. Nevertheless, the incidence of such sudden death appears to be extremely low, given that well over 10 000 renal transplant patients are likely to have been treated with pulse steroids.

Severe fatal infections have also been reported (Clarke and Salaman, 1974; Muusche et al, 1976). However, these are rare, and have occurred in transplant patients on daily doses of azathioprine, often following continued, long-term use of 1 g pulses. *In vitro* studies indicate, however, that methylprednisolone pulses fail to reduce bacterial phagocytosis or killing by human neutrophils (Webel et al, 1974).

Other reported complications include transient arthralgias and synovitis, hyperglycaemia, pancreatitis, gastrointestinal bleeding, visual disturbance and acute psychosis (Bailey and Armour, 1974; Newmark et al, 1974; Bennett and Strong, 1975; Fan et al, 1978). Reports of complications occurring in patients enrolled in recent trials of pulse therapy suggest the overall safety of this mode of treatment in rheumatoid arthritis. It must be said, however, that there is little underlying rationale for such therapy, and it should be regarded at present as experimental, with further controlled studies required.

LOCAL CORTICOSTEROID INJECTION THERAPY

Since their introduction in 1950, the value of intra-articular and local soft-tissue corticosteroid injections in the suppression of inflammatory symptoms has been confirmed in numerous studies (Gray et al, 1981). Numerous long-acting steroid ester preparations have been developed to enhance anti-inflammatory activity and reduce hormal side-effects. Although inconclusive, present evidence suggests that the triamcinolone preparations are most potent. Duration of action is probably related to insolubility and therefore, prolonged retention at the site of injection. That these agents exert a marked systemic effect is shown by joint improvement at distant sites from the injection and by suppression of the hypothalamic–pituitary–adrenal axis (Ward and Mason, 1953; Kochler et al, 1974). The major adverse consequences of steroid injections are listed in Table 3, and discussed in greater detail below.

Table 3. Adverse effects of local corticosteroid injection.

1. Infectious arthritis

2. Tendon rupture

3. Destructive arthritis

4. Postinjection synovitis

5. Cutaneous atrophy

6. Cartilage damage

Infectious arthritis

Infectious arthritis is a potentially serious, but extremely rare, complication of intra-articular steroid injection. No infectious complications were recorded in a review of practice in the Department of Orthopaedic Surgery at the Mayo Clinic in 1976 (Fitzgerald, 1976). Hollander (1969), auditing complications in the Arthritis Center of the Unversity of Pennsylvania, found 14 infected joints in 4000 patients who received a total of more than

100 000 injections. This was an incidence of less than one infection every 7000 injections. The experience of the Arthritis Division at the University of Miami has been even more encouraging, with 2 cases of septic arthritis in nearly 100 000 intra-articular injections (Gray et al, 1981).

The importance of rigorous aseptic and atraumatic technique in performing steroid injections, however, cannot be overemphasized. The usual organism isolated is *Staphylococcus aureus* rather than skin commensals, suggesting that bacteria are not directly introduced into the joint cavity (Gowans and Graniere, 1959). Articular trauma, or the introduction of steroids, may render the joint susceptible to haematogenous spread from distant skin lesions. Gram-negative infections are infrequent, usually occurring in patients with pre-existing urinary tract foci. Septic bursitis has been reported in 2 of 25 patients who had injection treatment of olecranon bursitis (Canoso and Sheckman, 1979). The reason for this unexpectedly high rate of infection is not clear.

Tendon rupture

There are several reports of tendon and ligament rupture following corticosteroid injection (Lee, 1957; Ismail et al, 1967; Sweetnam, 1969; Freiberg and Weinstein, 1972). Most frequently encountered are ruptures of the wrist extensors, supraspinatus, biceps and Achilles tendons. As with infection, this complication of injection therapy is also rare. Gray et al (1978) found no instance of rupture in over 300 injections for rheumatoid flexor tenosynovitis, and McKenzie (1972) noted no significant adverse effects after treatment of de Quervain's tenosynovitis.

Tendon rupture may occur spontaneously or as a result of trauma, and controlled studies of steroid treatment in primates have documented a significant reduction in the tensile strength of the anterior cruciate ligament (Noyes et al, 1977). Attention to injection technique is again important. Forceful injection into the substance of a tendon should always be avoided, and care should be taken in gentle filling of the tendon sheath.

Destructive arthritis

Case reports from two decades ago suggested that repeated intra-articular injections could result in an accelerated, destructive arthropathy, indistinguishable from a Charcot joint (Chandler et al, 1959; Sweetnam et al, 1960; Steinberg et al, 1962; Alarcon-Segovia and Ward, 1966; Bentley and Goodfellow, 1969). Hollander et al (1961) reported such osteonecrosis in around 0.8% of 8000 individuals who received multiple hip and knee injections over many years. Balch et al (1977) found similar changes in 2 of 65 knee joints treated with between 15 and 167 injections over a period of 4–12 years.

Potential mechanisms for this condition include the analgesic effect of steroid injections, a direct biochemical action on cartilage and ischaemic necrosis. In many instances, however, the effects of steroid injections are difficult to disentangle from the natural history of the arthropathies for which those injections were given. The judicious use of steroid injections, with at least a month between injections and a rest period of 24–48 hours afterwards, has probably substantially reduced the incidence of this complication.

Postinjection synovitis

An acute, self-limiting synovitis occurs in up to 10% of joints injected with steroid (Hollander et al, 1961; McCarty and Hogan, 1964; Keagy and Keim, 1967; Fitzgerald 1976). The frequency of this flare depends upon the dose and preparation of steroid used, and the technique of administration. Symptoms usually develop within a few hours after injection and subside over 24–48 hours. Arthrocentesis is mandatory to exclude infection, and synovial fluid analysis often reveals a leucocytosis greater than 100 000.

The intra-articular microcrystalline steroid preparations have certain properties in common with monosodium urate and calcium pyrophosphate crystals: they are relatively insoluble in water and are ingested by macrophages. Postinjection synovitis, in some cases, may represent a true crystal synovitis, attributable to these crystals (McCarty and Hogan, 1964).

Cutaneous complications

Dermal and subcutaneous atrophy often occur at the site of steroid injections, most probably as a result of leakage along the needle track (Cassidy and Bole, 1966; Steinbrocker and Neustadt, 1972). Such atrophic and pigmentary changes may reverse spontaneously over the course of a few months, or last for several years.

Flushing of the face, neck and trunk, accompanied by headache and malaise, constitute a recognized (though rare) reaction to triamcinolone injections (Gottleib and Riskin, 1980). Although these symptoms are transient, they may be sufficiently severe to warrant a change in the local steroid formulation.

Cartilage destruction

Perhaps the greatest concern over the widespread use of intra-articular corticosteroid injections is about the effect that these agents might have on hyaline cartilage. Evidence of this deleterious effect has come largely from animal models and *in vitro* studies.

The morphology, proliferation and biological functions of fibroblasts grown in tissue culture are profoundly altered by the presence of corticosteroids (Berliner and Nabors, 1967; Harvey et al, 1974; Nacht and Garzon, 1974). Notable among these biological functions is the synthesis of mucopolysaccharide, collagen and DNA. The effects of steroids on these functions are dose-dependent.

Intra-articular steroid injections to young rabbits have shown reductions in radiolabelled sulphur and glycine utilization in the injected joint when compared with the contralateral joint (Mankin and Conger, 1966a, 1966b).

The major effect seems to be that of a reduction in protein synthesis. Articular cartilage in these animals manifests gross as well as microscopic abnormalities, which appear to be irreversible (Salter et al, 1967; Salter and Murray,1969).

Studies in primates and *in vitro* human systems have failed to demonstrate these effects. When one to six intra-articular steroid injections were given into the knee joints of monkeys, similar minor changes (cartilage clefts, decreased chondrocyte number) were found in steroid-treated animals and in non-treated controls (Gibson et al, 1977). In a study of human cartilage explants in culture, hydrocortisone-incubated and control samples showed similar galactosamine, glucosamine and hyaluronic acid contents (Jacoby, 1967).

In summary, the findings from studies in smaller mammals of steroid-induced impairment of cartilage synthesis are not borne out by those in primates. It is likely that the putative adverse consequence of intra-articular steroids is outweighed by their anti-inflammatory properties which might lead to a reduction in joint destruction.

CONCLUSION

Corticosteroids are invaluable therapeutic agents in the management of a number of rheumatic diseases. It is perhaps a matter more of historical setting, rather than objective analysis, that has raised suspicion of these agents among practising clinicians over the last two decades. Of the large number of adverse effects that have been ascribed to corticosteroids, critical appraisal of the evidence suggests that in many instances this is far less conclusive than we would wish. Furthermore, when evidence does point towards an increased risk of a particular adverse effect, the magnitude of this increase is often small, and outweighed by the potential benefits of this group of drugs in diseases often associated with poor long-term outcomes.

Among the most frequently occurring adverse consequences of orally administered steroids are their effects on metabolism, connective tissue (particularly bone, muscle and the eye) and growth in childhood. Suppression of the hypothalamic–pituitary–adrenal axis, susceptibility to infection, gastrointestinal and central nervous system complications are much less of a problem in day-to-day rheumatological practice. The widespread use of pulsed intravenous steroid therapy in the last decade has led to the hypothesis that this route of administration might be attended by a different profile of adverse effects. This must remain speculative until further evidence becomes available. Finally, a large body of evidence suggests that local steroid injections, whether into joints or soft tissues, are safe, provided that sound technique is adopted and joints are not injected too frequently.

Caution should undoubtedly be exercised in the administration of drugs with wide-ranging actions, such as the corticosteroids. Nevertheless, the evidence currently available suggests that when corticosteroids are used judiciously their potential benefits outweigh their adverse effects.

REFERENCES

Aaron H (1968) Adverse ophthalmic effects of corticosteroids. *Medical Letter on Drugs and Therapeutics* **10**: 21–22.

Ackerman G & Nolan C (1968) Adrenal cortical responsiveness after alternate-day corticosteroid therapy. *New England Journal of Medicine* **278**: 405–409.

Adinoff AD & Hollister JR (1983) Steroid induced fractures and bone loss in patients with asthma. *New England Journal of Medicine* **309**: 265–268.

Afifi AK, Berman RA & Harvey MC (1968) Steroid myopathy: clinical, histologic observations. *Johns Hopkins Medical Journal* **123**: 158.

Alarcon-Segovia D & Ward LE (1966) Marked destructive changes occurring in osteoarthritis finger joints after intra-articular injection of corticosteroids. *Arthritis and Rheumatism* **9**: 443–449.

Alavi IA, Sharma BK & Pillary VK (1971) Steroid-induced diabetic ketoacidosis. *American Journal of Medical Science* **262**: 15.

Allebeck P (1982) Increased mortality in rheumatoid arthritis. *Scandinavian Journal of Rheumatology* **11**: 81–86.

Allison F, Smith MR & Wood WB (1955) Studies on the pathogenesis of acute inflammation. II. The action of cortisone on inflammatory response to thermal injury. *Journal of Experimental Medicine* **102**: 669–676.

Als OS, Gotfredsen A & Christiansen C (1983) Relationship between local and total bone mineral in patients with rheumatoid arthritis and normal subjects. *Clinical Rheumatology* **2**: 265–271.

Als OS, Gotfredsen A & Christiansen C (1985) The effect of glucocorticoids on bone mass in rheumatoid arthritis patients. *Arthritis and Rheumatism* **28**: 369–375.

Axelrod L (1976) Glucocorticoid therapy. *Medicine* **55**: 39–65.

Bailey RR & Armour P (1974) Acute arthralgia after high-dose intravenous methylprednisolone (letter). *Lancet* **ii**: 1014.

Balch HW, Gibson JMC, El-Ghobarey AF, Bain LS & Lynch MP (1977) Repeated corticosteroid injections into knee joints. *Rheumatology and Rehabilitation* **16**: 137–140.

Balfour-Lynn L (1986) Growth and childhood asthma. *Archives of Diseases in Childhood* **61**: 1049–1055.

Barnal E (1984) Bilateral sport rupture of Achilles tendon on long-term systemic steroid therapy. *British Journal of Sports Medicine* **18**: 128–129.

Baylink DJ (1983) Glucocorticoid-induced osteoporosis. *New England Journal of Medicine* **309**: 306–308.

Beisel WR & Rapoport MI (1969) Adrenocortical function and infectious illness. *New England Journal of Medicine* **280**: 541–546.

Bennett WM & Strong D (1975) Acute arthralgia after high-dose steroids (letter). *Lancet* **i**: 332.

Bentley G & Goodfellow JW (1969) Disorganisation of the knees following intra-articular hydrocortisone injections. *Journal of Bone and Joint Surgery* **51B**: 498–502.

Beresford JN, Gallagher JA, Poser JW & Russell RGG (1984) Production of osteocalcin by human bone cells in vitro. Effects of $1,25(OH)_2D_3$, parathyroid hormone and glucocorticoids. *Metabolism of Bone Disease and Related Research* **5**: 229–234.

Beresford JN, Gallagher JA & Russell RGG (1986) 1,25-Dihydroxyvitamin D_3 and human bone derived cells in vitro. Effects on alkaline phosphatase, type 1 collagen and proliferation. *Endocrinology* **119**: 1776–1785.

Berliner DL & Nabors CJ (1967) Effects of corticosteroids on fibroblast functions. *Journal of the Reticuloendothelial Society* **4**: 284–313.

Bihari M & Grossman BJ (1968) Posterior subcapsular cataracts. Related to longterm corticosteroid treatment in children. *American Journal of Diseases of Children* **116**: 604–608.

Black R, Oglesby R, von Sallmann L et al (1960) Posterior subcapsular cataracts induced by corticosteroids in patients with rheumatoid arthritis. *Journal of the American Medical Association* **174**: 166–171.

Blerau R & Weingarten C (1964) Diabetic acidosis secondary to steroid therapy. *New England Journal of Medicine* **271**: 836.

Bodman S & Condemi J (1967) Mediastinal widening in iatrogenic Cushing's syndrome. *Annals of Internal Medicine* **67**: 399–403.

Boland EW & Headley NE (1950) Management of rheumatoid arthritis with smaller (maintenance) doses of cortisone acetate. *Journal of the American Medical Association* **144:** 365–372.

Bollet AJ, Black R & Bunim JJ (1955) Major undesirable side-effects resulting from prednisolone and prednisone. *Journal of the American Medical Association* **158:** 459–463.

Bond W (1977) Toxic reactions and the side effects of glucocorticoids in man. *American Journal of Hospital Pharmacy* **34:** 479–485.

Boston Collaborative Drug Surveillance Group (1972) Acute adverse reactions to prednisone in relation to dosage. *Clinical Pharmacology Therapeutics* **13:** 694–698.

Bulkley BH & Roberts WC (1975) The heart in systemic lupus erythematosus and the changes induced in it by corticosteroid therapy. *American Journal of Medicine* **58:** 243–264.

Burde RM & Becker B (1970) Corticosteroid-induced glaucoma and cataracts in contact lens wearers. *Journal of the American Medical Association* **213:** 2075.

Byron MA & Mowat AG (1985) Corticosteroid prescribing in rheumatoid arthritis—the fiction and the fact. *British Journal of Rheumatology* **24:** 164–166.

Byyny R (1976) Withdrawal from corticosteroid therapy. *New England Journal of Medicine* **295:** 30–32.

Canoso JJ & Sheckman PR (1979) Septic subcutaneous bursitis: report of sixteen cases. *Journal of Rheumatology* **6:** 96–102.

Carone F & Liebon A (1957) Acute pancreatic lesion in patients treated with ACTH and adrenal corticoids. *New England Journal of Medicine* **257:** 690–697.

Carpenter W & Bunney W (1971) Behavioural effects of cortisol in man. *Seminars in Psychology* **3:** 421–434.

Cassidy JT & Bole GG (1966) Cutaneous atrophy secondary to intra-articular corticosteroid administration. *Annals of Internal Medicine* **65:** 1008–1018.

Chai H, Weltman D, Spaulding H et al (1975) Posterior polar cataracts and steroid therapy in children. *Journal of Allergy and Clinical Immunology* **55:** 123–127.

Chandler GN, Jones DT, Wright V & Hartfall SJ (1959) Charcot's arthropathy following intra-articular hydrocortisone. *British Medical Journal* **1:** 952–953.

Chesney RW, Mazess RB, Hamstra AJ, DeLuca HF & O'Reagan S (1978) Reduction of serum 1,25-dihydroxyvitamin D, in children receiving glucocorticoids. *Lancet* **ii:** 1123–1125.

Chyun YS & Raisz LG (1982) Opposing effects of prostaglandin E2 and cortisol on bone growth in organ culture. *Clinical Research* **30:** 387A.

Claman HN (1972) Corticosteroids and lymphoid cells. *New England Journal of Medicine* **287:** 388–397.

Claman HN (1983) Glucocorticosteroids. II The clinical responses. *Hospital Practice* **18:** 143–146.

Clarke AG & Salaman JR (1974) Methylprednisolone in the treatment of renal transplant rejection. *Clinical Nephrology* **2:** 230–234.

Cohen B, Som P, Haffner P et al (1981) Steroid exophthalmos. *Journal of Computer Assisted Tomography* **6:** 907–908.

Conklin J, Alderson P & Thomas M (1983) Comparison of bone scan and radiograph sensitivity in detection of steroid-induced ischaemic necrosis of bone. *Radiology* **147:** 221–226.

Conn HO & Blitzer BL (1976) Nonassociation of adrenocorticosteroid therapy and peptic ulcer. *New England Journal of Medicine* **294:** 473–479.

Conn HO & Poynard T (1985) Adrenocorticosteroid administration and peptic ulcer: a critical analsyis. *Journal of Chronic Disease* **38:** 457–468.

Cooper C, Barker DJP & Wickham C (1988a) Physical activity, muscle strength and calcium intake in fracture of the proximal femur in Britain. *British Medical Journal* **297:** 1443–1446.

Cooper C, Poll V, Mclaren M, Daunt SO'N & Cawley MID (1988b) Alterations in appendicular skeletal mass in patients with rheumatoid, psoriatic and osteo arthropathy. *Annals of the Rheumatic Diseases* **47:** 481–484.

Crews SJ (1965) Adverse reactions to corticosteroid therapy in the eye. *Proceedings of the Royal Society of Medicine* **58:** 533.

Curtess PH, Clark WS & Herndon CH (1954) Vertebral fractures resulting from prolonged cortisone and corticotrophin therapy. *Journal of the American Medical Association* **156:** 467–479.

Cushing H (1932) The basophil adenomas of the pituitary and their clinical manifestations. *Bulletin of Johns Hopkins Hospital* **50:** 137–195.

Cushman P (1970) Glucocorticoids and the gastrointestinal tract. Current status. *Gut* **11:** 534.

David D & Berkowitz J (1969) Ocular effects of topical and systemic corticosteroids. *Lancet* **i:** 149–151.

David D, Grieco M & Cushman P (1970) Adrenal corticosteroids after 20 years. *Journal of Chronic Disease* **22:** 637–711.

Dayton MT, Kleckner SC & Brown DK (1987) Peptic ulcer perforation associated with steroid use. *Archives of Surgery* **122:** 376–380.

Dixon R & Christy N (1980) On the various forms of corticosteroid withdrawal syndrome. *American Journal of Medicine* **68:** 224–230.

Dujovne CA & Azarnoff DL (1975) Clinical complications of corticosteroid therapy: a selected review. In Azarnoff DL (ed.) *Steroid Therapy*, pp 27–41. London: WB Saunders.

Duncan H (1972) Osteoporosis in rheumatoid arthritis and corticosteroid induced osteoporosis. *Orthopedic Clinics of North America* **3:** 571–583.

Elliot FE (1987) Adverse effects of corticosteroid therapy (editorial). *Journal of Allergy and Clinical Immunology* **80:** 515–517.

Fan PT, Yu DTY, Clemens PJ, Fowlston S, Eisman J & Bluestone R (1978) Effect of corticosteroids on the human immune response; comparison of one and three daily 1 g intravenous pulses of methylprednisolone. *Journal of Laboratory and Clinical Medicine* **91:** 625–634.

Fauci AS, Dale DC & Balow JE (1976) Glucocorticosteroid therapy: mechanisms of action and clinical considerations. *Annals of Internal Medicine* **84:** 304–315.

Felson DT & Anderson JJ (1987) Across-study evaluation of association between steroid dose and bolus steroids and avascular necrosis of bone. *Lancet* **i:** 902–905.

Fitzgerald RH (1976) Intrasynovial injection of steroids: uses and abuses. *Mayo Clinic Proceedings* **51:** 655–659.

Forster PJG, Grindulis KA, Neumann V, Hubbell S & McConkey B (1982) High dose intravenous methyl prednisolone in rheumatoid arthritis. *Annals of the Rheumatic Diseases* **41:** 444–446.

Freiberg RA & Weinstein A (1972) The scallop sign and spontaneous rupture of finger extensor tendons in rheumatoid arthritis. *Clinical Orthopaedics* **83:** 128–130.

Freiberger RH, Kammerer WH & Rivelis AL (1958) Peptic ulcers in rheumatoid patients receiving corticosteroid therapy. *Radiology* **71:** 542–547.

Fritz K & Weston W (1984) Systemic glucocorticoid therapy of skin disease in children. *Pediatric Dermatology* **1:** 236–245.

Furst C, Smiley W & Ansell B (1966) Steroid cataract. *Annals of the Rheumatic Diseases* **25:** 364–367.

Gallant C & Kenny P (1986) Oral glucocorticoids and their complications. *Journal of the American Academy of Dermatology* **14:** 161–177.

Gedda PO & Moritz U (1958) Peptic ulcer during treatment of rheumatoid arthritis with cortisone derivatives. *Acta Rheumatologica Scandinavica* **4:** 249–256.

Gennari C & Imbimbo B (1985) Effects of prednisone and deflazacort on vertebral bone mass. *Calcified Tissue International* **37:** 592–593.

Gibson T, Burry HC, Poswillo D & Glas J (1977) Effect of intra-articular corticosteroid injections on primate cartilage. *Annals of the Rheumatic Diseases* **36:** 74–79.

Glaser GH (1953) Psychotic reactions induced by corticotropin (ACTH) and cortisone. *Psychosomatic Medicine* **15:** 280.

Glenn F & Grafe W (1967) Surgical complications of adrenal steroid therapy. *Annals of Surgery* **165:** 1023–1032.

Godfrey S, Balfour-Lynn L & Tooley M (1978) A three- to five-year follow up of the use of the aerosol steroid beclomethasone dipropionate in childhood asthma. *Journal of Allergy and Clinical Immunology* **62:** 335–339.

Goggans F, Weisberg L & Koran L (1983) Lithium prophylaxis of prednisone psychosis: a case report. *Journal of Clinical Psychiatry* **44:** 111–112.

Golding DN & Begg TB (1960) Dexamethasone myopathy. *British Medical Journal* **2:** 1129.

Gottlieb N (1980) Temporal fat pad sign during corticosteroid treatments. *Archives of Internal Medicine* **140:** 1507–1508.

Gottlieb NL & Riskin WG (1980) Complications associated with locally injected microcrystalline corticosteroid esters. *Journal of the American Medical Association* **243:** 1547–1548.

Gowans JDC & Graniere PA (1959) Septic arthritis: its relation to intra-articular injections of hydrocortisone acetate. *New England Journal of Medicine* **261:** 502–503.

Gray RG, Kiem IS & Gottlieb NL (1978) Intratendon sheath corticosteroid treatment of rheumatoid arthritis-associated and idiopathic hand flexor tenosynovitis. *Arthritis and Rheumatism* **21:** 92–96.

Gray RG, Tenenbaum J & Gottlieb NL (1981) Local corticosteroid injection treatment in rheumatic disorders. *Seminars in Arthritis and Rheumatism* **10:** 231–254.

Grieco MH (1984) The role of corticosteroid therapy in infection. *Hospital Practice* **18:** 131–143.

Haanaes QC & Bergman A (1983) Tuberculosis in patients treated with corticosteroids. *European Journal of Respiratory Diseases* **64:** 294–297.

Hahn RJ (1978) Corticosteroid-induced osteoporosis. *Archives of Internal Medicine* **138:** 882–885.

Hahn TJ, Halstead LR & Baron DT (1981) Effects of short term glucocorticoid administration on intestinal calcium absorption and circulating vitamin D metabolite concentrations in man. *Journal of Clinical Endocrinology and Metabolism* **52:** 111–115.

Hall R, Popkin M, Stickney S et al (1979) Presentation of the steroid psychosis. *Journal of Nervous and Mental Diseases* **167:** 229–236.

Harvey W, Grahame R & Panayi GS (1974) Effects of steroid hormones on human fibroblasts *in vitro*. *Annals of the Rheumatic Diseases* **33:** 437–441.

Hench PS (1952) The reversibility of certain rheumatic and non-rheumatic conditions by the use of cortisone or of the pituitary adrenocorticotropic hormone. *Annals of Internal Medicine* **36:** 1–38.

Hirsh JG & Church AB (1961) Adrenal steroids and infection: the effect of cortisone administration on polymorphonuclear leukocyte functions and on serum opsonins and bactericidins. *Journal of Clinical Investigation* **40:** 794–798.

Hollander JL (1969) Intrasynovial corticosteroid therapy in arthritis. *Maryland State Medical Journal* **19:** 62–66.

Hollander JL, Jessar RA & Brown RR (1961) Intra-synovial corticosteroid therapy: a decade of use. *Bulletin on the Rheumatic Diseases* **11:** 239–240.

Hooyman JR, Melton LJ, Nelson AM, O'Fallon WM & Riggs BL (1984) Fractures after rheumatoid arthritis. A population-based study. *Arthritis and Rheumatology* **27:** 1353–1361.

Horber FF, Hoppeler H & Herren D (1986) Altered skeletal muscle ultrastructure in renal transplant patients on prednisone. *Kidney International* **30:** 411–416.

Hunt R, Ehrlich P, Garcia J et al (1969) Effects of vitamin A on reversing the inhibitory effect of cortisone on healing of open wounds in animals and man. *Annals of Surgery* **170:** 633–640.

Ismail AM, Balakrishman R & Rajakumar MK (1967) Rupture of patellar ligament after steroid infiltration: report of a case. *Journal of Bone and Joint Surgery* **51B:** 503–505.

Jacoby RK (1976) The effect of hydrocortisone acetate on adult human articular cartilage. *Rheumatology* **3:** 384–389.

Jee WSS, Park HZ, Roberts WE & Kenner GH (1970) Corticosteroid and bone. *American Journal of Anatomy* **129:** 477–481.

Judge T (1960) Scorbutic arthritis complicating triamcinolone therapy. *British Medical Journal* **1:** 329.

Kalbak K (1972) Incidence of arteriosclerosis in patients with rheumatoid arthritis receiving long-term corticosteroid therapy. *Annals of the Rheumatic Diseases* **31:** 196–200.

Kaplan MH, Armstrong D & Rosen P (1974) Tuberculosis complicating neoplastic disease. *Cancer* **33:** 850–855.

Kass EH & Finland M (1958) Corticosteroids and infectious diseases. *Advances in Internal Medicine* **9:** 45–80.

Keagy RD & Keim HA (1967) Intra-articular steroid therapy: repeated use in patients with chronic arthritis. *American Journal of Medical Science* **253:** 45–51.

Kern F, Clark GM & Lukens JG (1957) Peptic ulceration occurring during therapy for rheumatoid arthritis. *Gastroenterology* **33:** 25–33.

Klein RG, Arnaud SB, Gallagher JC, DeLuca HF & Riggs BL (1977) Intestinal calcium absorption in exogenous hypercortisonism. *Journal of Clinical Investigation* **6:** 253–259.

Klinefelter, H, Winkerwerden W & Bledsoe T (1979) Single daily dose prednisone therapy. *Journal of the American Medical Association* **241:** 2721–2723.

Kochler BE, Urowitz M & Killinger DW (1974) The systemic effects of intra-articular corticosteroid. *Journal of Rheumatology* **1:** 117–125.

Landon J, Snitcher E & Rees L (1976) The use and interpretation of tests for steroid-impaired hypothalamic–pituitary–adrenal cortical function. *British Journal of Dermatology* **94:** 61–65.

Lee HB (1957) Avulsion and rupture of the tendo-calcaneus after injection of hydrocortisone. *British Medical Journal* **2:** 395.

Leiberman P, Patterson RP & Kunski R (1972) Complication of long-term steroid therapy for asthma. *Journal of Allergy and Clinical Immunology* **49:** 329–336.

Liebling MR, Leib E, McLaughlin K et al (1981) Pulse methylprednisolone in rheumatoid arthritis. *Annals of Internal Medicine* **94:** 21–26.

Loeb J (1976) Corticosteroids and growth. *New England Journal of Medicine* **295:** 547–552.

Lorenzen I & Hansen LJ (1967) Effect of glucocorticoids on human vascular connective tissue. *Vascular Disease* **4:** 335–341.

Lubin RI, Misbach WD, Zemke, EM et al (1951) Acute perforation of duodenal ulcer during ACTH and cortisone therapy. *Gastroenterology* **18:** 308–312.

Lucky A (1984) Principles of the use of glucocorticoids in a growing child. *Pediatric Dermatology* **1:** 226–235.

Luengo M, Picado C, Guanbens N, Del Rio L, Brancos MA & Montserrat JM (1987) Bone loss in chronic corticodependent asthma. In Christiansen C, Johansen JS, Riis BJ (eds) *Osteoporosis*, pp 1068–1069. Copenhagen: Osteopress.

Lukert BP & Raisz LG (1990) Glucocorticoid-induced osteoporosis: pathogenesis and management. *Annals of Internal Medicine* **112:** 352–364.

Lund B, Storm TL et al (1985) Bone mineral loss, bone histomorphometry and vitamin D metabolism in patients with rheumatoid arthritis on long-term glucocorticoid treatment. *Clinical Rheumatology* **4:** 143–149.

MacGregor RR, Spagnuolo PJ & Lentnek AL (1974) Inhibition of granulocyte adherence to ethanol, prednisone and aspirin, measured with an assay system. *New England Journal of Medicine* **291:** 642–646.

Mankin HJ & Conger KA (1966a) The acute effects of intra-articular hydrocortisone on articular cartilage in rabbits. *Journal of Bone and Joint Surgery* **48A:** 1383–1388.

Mankin HJ & Conger KA (1966b) The effect of cortisol on articular cartilage of rabbits. 1. Effect of a single dose of cortisol on glycine-C^{14} incorporation. *Laboratory Investigation* **15:** 794–800.

McCarty DJ & Hogan JM (1964) Inflammatory reaction after intrasynovial injection of microcrystalline adrenocorticosteroid esters. *Arthritis and Rheumatism* **7:** 359–367.

McConkey B, Fraser GM & Bligh AS (1962) Osteoporosis and purpura in rheumatoid disease: prevalence and relation to treatment with corticosteroids. *Quarterly Journal of Medicine* **31:** 419.

McKenzie MM (1972) Conservative treatment of de Quervain's disease. *British Medical Journal* **4:** 659–660.

Messer J, Reitman D, Sacks HS, Smith H & Chalmers TC (1983) Association of adrenocorticosteroid therapy and peptic ulcer disease. *New England Journal of Medicine* **309:** 21–24.

Million R, Kellgren JH, Poole P & Jason MIV (1984) Long-term study of management of rheumatoid arthritis. *Lancet* **i:** 812–816.

Murray AB, Fraser B, Hardwick DF & Pirie G (1976) Chronic asthma and growth failure in children. *Lancet* **ii:** 197.

Muusche MM, Ringoir SMG & Lameire NN (1976) High intravenous doses of methylprednisolone for acute renal rejection. *Nephrology* **16:** 287–291.

Nacht S & Garzon P (1974) Effects of corticosteroids on connective tissue and fibroblasts. *Advances in Steroid Biochemistry and Pharmacology* **4:** 157–187.

Nashel DJ (1986) Is atherosclerosis a complication of longterm corticosteroid treatment? *American Journal of Medicine* **80:** 925–929.

Neumann V, Hopkins R, Dixon J, Watkins A, Bird H & Wright V (1985) Combination therapy with pulsed methylprednisolone in rheumatoid arthritis. *Annals of the Rheumatic Diseases* **44:** 747–751.

Newmark KJ, Mitra S & Berman LB (1974) Acute arthralgia following high-dose intravenous methylprednisolone therapy (letter). *Lancet* **i:** 229.

Noyes FR, Grood ES, Nussbaum NL & Cooper SM (1977) Effect of intra-articular corti-costeroids on ligament properties: a biomechanical and histologic study in rhesus knees. *Clinical Orthopaedics* **123**: 197–209.

Olefsky J & Kimmerling G (1976) Effects of glucocorticoids on carbohydrate metabolism. *American Journal of Medical Science* **271**: 202–210.

Oppenheimer EH & Boitnott JK (1960) Pancreatitis in children following adrenal cortico-steroid therapy. *Johns Hopkins Medical Journal* **107**: 297.

Paganini-Hill A, Ross RK, Gerkins VR & Henderson BE (1981) Menopausal estrogen therapy and hip fractures. *Annals of Internal Medicine* **95**: 28–31.

Peck WA (1984) The effects of glucocorticoids on bone cell metabolism and function. *Advances in Experimental Medicine and Biology* **171**: 111–119.

Pincus T, Callahan LF, Sale WG, Brooks AL, Payne LE & Vaughn WK (1984) Severe functional declines, work disability, and increased mortality in seventy-five rheumatoid arthritis patients studied over nine years. *Arthritis and Rheumatism* **27**: 868–872.

Prior P, Symmons DPM, Scott DL, Brown R & Hawkins CF (1984) Cause of death in rheumatoid arthritis. *British Journal of Rheumatology* **23**: 92–99.

Radia M & Furst DE (1988) Comparison of three pulse methyl prednisolone regimens in the treatment of rheumatoid arthritis. *Journal of Rheumatology* **15**: 242–246.

Rasker JJ & Cosh JA (1981) Cause and age at death in a prospective study of 100 patients with rheumatoid arthritis. *Annals of the Rheumatic Diseases* **40**: 115–120.

Rees RB (1981) Oral vs parenteral corticosteroids: a clinical controversy. *Journal of the American Academy of Dermatology* **5**: 602–604.

Reid DM (1990a). In Francis RM (ed.) *Osteoporosis: Pathogenesis and Management*, pp 103–144. London: Kluwer.

Reid DM (1990b) Corticosteroid-induced osteoporosis. In Smith R (ed.) *Osteoporosis 1990*, pp 99–117. London: Royal College of Physicians.

Reid DM, Kennedy NSJ, Smith MA, Tothill P & Nuki G (1982) Total body calcium in rheumatoid arthritis: effects of disease activity and corticosteroid treatment. *British Medical Journal* **285**: 330–332.

Reid DM, Nicoll J, Kennedy NSJ et al (1984) Bone mass in rheumatoid arthritis, polymyalgia rheumatica and asthma: disease determines susceptibility to corticosteroid induced osteoporosis. In Christiansen C, Arnaud CD, Nordin BEC, Parfitt AM, Peck WA & Riggs BL (eds) *Osteoporosis*, pp 217–218. Copenhagen: Department of Clinical Chemistry, Glostrup Hospital.

Reid DM, Kennedy NSJ, Smith MA et al (1986) Bone loss in rheumatoid arthritis and primary generalised osteoarthrosis: effects of corticosteroids, suppressive antirheumatic drugs and calcium supplements. *British Journal of Rheumatology* **25**: 253–259.

Reid IR, King AR, Alexander CJ & Ibbertson HK (1988) Prevention of steroid-induced osteoporosis with (3-amino-1-hydroxypropylidene)-1,1-biphosphonate (APD). *Lancet* **i**: 143–147.

Reimer LG, Morris HG & Ellis EF (1975) Growth of asthmatic children during treatment with alternate-day steroids. *Journal of Allergy and Clinical Immunology* **55**: 224–231.

Richards J, Santingo S & Klaustermeyer W (1980) Aseptic necrosis of the femoral head in corticosteroid treatment pulmonary disease. *Archives of Internal Medicine* **140**: 1473–1475.

Riemenschneider JA, Wilson JR & Vernier RL (1968) Glucocorticoid-induced pancreatitis in children. *Pediatrics* **41**: 428.

Rimza M (1978) Complications of corticosteroid therapy. *American Journal of Diseases of Children* **132**: 806–810.

Rinehart JJ, Sagone AL, Balcerzak SP et al (1975) Effects of corticosteroid therapy on human monocyte function. *New England Journal of Medicine* **292**: 236–241.

Ritchie EA (1956) Toxic psychosis under cortisone and corticotropin. *Journal of Mental Science* **102**: 830.

Rodan GA & Martin TJ (1981) Role of osteoblasts in hormonal control of bone resorption—a hypothesis. *Calcified Tissue International* **33**: 349–351.

Rooklin A, Lampert S & Jaeger E (1978) Posterior subcapsular cataracts in steroid-requiring asthmatic children. *Journal of Allergy and Clinical Immunology* **63**: 383–386.

Rosenberg EF (1958) Rheumatoid arthritis. Osteoporosis and fractures related to steroid therapy. *Acta Medica Scandinavica* **341**: 211–224.

Rosenblum AA & Rosenblum P (1964) Anaphylactic reactions in adrenocorticotropin hormone in children. *Journal of Pediatrics* **64**: 387.

Rosenfeld S, Marmorston J, Sobel H & White AE (1960) Enhancement of experimental atherosclerosis by ACTH in the dog. *Proceedings of the Society of Experimental Biology and Medicine* **103**: 83–86.

Salassa R, Bennett W, Keating F et al (1953) Post-operative adrenal cortical insufficiency. *Journal of the American Medical Association* **152**: 1509–1515.

Salter RB & Murray O (1969) Effects of hydrocortisone on musculoskeletal tissues. *Journal of Bone and Joint Surgery* **51B**: 195.

Salter RB, Gross A & Hamilton-Hall J (1967) Hydrocortisone arthropathy: an experimental investigation. *Canadian Medical Association Journal* **97**: 374–377.

Schaadt O & Bohr H (1984) Bone mineral in lumbar spine, femoral neck and femoral shaft measured by dual photon absorptiometry with 153-gadolinium in prednisone treatment. *Advances in Experimental Medicine and Biology* **171**: 201–208.

Schatz M, Patterson R, Kloner R et al (1976) The prevalence of tuberculosis and positive tuberculin skin tests in a steroid-treated asthmatic population. *Annals of Internal Medicine* **84**: 261–265.

Shiono H, Ooonishi M, Yamaguchi M et al (1977) Posterior subcapsular cataracts associated with long-term oral corticosteroid therapy. *Clinical Pediatrics* (Philadelphia) **16**: 726–728.

Shohat M, Shohat T, Kedem R, Mimouni M & Danon YI (1987) Childhood asthma and growth outcome. *Archives of Diseases in Childhood* **62**: 63–65.

Shubin H (1965) Long-term administration of corticosteroids in pulmonary disease. *Diseases of the Chest* **48**: 287–290.

Smyllie HC & Connolly CK (1968) Incidence of serious complications of corticosteroid therapy in respiratory disease: a retrospective survey of patients in the Brompton Hospital. *Thorax* **23**: 571–581.

Smyth GA (1951) Activation of peptic ulcer during pituitary adrenocorticotropic hormone therapy: report of three cases. *Journal of the American Medical Association* **145**: 474–477.

Staples P, Gerding D, Decker J et al (1974) Incidence of infection in systemic lupus erythematosus. *Arthritis and Rheumatism* **17**: 1–10.

Steinberg CLR, Duthie RD & Piva AE (1962) Charcot-like arthropathy following intra-articular hydrocortisone. *Journal of the American Medical Association* **181**: 851–854.

Steinbrocker O & Neustadt DH (1972) *Aspiration and Injection Therapy in Arthritis and Musculoskeletal Disorders*, p 20. New York: Harper & Row.

Sterioff S, Oringer MB & Cameron JL (1974) Colon perforation associated with steroid therapy. *Surgery* **75**: 56.

Storrs FJ (1979) Use and abuse of systemic corticosteroid therapy. *Journal of the American Academy of Dermatology* **1**: 95–105.

Stubbs SS & Morrell RM (1973) Intravenous methylprednisolone sodium succinate; adverse reactions reported in association with immunosuppressive therapy. *Transplantation Proceedings* **5**: 1145–1146.

Stumpf HH, Wilens SL & Somoza C (1956) Pancreatic lesions and peripancreatic fat necrosis in cortisone-treated rabbits. *Laboratory Investigation* **5**: 224.

Sutton RD, Benedeck TG & Edwards GA (1963) Aseptic bone necrosis and corticosteroid therapy. *Archives of Internal Medicine* **112**: 594.

Sweetnam DR (1969) Corticosteroid arthropathy and tendon rupture. *Journal of Bone and Joint Surgery* **51B**: 397–398.

Sweetnam DR, Mason RM & Murray RO (1960) Steroid arthropathy of the hip. *British Medical Journal* **1**: 1392–1394.

Vandenbroucke JP, Hazxevoet HM & Cats A (1984) Survival and cause of death in rheumatoid arthritis: a 25-year prospective follow-up. *Journal of Rheumatology* **11**:158–161.

Verstraeten A & Dequeker J (1986) Vertebral and peripheral bone mineral content in post menopausal patients with rheumatoid arthritis: effect of low dose corticosteroids. *Annals of the Rheumatic Diseases* **45**: 852–857.

Virkkunen M & Lehtinen L (1958) Side effects of corticosteroids. Observations after five years continuous use. *Acta Medica Scandinavica* **341**: 205–210.

Ward LE & Mason HL (1953) Systemic effects from hydrocortisone acetate administered intra-articularly to rheumatoid patients. *Journal of Laboratory and Clinical Medicine* **42**: 961–962.

Webel ML, Ritts RE, Taswell HR, Donadio JV & Woods JE (1974) Cellular immunity after intravenous administration of methylprednisolone. *Journal of Laboratory and Clinical Medicine* **83:** 383–392.

Weisberg L & Chutorian A (1977) Pseudotumor cerebri in congenital adrenal hyperplasis. *American Journal of Diseases of Children* **113:** 1243–1248.

Weiss MM (1989) Corticosteroids in rheumatoid arthritis. *Seminars in Arthritis and Rheumatism* **19:** 9–21.

9

Fibromyalgia—which is the best treatment? A personalized, comprehensive, ambulatory, patient-involved management programme

ALFONSE T. MASI
MUHAMMAD B. YUNUS

A basic tenet of medicine is that proper management and care of a patient requires knowledge of what condition is being treated, some understanding or concept of its pathogenesis and a personalized approach to the particular problems or concerns. An integrative perspective of fibromyalgia management is presented here; this approach incorporates considerations of disordered physiological, psychological and social dynamics, which should be addressed cooperatively by patients and care-givers. Further research is required to determine which of the proposed comprehensive approaches might be more effectively utilized with particular patients (or subsets of patients) suffering from this common malady.

WHAT IS FIBROMYALGIA?

Fibromyalgia (L. *fibra*, fibre; Gr. *mys*, muscle, Gr. *algos*, pain + *ia*, condition) literally means a painful condition of fibromuscular tissues. It may be one of man's oldest chronic, painful conditions, as indicated in the Old Testament description of Job suffering deep pain, disturbed sleep and exhaustion (Smythe, 1989a), during the period of his repeated personal calamities. Of note, Job's trials ended at last; his faith was rewarded and sufferings ended.

The term 'muscular rheumatism' was often used in the European literature, since at least the seventeenth century (Reynolds, 1983). Sir William Gowers (1904) introduced the term 'fibrositis' to describe muscular rheumatism of the back. However, the latter term is a misnomer (Bennett, 1981), since it implies inflammation, which is absent in this condition (Bengtsson and Henriksson, 1989; Yunus and Kalyan-Raman, 1989). Also, it does not designate the important 'myalgia' component, which seems to be the most likely cause of musculoskeletal pain in fibromyalgia (Bennett, 1989a). Since the aetiology and pathogenesis are unknown, the term 'fibromyalgia syndrome' (FMS) is often used (Yunus, 1983).

Nosologically, this entity is a form of non-articular rheumatism. It is

Baillière's Clinical Rheumatology—
Vol. 4, No. 2, August 1990
ISBN 0–7020–1480–X

A. T. MASI & M. B. YUNUS

classified by the American College of Rheumatology (ACR), previously the American Rheumatism Association (ARA), as a generalized myofascial pain syndrome (Schumacher, 1988). Fibromyalgia is also defined as a chronic pain syndrome according to the International Association for the Study of Pain Subcommittee on Taxonomy (1986).

Clinically, fibromyalgia is characterized by chronic, mainly symmetrical, widespread, 'deep', musculoskeletal aching pain and stiffness as well as various systemic manifestations, e.g. poor sleep, fatigue and a variety of functional disorders, plus characteristic, localized soft tissue *tender points* (Bennett, 1989a; Smythe, 1989b; Wolfe, 1989; Yunus et al, 1989a). Symptoms are usually aggravated by cold and damp, poor sleep and many other physical and psychological factors, as indicated below.

FIBROMYALGIA SYNDROME OR MYOFASCIAL PAIN SYNDROME?

For classification purposes, fibromyalgia syndrome (FMS) should be differentiated from the host of localized or regional forms of myofascial pain syndrome (MPS), affecting one or a few areas (Sola, 1981; Travell and Simons, 1983; Simons, 1986; Campbell, 1989; Smythe and Sheon, 1990).

Is MPS a *forme fruste* of FMS?

The relationship of regional MPS to FMS is unclear (Simons, 1986; Campbell, 1989; Smythe and Sheon, 1990), but a small proportion of generalized FMS patients have a localized onset, similar to MPS, which then becomes widespread. Asymmetric, localized manifestations are typical of MPS, especially when initiated by injury or strain mechanisms. In MPS, local mechanical factors are predominant, whereas in FMS the centrally acting modulating factors are very important (Smythe and Sheon, 1990).

Methods used to treat MPS effectively may be applied to relieve certain localized, disabling musculoskeletal manifestations of FMS (see below). However, the management of FMS is not primarily addressed in this fashion. Rather, it requires a more comprehensive, ongoing, rehabilitation-oriented management programme than is typically needed in MPS.

Trigger points versus tender points

A characteristic feature of regional MPS is the *trigger point*. It is a distinctly localized area of tenderness to firm, fingertip palpation, like the tender point of FMS. Both may occur in reportedly palpable, taut muscle bands. However, the trigger point also refers pain to a separate and distant reference zone or target area of the body (like a trigger which shoots a bullet to a distant target), and usually restricts range of motion (Sola, 1981; Simons, 1986).

Many trigger points are located in areas in which acupuncture points are also found (Melzack et al, 1977; Melzack, 1981). Myofascial trigger points may be caused by localized muscle injury, e.g. strain, overuse, chilling of a fatigued muscle, dyskinesia, dystonia or by referred nerve root injury. As in FMS, host factors may be predisposing, e.g. general fatigue, muscular deconditioning and psychological stress. Following the muscle injury, protracted pain may sustain itself, in spite of control or elimination of the initiating stimuli; this is believed to be caused by a continuing, reflex pain cycle which may even recruit additional trigger points (Sola, 1981). Such trigger points, therefore, may be considered to be playing a primary role in MPS. Their elimination usually results in interruption of this cycle, and dramatic relief of the localized and referred pain (Sola, 1981). However, in FMS, the many tender points found are considered to be playing a secondary or 'sentinel' role, i.e. reflecting a more general chronic pain state, rather than being the primary factor. Unless such tender points in FMS are unusually severe or disabling, i.e. significantly restricting motion, their elimination rarely results in more than mildly or moderately beneficial response, analogous to secondary trigger points found in MPS (Sola, 1981).

CLASSIFICATION OF FIBROMYALGIA SYNDROMES

Symptomatic and musculoskeletal findings in primary, concomitant and secondary forms of fibromyalgia are similar (Yunus et al, 1988; Wolfe et al, 1990). Nevertheless, for purposes of clinical diagnosis and therapy, fibromyalgia syndromes should be appropriately classified (Yunus, 1983, 1988; Smythe and Sheon, 1990).

1. *Primary fibromyalgia syndrome* occurs in the absence of an associated or underlying rheumatologic or other significant condition.
2. *Concomitant or associated fibromyalgia* occurs with another significant condition, e.g. osteoarthritis, which, however, cannot explain the overall fibromyalgia manifestations.
3. *Secondary fibromyalgia* occurs in the presence of an underlying condition, e.g. rheumatoid arthritis, polymyalgia rheumatica, systemic lupus erythematosus, hypothyroidism or Lyme disease (Hench, 1989; Sigal, 1990), which presumably is the cause of the fibromyalgia, the symptoms of which may often remit significantly when the primary disorder is treated (Smythe and Sheon, 1990).

This discussion focuses on primary fibromyalgia syndrome (PFS) or simply 'fibromyalgia'. It does not address specific problems of associated or secondary fibromyalgia; these conditions should be managed with measures directed at the fibromyalgia aspects, as outlined below, as well as at the concomitant or underlying disorder. Secondary fibromyalgia should be diagnosed promptly and its underlying (primary) condition treated.

PATHOPHYSIOLOGIC CONCEPTS OF FIBROMYALGIA (A 'DYSFUNCTIONAL SYNDROME') AS RELATED TO MANAGEMENT

Proper management of FMS ultimately depends upon understanding its

Table 1. Simplified framework of pathophysiological theories in fibromyalgia.*

Phenomenological levels	Muscle injury (Bennett, 1989b)	Non-restorative sleep (Moldofsky, 1989a)	Psychophysiological (Blumer & Heilbronn, 1982)
Preconditioners	Enhanced predisposition to muscle microtrauma	Neurohumoral/other contributors to non-restorative sleep disorder	'Masked' depression, unbearable guilt and anguish
Stressors	Too much/too little physical activity	Factors altering sleep physiology, e.g. presence of alpha-delta sleep	Pain-prone personality, 'solid citizen', self-sacrifice, 'ergomania'
Tissue effects	Muscle microtrauma and local sarcomere injury	Increased pain transmission (e.g. substance P)	Central pain perception
Symptoms	Myalgia, sleep disturbance, fatigue	Myalgia, fatigue	Continuous pain, 'anhedonia', misery, insomnia, fatigue
Physical findings	Deconditioned status	Deconditioned status	'Anergia' or 'burned-out', detached, passive
Psychological reactions	Anxiety/fatigue	Heightened sensitivities	Hypochondriacal preoccupations, denial
Behavioural patterns	Inactivity, avoidance	Complaining	Passive-dependent, suffering, invalid role

* Theories are not mutually exclusive nor are mechanisms necessarily unidirectional.

scope and pathogenesis (Bennett, 1989b). It is not a 'disease', in the sense of a specific illness with a definite, recognizable pathophysiological mechanism. Rather, it is a 'dysfunctional syndrome' with a broad spectrum of manifestations (Yunus et al, 1989a), which may involve the musculoskeletal, neuropsychiatric, autonomic and other systems of the body. As such, FMS is a disordered state of being, which deserves remedy. Specific attention should be directed to its chronic, diffuse pain and frequent emotional manifestations, as well as physical or behavioural dysfunctions. Individual patients may present with diverse subjective, psychological and behavioural abnormalities, often related to their psychosocial milieu (Turk and Flor, 1989). Accordingly, patients may be subgrouped and treated more effectively within a 'multiaxial taxonomy' concept, including clinical, psychosocial and behavioural characteristics (Turk and Flor, 1989). As with chronic pain syndromes generally, patients are best managed individually (Reuler et al, 1980).

Multifactorial causation

Consensus, at this time, supports a complex interrelationship among presumed contributory factors (Yunus, 1988; Bennett, 1989a,b; Smythe, 1989b). Nevertheless, one may attempt to view the broad range of phenomena in fibromyalgia within a simplified framework of three popular pathophysiological theories (Blumer and Heilbronn, 1982; Moldofsky, 1989a; Bennett, 1989b), for purposes of developing conceptual models of potential usefulness in management (Table 1). Importantly, these simplified hypotheses are not mutually exclusive, but tend to be synergistic. Accordingly, comprehensive therapy is often indicated in this condition.

Phenomenological levels

The schematic levels (Table 1) could be considered 'hierarchies' of events, if, in fact, the sequences were typically from top to bottom. However, the presumed consequences of the 'tissue effects', e.g. symptoms, physical findings, psychological reactions or behavioural patterns, may 'cycle-back' and influence or amplify the 'higher level' stressors or preconditioning factors, if not the tissue effects themselves. Such 'amplification' mechanisms may lead to greater tissue reactions or may spill over into other hierarchies, thereby activating those pathways. Thus, each of these theories may, in actuality, involve multidirectional and multidimensional mechanisms to some extent. Accordingly, management priorities for the individual patient will vary, depending upon observed features (at the various phenomenologic levels) and the therapist's interpretation of the presumed major pathophysiological mechanisms operating.

Peripheral mechanisms

Peripherally, the origin of the aching pain and stiffness in fibromyalgia seems to be in the muscle or musculotendinous junctions, but the mechanisms, including presumed muscle microtrauma, are unknown (Bennett,

1989b,c). This example is but one type of potential 'biomechanical dys-function' contributing to fibromyalgia. Also, it indicates one possible type of 'somatic' aetiology as opposed to a polar 'psychophysiological' theory (Blumer and Heilbronn, 1982). Microinjury of unfit muscles might be related to biochemical changes in the sarcolemmal membrane, which could be revealed by molecular biology techniques (Bennett, 1989b,c). If such were found, more specific therapy might become available in the future. Other possible derangements of muscle function in FMS must also be considered (e.g. length and tonus controls, spinal myotatic reflex systems, intrafusal spindle receptors and their afferent and gamma motor efferent neuron functions, as well as reciprocal, reflex inhibition of antagonist muscles) in addition to effects of fatigue and CNS modulators (Korr, 1986; Emre and Mathies, 1988; Mau, 1988; Newham, 1988). All of these muscle-related factors need further study in FMS and discoveries may contribute to future management.

Disturbed sleep and neurohumoral mechanisms

The second type of theory emphasizes sleep–wake cycle disturbances, which are prominent in fibromyalgia, whether they result from or mainly contribute to the peripheral manifestations (Moldofsky et al, 1975, 1983; Moldofsky and Lue, 1980; Moldofsky, 1982, 1989a,b). Fibromyalgia patients usually complain of sleep problems, specifically light, non-refreshing sleep associ-ated with the polysomnographic finding of 'alpha-delta' sleep. Endogenous, neurohormonal imbalances may contribute to such altered sleep in fibro-myalgia (Russell, 1989), possibly because of brain serotonin deficiency (Moldofsky, 1982). Pain modulation generally may be altered by biogenic amines (Harvey et al, 1975) or by pain-related neuropeptides, e.g. substance P (Vaerøy et al, 1989).

Psychophysiological mechanisms

The third type of theory proposes that some fibromyalgia patients are 'pain-prone', i.e. they develop or 'amplify' their pain by virtue of depression (Blumer and Heilbronn, 1982). Alternatively, FMS may be only one dis-order within a spectrum of 'generalized pain intolerance' (Quimby et al, 1988). Anxiety, tension, compulsion, preoccupation and certain other personality or behavioural traits are believed to increase pain in fibro-myalgia (Quimby et al, 1988; Hudson and Pope, 1989). Interestingly, American Psychiatric Association (1987) criteria for generalized anxiety disorder include many musculoskeletal (e.g. aches, soreness, tension) and other manifestations (e.g. fatigue, sleeplessness, irritability and excessive worry) often found in FMS, particularly in the more severe and less responsive patients.

Onset and perpetuation of FMS

Multiple factors probably conspire to precipitate the onset of FMS in most

FIBROMYALGIA: PROBABLE CONTRIBUTORY FACTORS

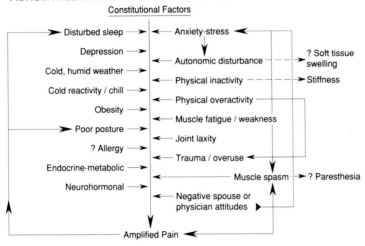

Figure 1. Interacting physical, metabolic, psychological and behavioural factors that may precipitate the development of fibromyalgia and accentuate its severity, in the constitutionally predisposed person. The objectives of management are to reduce or eliminate as many as possible of these negative, contributory factors and to increase the positive, protective factors.

patients (Figure 1). Then, the process tends to self-perpetuate (pain causing muscle tensing or 'spasms' which causes more pain), unless favourable modulating factors are marshalled. However, direct evidence of neuro-muscular hyperexcitability in FMS (Vitali et al, 1989) is unconfirmed (Zidar et al, 1990). Patients seem to have their own personal combinations ('fingerprints') of major predisposing and contributory factors, some of which are outlined in Table 1 and Figure 1.

Is FMS a band in the spectrum of dysfunctional syndromes?

Conceptually, FMS is similar to irritable bowel syndrome, functional head-ache syndrome and primary dysmenorrhoea syndrome; all are painful functional disorders, affecting either skeletal or smooth muscle tissues, with varying degrees of psychological manifestations (Yunus et al, 1989a), possibly suggesting a component of autonomic dysfunction. These con-ditions, along with major affective and other psychiatric disorders, may belong to a family of 'affective spectrum disorders', that may share common pathophysiological features (Hudson and Pope, 1989). Furthermore, it has been proposed that some forms of anxiety and depression may represent different phenotypic manifestations of the same genetic predisposition, depending upon varying environmental conditions (Paul, 1988). Specific-ally, uncontrollable stress contributed to higher self-ratings of helplessness, tension, anxiety and depression, than controllable stress in a small sample of healthy human volunteers (Breier et al, 1987).

An intriguing syndrome with similar muscular and neuropsychiatric manifestations to fibromyalgia is 'spasmophilia' (Agnoli et al, 1985), which is believed to be an idiopathic form of normocalcaemic 'tetany'. This syndrome may be related to chronic hyperventilation (Nixon, 1989), which also has prominent muscular aches, pains and fatigue, and is proposed to result from long-term, increased arousal mechanisms, overwhelming the body's performance abilities. Little information is available on the effects of β-adrenergic blocking agents on spasmophilia or FMS, but controlled trials would seem to be relevant to management.

CONCEPTS OF CHRONIC PAIN AS RELATED TO FIBROMYALGIA MANAGEMENT

Fibromyalgia may be considered as a form of chronic ('intractable') benign pain, of varied severity. Chronic pain is a complex, personal experience which includes emotional and behavioural responses (Fordyce, 1988). It is not simply a neurophysiological, 'hard-wired' sensory phenomenon (Garrett, 1989; Wall and Melzack, 1989). Elements and features of the neurophysiological and psychosocial components of chronic pain may be outlined (Table 2) in an attempt to develop a conceptual framework for patient management.

Different pain or suffering features in fibromyalgia may relate to particular neurophysiological mechanisms (e.g. first, second or third order neuron processing) or to factors influencing psychological reactions (e.g. social and environmental experiences.)

Nociception

This peripheral sensory process by receptors and free nerve endings is the starting point of pain impulse transmission, at least with acute injury or trauma. Nociception may not be the most important contributor to many forms of chronic pain. However, it might contribute importantly in some FMS patients, e.g. those with more localized, peripheral manifestations, particularly if induced by physical mechanisms (Littlejohn, 1989; Smythe, 1989b).

Spinothalamic pain impulse transmission and modulation

This more complex 'intermediary' process may be a more important contributor in other FMS patients. Possibly, altered sleep physiology (Moldofsky, 1982) or imbalances between dorsal horn algogenic factors—e.g. substance P—and descending track pain modulators—e.g. enkephalins (Russell, 1989) and other 'endocoids' (Lal et al, 1985)—may predispose certain individuals to FMS.

Cortical, cognitive and emotional mechanisms

Some people may have mainly higher-level CNS reasons for chronic pain perception (Blumer and Heilbronn, 1982). Such hypothesis assumes that the chronic pain is a somatic expression of unresolved psychic pain. Chronic pain and suffering may be evoked by a broad spectrum of social and environmental factors (Fordyce, 1976, 1988), which are sensitive to learning and anticipated socioenvironmental consequences (see below).

Concepts of the pathophysiology of fibromyalgia and mechanisms of chronic pain perpetuation may be helpful in managing individual patients.

SEVERITY GRADIENT AND CONTRIBUTORY FACTORS IN FIBROMYALGIA

A considerable severity gradient (Figure 2) exists between the mildest and most severe fibromyalgia patients (Masi and Yunus, 1986). Also, each patient has various types and degrees of contributory factors which may aggravate the condition (see Figure 1): physical (e.g. deconditioning, obesity, repetitive straining occupations, joint hypermobility, muscle

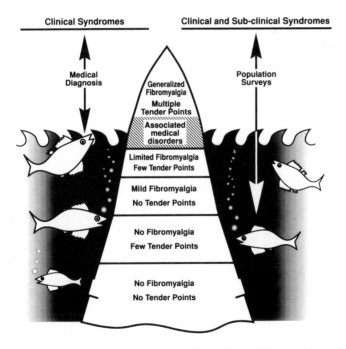

Fibromyalgia: its biological gradient and detection.

Figure 2. An 'iceberg' analogy to illustrate the severity gradient of fibromyalgia syndromes in the population. A minority of the total persons affected by such manifestations have a generalized form with widespread pain and multiple tender points (either primary or associated with medical disorders) and represent the peak of the iceberg. The majority of people with fibromyalgia manifestations have limited findings and do not come to medical attention. Regional myofascial pain syndrome (MPS) probably overlaps with the milder and limited fibromyalgia groups.

Table 2. Schematic framework of chronic pain mechanisms in fibromyalgia and their potential management.

Characteristics and elements	Component mechanisms contributing to chronic pain phenomena			
	Peripheral nociception	Spinothalamic processing and transmission	Pain perception and affective responses	Suffering and pain behaviours
Definitions	First-order free nerve ending and receptor responses to tissue injury or irritation: a physical sensation perceived as sharp and localized from skin, but as burning and poorly localized from deeper tissues, including muscles	Second-order neuron processing and transmission of impulses through dorsal horn to brain stem and thalamus: involves a complex inhibition ('gating') by afferent large (A-beta) fibre stimulation and modulation by descending fibres from brain stem	Third-order neuron impulse projection from specific thalamic nuclei to sensory, motor association and other cortical nuclei; poorly localized burning pain is projected to the limbic system	Dysphoric and dysfunctional responses resulting from chronic pain as well as psychosocial stresses in susceptible persons
Stimuli, initiators or inhibitors	Chemical algogenic factors; serotonin, acetylcholine, bradykinin, K^+ ion (>20 mmol/l), H^+ ($<$pH 6), released in mechanical, ischaemic or thermal injury	Neurotransmitters; substance P, in substantia gelatinosa (lamina II) of dorsal horn, and neuromodulators (at least acute phases); enkephalin and somatostatin locally, in response to brain activity	Electrical stimulation of the thalamus can elicit pain, but rarely of the cortex, suggesting that nociceptive impulse transmission ends at the thalamus (although processed in cortical centres)	Aversive stimuli, e.g. psychological or environmental factors, may cause continuing pain perception, especially when accompanied by emotional reactions in persons with ineffective coping abilities
Receptors, conductors or mechanisms	Primary afferent neurons; thinly myelinated A-delta (1–5 μm diameter) and unmyelinated C-fibres (0.25–1.5 μm diameter). The latter is associated with dull, diffuse, more deeply perceived 'burning' sensations	Axons cross the cord and impulses rise via the spinothalamic pathways to brain stem, non-specific and specific (VPL) thalamic nuclei, without synapses in the fast-conducting tracts and with polysynaptic connections in the slow-conducting tracts, plus spinoreticular pathways	Short and long latency cortical evoked potentials are recorded after nociceptive stimuli; the long latency potentials correlate with reported pain intensity modelling	Predisposed individuals with anxiety, depression, somatocizing or other psychological traits or persons who have learned such behaviour from family or environmental exposures

Effects	Impulses enter the spinal cord through dorsal roots and terminate widely in the dorsal horn via Lissauer's tract, over 2 or 3 segments above and below entry	Nociception is believed to be relayed by 2 (of 4) types of neurons (high-threshold, and wide, dynamic-range neurons) to specific thalamic nuclei, e.g. post central gyrus (sharp, localized pain); non-specific thalamic nuclei (non-specific pain and 'feel') and limbic system (dull, poorly localized pain)	Complex perceptual experience with intricate cognitive and emotional components, which are largely undefined, especially regarding the dull, burning, throbbing, poorly localized pain	Physical and psychological impairments may develop out of proportion to the tissue injury; more likely with deep, poorly localized pain than superficial, well-localized pain. Objective and self-reports of pain correlate with depression measures
Function	Signalling injury or disease. Useful in acute phase, often counterproductive in chronic phase	Send information to multiple sensory, limbic, motor and autonomic response areas which process the sensation as pain and allow physiological response, including motor and autonomic	Allows refined conscious awareness of pain as well as aversive and emotional responses (the latter possibly relayed within thalamofrontal tracts)	Stimulates anticipatory threats to well-being and dependency, but can often become counterproductive
Management	Remedy factors producing stimuli, use analgesic/ anti-inflammatory agents effective at the peripheral level or interrupt pathway with injection, physical conditioning manipulation or physical therapy	Increase pain inhibitors (e.g. serotonin and enkephalin) with improved sleep and diminish pain-promotors (e.g. noradrenaline from exaggerated sympathetic responses) with anxiety control. Other potential therapy might include massage, acupuncture, TENS and possible spinal opioid analgesia in hyperacute cases	Although narcotics may reduce cortical evoked potentials to pain, they are not indicated in FMS. Theoretically, promoting endogenous opiate-like peptides may modulate pain sensation or affective responses, e.g. by physical conditioning, cognitive and biofeedback therapy	Rehabilitation, including cognitive and behavioural management, in a structured, interactive, patient-involved programme. Antidepressant treatment may also be indicated and helpful in a proportion of chronic pain patients

hypertonicity, postural abnormalities); emotional (e.g. anxiety, depression, somatiform tendencies) or socioenvironmental (e.g. unemployment, over-work, overcommitment and other stressed lifestyles). Such individual factors are not 'causal', in the sense that elimination of any one of them will cure the condition. However, collectively, they operate as perpetuating or amplifying mechanisms (Figure 1), and as such, they should be recognized and remedied. It is important to recognize that a patient can fluctuate within the severity gradient and that the objective of management is to maintain the best status.

WHICH IS THE BEST TREATMENT OF FIBROMYALGIA?

No specific treatment will be best for everyone presenting with manifold fibromyalgia complaints (Turk and Flor, 1989). Nor will a particular approach satisfy the complex concerns and needs of such varied sufferers (Bennett, 1989a; Bradley, 1989; Goldenberg, 1989a,b; McCain, 1989; Smythe, 1989b). Knowledge of the relative contributions of physical, neuro-physiological, psychological, socioenvironmental and behavioural mechan-isms (if not also familial) to the onset and course of fibromyalgia is lacking (Smythe, 1989b).

Accordingly, the care-giver, often the physician coordinator, can most effectively approach management of a client in a personalized, compre-hensive, patient-involved manner. In this way, one may attempt to address directly and diminish those major factors believed to be contributing to that particular patient's fibromyalgia. Thereby, one hopes to engender greater patient motivation in managing this chronic condition. The experienced, caring physician (Reuler et al, 1980) or other care-giver (Hadler, 1986) understands the importance of providing individualized therapy for chronic conditions.

This article offers a clinical, intuitive perspective of the multifaceted process of management in fibromyalgia. Little understanding exists of the relative benefits and limitations of the various modalities. Further research must establish scientific justification for future therapy of this mysterious disorder.

THE THERAPEUTIC HISTORY (STUDYING THE 'PERSON IN THE PATIENT')

Fibromyalgia is usually readily recognizable by its pattern of symptoms and physical findings (Yunus et al, 1981; Campbell et al, 1983; Wolfe, 1989). Nevertheless, the process of taking a personalized history allows assessment of the patient's individual manifestations, psyche and living circumstances, which may contribute directly to therapy (Turk and Flor, 1989). Studying the 'person in the patient' reflects back to the old idea that the patient's nature has a good deal to do with the nature of the illness (Wolf, 1990). Furthermore, integrating the history into a coherent 'story about the patient' allows core problems and issues to be put into a perspective which might be more effectively addressed than would be possible with only fragmented clinical data.

Therapy begins ideally with the first encounter, the initial, inviting greetings and mutual introductions. Positive patient–physician relationships may not materialize unless one makes such conscious efforts. Fibromyalgia patients are often hypersensitized to physicians' attitudes, based upon frequent prior encounters, often negative (Yunus, 1988; Smythe, 1989b). Patients often fear that their concerns will not be understood or seriously addressed. To complicate matters, busy, time-pressured physicians often become frustrated by the extensive musculoskeletal, systemic and emotional complaints of many fibromyalgia patients, frequently presented in a disconnected, anxious fashion. Frustrations on either side should not be allowed to develop. Concerned listening skills, empathy and supportive attitudes help to promote positive physician–patient relationships, which aid in management.

Logistics of obtaining personalized information

Practice circumstances will dictate the logistics of obtaining a therapeutic medical history, e.g. the time available, use of open-ended interviewing techniques versus structured questionnaires and the availability of associates (i.e. non-physician health workers) to help obtain and summarize the detailed information. Grading of pain, global severity and dysfunctions, e.g. on a scale of 0–10, is useful in evaluating initial severity and following subsequent progress. Whatever system of data collection is effective should be utilized.

The comments following reflect the anamnesis of patients with mild or severe fibromyalgia; the large intermediate group falls between these extremes (Masi and Yunus, 1986).

Mild fibromyalgia

Many fibromyalgia patients present with relatively limited manifestations and usually are emotionally stable. Their medical history can usually be obtained effectively in a single encounter, as might be done with most other patients having similar functionally related complaints, such as irritable bowel syndrome or functional headache syndrome, which overlap with fibromyalgia (Yunus et al, 1989a).

Such mildly affected patients usually have adequate or normal function and are often more concerned about the cause of the pain, rather than its elimination. They often state, 'I can live with this (mild) pain, if I know it is not serious'. They are frequently concerned about the possibility of having cancer, rheumatoid arthritis or lupus, which may have affected a family member. The history uncovers such private concerns and helps to establish a firm, convincing diagnosis, which is in itself therapeutic. It also provides a database for personalized education about the patient's fibromyalgia syndrome and helps in outlining appropriate behavioural changes, needed in rehabilitation.

Severe fibromyalgia

Fortunately, relatively few fibromyalgia patients have marked manifestations, which include psychological disturbances and multiple somatic complaints (Yunus et al, 1990). In such patients, the personalized medical history can be profoundly complex. Its documentation often requires more time than is scheduled during an initial visit. Nevertheless, the diagnosis of fibromyalgia can usually be inferred quickly from a brief evaluation, especially in apparently healthy people (Smythe, 1989b; Yunus et al, 1989b; Wolfe et al, 1990). Often, these patients have a chief complaint of 'hurting all over', admit to anxiety, stress and depression, and describe symptoms of other functional disorders, such as irritable bowel syndrome (alternating diarrhoea, constipation and abdominal cramping, alleviated by bowel movements). Such history, combined with the presence of multiple, mainly symmetrical, specific soft tissue tender points on physical examination, is typical of fibromyalgia (Yunus et al, 1989b).

An abbreviated clinical history, however, does not usually provide sufficient information to convince patients that their complex condition can 'all be explained by fibromyalgia'. Doubt is particularly likely among patients who have consulted several physicians previously and were not offered a unified diagnosis. Also, many patients will not be reassured until they believe that their physician understands and knows about their 'complete' condition.

With such complex, severe fibromyalgia, a full information base need not be acquired or analysed on the first visit or necessarily by one care-giver. The process may be accomplished over several visits or by several care-givers, working as a supportive team. Ideally, a single therapist should have responsibility as the coordinator, in order to synthesize the information and communicate the relevant aspects to the concerned patient. In a family physician setting, the care-givers may already have a long-standing relationship with the patient, and an extensive database. Nevertheless, it is important to review and synthesize the relevant aspects for the patient, in order to establish a convincing and reassuring diagnosis.

PHYSICAL EXAMINATION

An astute examination can identify physical factors contributing importantly to fibromyalgia manifestations, e.g. weak, flabby muscles (Bennett, 1989b,c), joint hyperlaxity (Beighton et al, 1989; Grahame, 1990), muscle imbalances, hypertonicity, contractures or stiffness (Siegler and Beck, 1989), poor posture (Smythe, 1989b) or obesity. Once recognized, such physical conditions can often be improved by patient involvement in a prescribed aerobic conditioning (McCain , 1989; McCain et al, 1989) or strengthening programme (Kessler and Hertling, 1988; Kaplan and Tanner, 1989). Also, dramatic relief can sometimes be provided by detecting and eliminating a previously unrecognized, disabling tender point or trigger point, by either muscle stretching manoeuvres (Travell and Simons, 1983; Simons, 1986) or localized depot steroid injection (Masi, 1987; Yunus, 1988; Smythe and Sheon, 1990).

Patients vary greatly in the number and intensity of their tender points, which may not correlate with severity of symptoms or number of symptom sites (Yunus et al, 1989a). Nevertheless, tender point examination may be a useful gauge, although approximate, of a particular patient's subsequent course under therapy. Often, a patient will exhibit either less intense or fewer tender points, as the condition improves symptomatically over time, and tender points tend to increase as the condition worsens.

Unfortunately, there is a scarcity of objective, clinical measures to test degrees of muscle fitness (Jacobsen and Danneskiold-Samsøe, 1987, 1989; Bennett et al, 1989; Klug et al (1989) or dysfunction in fibromyalgia patients. However, isokinetic, dynamometer muscle strength measurements were found to be lower in PFS patients with a large number of tender points than in healthy, matched controls (Jacobsen and Danneskiold-Samsøe, 1989). Future research on normal versus fibromyalgia muscle function (Jacobsen and Danneskiold-Samsøe, 1987, 1989; Bennett et al, 1989) promises to improve the accuracy of the physical examination in this condition, beyond the present level of clinical assessment.

LABORATORY AND RADIOLOGICAL STUDIES

Essentially all routine testing in fibromyalgia is normal (Bennett, 1989a; Smythe, 1989b), including blood studies (Yunus et al, 1981), muscle histology and ultrastructure (Yunus and Kalyan-Raman, 1989), and bone and soft tissue scintigraphy (Yunus et al, 1989c). However, specialized research procedures, e.g. detecting altered oxygen (Lund et al, 1986) or decreased high-energy phosphate levels in tender muscles, either directly on biopsy (Bengtsson et al, 1986) or by nuclear magnetic resonance spectroscopy techniques (Kushmerick, 1989), suggest that ischaemia is a possible contributory factor (Bennett, 1989b). Immunofluorescent studies of skin reveal band-like, finely granular deposition of IgG (and albumin) at the basal lamina, consistent with 'enhanced vascular permeability' in some patients (Caro, 1989).

The relevance of laboratory or radiological procedures to management is limited. They can help to document the primary diagnosis, in the minority of patients when clinical manifestations are uncertain, or to reassure the anxious, unconvinced patient. Usually, a minimal battery of screening studies, e.g. complete blood count and erythrocyte sedimentation rate, may be advisable, especially in older patients. Associated osteoarthritis may also be found in such patients on roentgenography (Yunus et al, 1988), but this procedure would not usually be indicated for management.

CONSIDERATIONS IN THE MANAGEMENT OF FIBROMYALGIA SYNDROME

Effective management of this condition (Table 3) depends greatly upon the

Table 3. Outline considerations in management of fibromyalgia syndrome.

1. Firmly establish the diagnosis and convince the patient of its benign nature
2. Educate the patient about the nature of fibromyalgia and its major interacting, multifactorial mechanisms
3. Reassure the patient that improved function and quality of life usually may be achieved, although some degree of discomfort may persist
4. Offer emotional support and guide the patient in behavioural modifications, i.e. remedying aggravating factors and enhancing relieving ones, with focus on performance goals rather than pain or suffering
5. Remedy physical perpetuating or aggravating factors, e.g. unfitness, occupational strains, poor posture, ligamentous laxity, obesity or muscle tensing with body cooling
6. Utilize physical therapy and specific stretching exercises, e.g. for neck, shoulder or lower back, as needed for symptom relief and preconditioning
7. Promote physical conditioning with prescribed, graduated exercises
8. Improve sleep quality, including hygiene measures initially and medication with a low-dose tricyclic antidepressant before bedtime, if needed
9. Trial of simple analgesic agents, e.g. salicylates or NSAIDs, as needed
10. Inject disabling and particularly symptomatic tender points with local anaesthetics and corticosteroid preparations, and consider other physical measures to relieve such local problems
11. Provide psychologic therapy and consider consultation, if necessary
12. Help the patient commit herself or himself to major management responsibility for self-rehabilitation, pain control and improved function

physician's astuteness in determining the major contributory factors (see Tables 1, 2 and Figure 1), as well as success in motivating the patient to achieve personalized therapy goals. Recent references may be consulted regarding additional perspectives on treatment of fibromyalgia (Hench and Mitler, 1986; Goldenberg, 1987, 1989a,b; Miller and Siefert, 1987; Wolfe, 1988; Bennett, 1989a; Bradley, 1989; McCain, 1989; McCain et al, 1989; Quimby et al, 1989; Smythe, 1989b) and regional myofascial pain syndromes (Travell and Simons, 1983; Campbell, 1989).

1. Establish the diagnosis

The first priority is to establish the diagnosis and convince the patient that the condition is real and not 'all in the head'. This step alone often provides considerable relief for desperate patients who have seen many physicians and have not yet been assured of their diagnosis, often fearing the worst. Belief in the reality of their diagnosis relieves both stress and pain.

2. Educate the patient and significant others

The patient should be educated about the nature of this condition in simple, understandable terms, as an integral part of the initial management. A simple handout explaining fibromyalgia and its interacting factors (as shown partly in Figure 1) is helpful. Mechanisms should be explained and the educational process reinforced during follow-up visits. The spouse or significant others should also be aware of the essential considerations so that they can help. The patient can be sent a copy of the consultation letter, which then could be shared with significant others, as appropriate. The patient should be encouraged to bring a supportive companion on follow-up visits.

Patients should appreciate how their particular contributory factors affect symptoms, e.g. poor sleep, lack of physical conditioning, work stresses, cold temperatures, emotional trauma and anxiety. Some factors are not evident initially, even after detailed evaluation. They may only be recognized in retrospect, be they physical or psychological.

Many patients fear that their anxiety or stress factors mean that the condition is 'all psychological' or 'all in the head'. Patients and care-givers should recognize that the described pain is as real as in a cancer patient (Reuler et al, 1980). Fibromyalgia is different from psychogenic pain (Yunus, 1988) and from pain described by malingerers. Fibromyalgia patients have consistent, reproducible symptoms and signs which persist over several visits (Yunus et al, 1989d). Although some FMS patients may demonstrate pain behaviour (Fordyce, 1976, 1988), they are not usually motivated by conscious secondary gains.

3. Provide reassurance

As in any illness, effective caring depends to a large extent on the ability to reassure patients and mobilize their rehabilitative potential. Compassionate but firm supportive care, provided in a non-threatening and non-judgmental manner, is often helpful. Physician experience and confidence in managing fibromyalgia patients tends to facilitate positive interactions. Such relationships may be one of the more effective modalities, although not proved statistically in clinical trials.

Absence of crippling or shortened longevity should be emphasized, as well as the usually good functional prognosis, in most patients. However, patients should understand that some degree of chronic discomfort usually continues, unless management is optimal. In most patients, such low-grade symptomatology does not interfere with a satisfying and productive quality of life.

4. Offer emotional support and guide behavioural modifications

Psychological factors

Psychological research into fibromyalgia has been somewhat conflicting (Goldenberg, 1989c). In a primary internal medicine setting, no significant difference was found in the psychological profile of fibromyalgia patients versus controls (Clark et al, 1985a). However, among fibromyalgia patients referred to rheumatologists, most investigators have found an elevation of Minnesota Multiphasic Personality Inventory (MMPI) scales for hysteria, depression and hypochondriasis, compared to either normals or rheumatoid arthritis patients. A minority of fibromyalgia patients qualify for classification as either being 'psychologically disturbed' by MMPI criteria (Ahles et al, 1984), or having a psychiatric diagnosis of an affective disorder (e.g. depression) or somatiform disorder (Ahles et al, submitted for publication).

Such psychologically disturbed patients have typical musculoskeletal mani-festations, comparable to other fibromyalgia patients, e.g. widespread aching pain and similar numbers of tender points. However, they tend to complain of greater severity of pain, as well as of increased anxiety, stress and depression (Yunus et al, 1990). Clinically, one suspects that such patients are more resistant to management and have greater dysfunction, but such longitudinal correlations have not yet been documented statistically.

Overall, fibromyalgia patients usually describe chronic stresses, involving their psychological, social or occupational relationships, which are believed to contribute to poor sleep (Moldofsky, 1989a,b) and other aspects of their symptom complex (Hudson and Pope, 1989; Turk and Flor, 1989). Also, patients often believe they are psychologically contributing to the process, either by not handling stresses adequately or by being oversensitized to the discomforts. Addressing such psychological concerns or behavioural patterns requires patience and persistence, both on the part of care-givers and patients.

Behavioural modifications

Direct enquiry helps to uncover the patient's individual manifestations and behaviour patterns. The management objectives are to 'accentuate the positive, eliminate the negative', which is a refrain from an old (circa 1950) American song. The longer the patient is able to cope successfully with the pains and dysfunctions, the more desensitized she or he becomes to them. Changing a mentality of 'I can't do it' to 'How can I do it?' is the key, especially in a setting which encourages performance not pain. The patient should focus on goals for living life more fully.

Accepting some pain. Successful behavioural management requires that patients accept some degree of chronic pain and be assured that performing normal activities will not cause tissue damage. Patients should learn that chronic pain modulation, to a considerable degree, lies within their own control. Importantly, they need to learn new behaviours which help to overcome disabilities that resulted from the chronic pain (Fordyce, 1976, 1988). The goal is to improve functioning, within programmed, preset levels, despite some pain. Patients should not feel defeated because they have not 'beaten the pain', but should be encouraged by gaining some degree of control.

Improvement usually occurs gradually with persistent efforts. Our patients who succeeded in managing their chronic pain (compared with those who did not) had definite functional goals which they were able to achieve. Some fibromyalgia patients may complain that even modest activity aggravates their pain. Nevertheless, these patients need to be encouraged to persist in their behavioural changes in order to increase their physical activities, within defined goals. Once achieved, the previous pain level often decreases. Care-givers, including family, should focus on performance, not pain or suffering, in the reactivation and rehabilitation process (Fordyce, 1976, 1988).

Accepting small benefits. Patients should be encouraged to accept and build upon relieving factors and not dismiss them as 'only temporary'. For example, stretching exercises, home massage (as well as professional massage or 'myotherapy'), hot baths or showers, local heat, moderate activities, a nap when exhausted, more restful sleep and prescribed relaxation, in overworked, tense persons, can all be beneficial. Even several minutes of relief, multiplied many times, can build up to hours, which may be used in productive activities, improved quality of life and achieving interim performance goals (Yunus, 1988).

Performing within reasonable limits. Patients should be encouraged to pace themselves with the objective of gradually increasing their physical capabilities. They must avoid 'pushing to their limits'. Trying to complete a job while feeling better, at the risk (from past experience) of flaring the condition, can be self-defeating. One should discourage an attitude of 'all or nothing', and adopt a philosophy of 'slow and steady' progress in developing functional abilities and goals. Learning how to gain satisfaction from relaxation is often difficult for persons with 'workaholic', 'over-achiever' attitudes, but it can be done with the help of supportive care-givers.

Fibromyalgia syndrome and chronic fatigue syndrome

A subgroup of fibromyalgia patients qualify for a classification of chronic fatigue syndrome (CFS) (Goldenberg et al, 1990). Any chronic psychiatric illness excludes such patients, by definition. It is well documented that patients with symptoms of persistent fatigue have a high frequency of affective disorders, particularly depression (Manu et al, 1988a,b). Care-givers should attempt to determine to what degree the fatigue in FMS is due to physical factors, e.g. poor muscular conditioning and non-restorative sleep (which may contribute to both fibromyalgia and some degree of reactive depression), versus a primary, psychodynamic abnormality (Blumer and Heilbronn, 1982). The former patients should be managed, at least initially, by their primary physician or rheumatologist, although greater time will usually be required for guidance, support and behavioural therapy. The latter patients should be diplomatically encouraged to have formal psychometric evaluation and psychological or psychiatric consultation, as indicated below.

5. Remedy perpetuating or aggravating physical factors

Physical problems, e.g. poor muscular fitness, ligamentous laxity, obesity and stooping posture, should be addressed. Strains at work (Littlejohn, 1989) or in recreation and other overuse, inconsistent use or misuse syndromes, can also contribute to pain and can be modified. Prolonged inactivity (e.g. during a long car ride) and exposure to cold, damp weather or cool indoor environments are frequent aggravating factors which can be appropriately corrected. Fibromyalgia patients seem to have an exaggerated response to cold and body cooling (Bennett, 1989c). Conscientious efforts to conserve body heat by layering garments, especially during sedentary periods or while sleeping in a cool room, are helpful in decreasing natural tendencies to muscle tightening under such circumstances (senior author's habit and advice).

Overloading activities

A perceptive history will usually reveal that various occupational strains (Littlejohn, 1989) or other physical factors may precipitate or aggravate the condition. Physical examination may reveal morphological abnormalities that may contribute to fibromyalgia, e.g. obesity or poor posture (see Figure 1), as well as ligamentous laxity (Grahame, 1990) or underdeveloped muscles, giving rise to poor neck or shoulder girdle strength, typically in some asthenic women. These factors may chronically overload incompetent muscle systems, causing fatigue, hypertonicity, possibly ischaemia and pain. Once developed, the process may self-perpetuate, due to other contributory factors (Figure 1).

Painful activities with unconditioned, tensed muscles will generally continue to be painful (Klug et al, 1989) and could lead to acute strains, spasms or tendinoligamentous sprains. Once developed, these may require days or weeks of rest and therapy for relief. It is believed that one usually cannot 'work through the problem' of a chronically overburdened or decompensated muscular system in fibromyalgia patients, unless aerobic conditioning can first be achieved (Klug et al, 1989). This is unlike the graded strengthening process in a young, fit athlete, following minor soft tissue injuries. Also, inactivity of an overloaded muscle system predisposes to further stiffness, pain and atrophy, which delays or complicates rehabilitation.

Analysis of dynamic loading and muscular competence factors is required to plan effective rehabilitation. Consultation from experts in industrial, sports or physical medicine may offer guidance in such problems. Sometimes, a solution is as simple as changing the position of a machine in relation to the worker, which may decrease a physical disadvantage such as working with the arms above shoulder level, and thereby relieve the symptoms.

Chronic pain from such localized strains can interfere with sleep and cause anxieties or tensions about job performance and security. Such factors may lead to generalized fibromyalgia, especially in the predisposed patient (see Figure 1). Correction of a significant physical perpetuating factor and general symptomatic supportive therapy often result in significant improvement of both the regional and more diffuse fibromyalgia manifestations. At times, a minor job adjustment is insufficient to remedy the problem, especially in the older, deconditioned patient. A major job transfer or disability retirement may be required in a minority of patients.

Postural fatigue

Poor posture may contribute to muscle strains and fatigue, particularly in the lower neck and lower back (Smythe, 1989b), thereby causing pain, and should be corrected. The C5–6 segment is the most unstable level in the vertebral column. Its support muscles may become overloaded in an attempt to splint the area chronically, in a patient with poor posture or other biomechanical abnormality in this location. Forward-stooped shoulders in the woman who is self-conscious about large breasts, or drooped head and neck in the shy person, can exert chronic muscular and ligamentous strains in the posterior neck and shoulder girdle areas and contribute to fibromyalgia symptoms (Smythe, 1989b). Poor sleeping posture, especially with pillows that hyperflex the neck, have been described as contributing to symptoms (Littlejohn, 1989; Smythe, 1989b). Deep soft-tissue stresses in vulnerable locations within the axial system, at both the lower neck and lower back, may cause strains or injuries. In turn, these factors can cause pain both within the adjacent dermatomes and throughout the respective upper and lower girdles and adjacent areas (Smythe, 1989b).

The relative contribution of such postural 'biomechanical factors' to the development of fibromyalgia versus other presumed contributory mechanisms (see Tables 1, 2 and Figure 1) is not known and deserves critical research. Nevertheless, postural abnormalities should be remedied with appropriate measures, such as improvement of sitting and standing postures, weight loss in obesity, posterior shoulder girdle muscle strengthening when needed, use of a neck pillow instead of a head pillow, and other measures (Smythe, 1989b).

Ligamentous laxity

Patients with joint hypermobility and ligamentous laxity (Beighton et al, 1989; Grahame, 1990), particularly younger females, may present with a history of chronic aching pains of the neck, shoulders and extremities (especially the lower extremities). These symptoms may have previously been intermittent and related to straining activities; however, at the time of presentation, symptoms may have become generalized, particularly following a period of greater stress or poor sleep. Such patients are often deconditioned physically and have asthenic rather than muscular physiques.

Mechanisms of muscular symptoms in such patients are not well known. Normal anatomical, postural relationships are maintained by both ligamentous binding and muscular tone, via muscle spindle impulse reflex mechanisms. One may speculate that if ligamentous binding is too lax, greater 'postural loading' will be transferred to muscles and may chronically overburden weak, deconditioned musculature. This situation is in contrast to well-trained ballet dancers or gymnasts, who often have joint hypermobility, but excellent muscular conditioning which can accommodate additional postural (or other) loading.

In our practice, fibromyalgia patients with ligamentous laxity are advised to engage in a graduated programme of muscle conditioning and strengthening, with preliminary stretching routines for fatigued, painful, 'tight' muscles (i.e. muscles that do not move through their intrinsic full range of motion). Importantly, 'warm-up' stretching exercises also relieve stiffness and musculotendinous contractions of antagonistic tissues. Hot baths, showers or other heat modalities may be useful in facilitating stretching. Consultation may be obtained from experts in physiatry, sports medicine or physical therapy, in order to prescribe specific stretching and strengthening exercise programmes and to monitor progress. However, basic understanding of body mechanics, exercise dynamics and patient motivation can be employed by the primary physician to improve symptoms in many such patients with milder ligamentous laxity and minor symptomatology. Accurate diagnosis and reassurance that such patients do not have a chronic inflammatory disorder such as rheumatoid arthritis offer considerable relief.

Weak muscles

Many patients presenting with fibromyalgia and physical perpetuating factors have weak muscles (Bennett, 1989a,b), either due to constitution or disuse. Occasionally in our practice, young adult women present with complaints of neck, shoulder girdle or upper arm aching pain, often unilateral, on the dominant side, which manifests during normal activities, e.g. an instructor writing on a chalkboard or a music teacher conducting a class. The local symptoms may have recently interfered with sleep and the localized myalgias then migrated to other areas. Such patients may have good posture and normal joint mobility, but have grossly underdeveloped, weak, unconditioned shoulder musculature, which fatigues easily. This presentation is similar to patients with occupational strains (Littlejohn, 1989). However, the precipitating activities are relatively minor and cause symptoms primarily because of the weak muscles, rather than any significant external overloading. Accurate assessment, reassurance and a graded, stretching and strengthening exercise programme often provide good results in the uncomplicated patient.

It is important to exclude underlying causes in these cases, such as cervical disc disease, cervical rib or even occult pleuritis or pericarditis, particularly in fibromyalgia patients whose symptoms started in an asymmetric, upper extremity area. Such organic, underlying mechanisms are usually suggested by a careful history and physical examination, but may require further diagnostic testing for confirmation.

Body heat and skeletal muscle tone

Fibromyalgia patients are believed to have an exaggerated chilling response to cold compared to a normal population (Bennett, 1989c). Also, resting tonus may be increased in painful, fatigued skeletal muscles, at least in trigger point areas (Simons, 1986). Almost all energy released by internal metabolism, including muscle contraction, is eventually converted into body heat (Guyton, 1986). Exact relationships between core body temperature and skeletal muscle resting tone are not well studied. However, body cooling increases muscular activity and tone, as compensatory temperature-increasing mechanisms. Clinical encounters and uncontrolled patient trials suggest that maintaining body warmth during sedentary periods by adding layers of clothing to conserve heat (which seems to be more effective than raising the room temperature) can ameliorate myalgias considerably, at least in some patients. Presumably, this diminishes a cycle of body cooling causing increased muscle tone which in turn causes myalgias and consequent decreased muscular activity. Further research is needed in this area. Nevertheless, these aspects deserve review in the personalized history and appropriate adjustments should be made, if necessary. Interestingly, hypothyroidism—a known cause of secondary fibromyalgia (Hench, 1989)— is characterized by tendency to hypothermia, skeletal muscle hypertonicity, myalgias and disturbed sleep.

Obesity

Significant overweight should be controlled with the aim of reducing mechanical stresses and for the general benefits of health, fitness and psychological well-being. However, the problem of obesity in fibromyalgia patients is often resistant, especially in those who may not be able to exercise sufficiently. The obesity may have developed or increased following onset of the fibromyalgia, as a result of inactivity, greater access to food at home, anxiety, depression or overeating caused by frustration. Importantly, use of a tricyclic antidepressant agent to promote sleep, especially when prescribed in higher than minimal doses (e.g. 10 mg or 25 mg amitriptyline, two hours before bedtime), may induce weight gain.

Compassionate understanding of such patients, offering moral support and specific, personalized guidance in controlling this difficult problem, is needed—not critical or judgmental admonishments. The former approach helps to develop a partnership in addressing the problem and increases patient motivation. The latter will often cause the patient to avoid further contact with the physician. Specific dietary guidance and even nutritional counselling may be advisable, as well as encouraging the patient to join a weight-reduction, group therapy programme.

6. Physical therapy modalities, including sample stretching activities

For temporary symptomatic relief, various forms of physical therapy may be used, including heat, massage and particularly stretching, which has been shown in a controlled trial of patients with chronic low back pain to improve reported pain scores (Deyo et al, 1990), although the study did not specifically include fibromyalgia. Regular stretching exercises are advised to keep muscles supple, which decreases stiffness and increases range of motion. These exercises can be done either at home or in a treatment centre initially. Patients should be encouraged to be generally active, and to take time for relaxation, trying to control stresses both at home and at work. Individual or group stretching programmes (including yoga and Tai Chi) are relaxing and are important preliminary therapy for the longer-acting, more effective modalities of aerobic conditioning and strengthening programmes.

Examples of general stretching routines

Walking for 30 minutes a day or warm-water activities, several times per week, can be recommended as first-line physical measures. Initially, these should be done in a relaxed fashion and, later, more briskly, as tolerated. Resistance exercises or active aerobics can precipitate muscle spasms, if engaged in prematurely, but can be performed in later stages of conditioning.

Examples of specific stretching routines

Twice-daily stretching of neck, shoulders and lower back for 5–15 minutes at a time may be advised to keep particular muscle groups supple. Stretching exercises should be slow and gradual, with smooth movements. In a hyper-acute phase, gentle massage and passive stretching may be indicated, or application of cold compresses. In the chronic phases, heat (e.g. a shower, bath or dry or moist pads) usually relieves muscle soreness for temporary periods of half an hour to an hour, and are helpful before stretching programmes.

Recognition of an acute tender or trigger point, e.g. at the suboccipital, subdeltoid, paraspinal or greater trochanteric areas, is most important, as it may inhibit any effective stretching exercises at the respective sites. In such cases, preliminary injection of the tender point will usually provide prompt relief of the acute pain and allow increased mobility. The area can then be stretched more effectively with a programme of prescribed exercises. Illustrated exercise hand-outs will improve patient understanding and compliance.

Other physical modalities to assist stretching

Anaesthetic spray and stretch techniques (Travell and Simons, 1983) as well as osteopathic manipulative treatment (Korr, 1978, 1986) may also relieve tender or trigger points. General myalgias may be helped by either ice packs (in acute cases) or heat (in more chronic cases) as well as by massage therapy (which may work by stimulating A-beta 'touch' fibres and block pain impulses by 'gate control'). Transcutaneous electrical nerve stimulation (TENS) is based upon the same 'gating' principle and is sometimes used in fibromyalgia for symptomatic benefits or to assist stretching. However, its efficacy is unproved, at least in chronic low back pain (Deyo et al, 1990). Physical therapy should be targeted to improve function and to facilitate rehabilitation, not simply for symptomatic relief.

7. Physical goals and conditioning

Inactivity increases stiffness, probably as a gelling phenomenon, and the patient should be encouraged to be active (Table 4). Physical activities tend to relieve tension, to improve muscle tone, strength and coordination, and to aid sleep. In a hyperacute, symptomatic phase, temporary inactivity may be indicated, but not for chronic management, as it will prolong rehabili-tation and relief of symptoms.

Well-defined physical activities and graded aerobic exercises increase physical fitness, and generally encourage a healthy mental attitude. Group exercises at a health or medical centre are useful. It is advisable to start

Table 4. Physical goals to help control fibromyalgia and fatigue.

- Become conditioned and stay in shape
- Maintain normal weight
- Practise good posture, sitting and standing
- Maintain relaxed and flexible muscles (regular stretching routines)
- Develop muscular conditioning and endurance (aerobic exercises)
- Strengthen weak or strained muscles, e.g. back muscles (resistance exercise programmes)
- Warm up before strenuous or straining activities
- Avoid overstraining, especially when fatigued

gently, avoiding high-impacting or strenuous exercises that consistently aggravate pain. If this occurs, the patient should stop before the pain becomes too uncomfortable and then gradually extend the exercise limits to reasonable pain tolerances.

Aerobic training

Cardiovascular fitness training, three times a week, over 20 weeks, decreased pain and tender points and improved global health and psychological status among fibromyalgia patients, in a recent controlled study (McCain et al, 1989). Vigorous exercise may work by increasing endorphins in the central nervous system (McCain, 1989).

Strength training and functional restoration

Although similar to aerobic cardiovascular fitness training, strengthening and functional restoration programmes emphasize correction of weakness and restoring function in specific areas (psychological as well as physical) with the primary goal of return to work, not relief of pain. Scant information is available on such programmes in fibromyalgia management. However, for general background orientation, physical medicine and rehabilitation literature may be consulted (Kessler and Hertling, 1988; Kaplan and Tanner, 1989). In resistant or acute cases, physiatric consultation may be advisable, with objectives of quantitating and restoring physical functions (e.g. work hardening). Such techniques are reported to be effective in chronic low back pain resulting from industrial injury (Mayer et al, 1987).

8. Promote restorative sleep

Deficiency of deep (stages 3 or 4) 'restorative' sleep is believed to be a major factor in this condition (Moldofsky et al, 1975; Moldofsky and Lue, 1980; Moldofsky, 1982, 1989a, b).

Natural measures

The importance of 'good quality' sleep should be emphasized and natural steps recommended initially, e.g. not 'taking worries to bed', allowing enough hours to sleep, having a quiet room and other 'sleep hygiene' measures (Fletcher, 1986). Other good sleep habits include going to bed earlier and at the same time each night, avoiding caffeine, taking a hot shower before bed, and sleeping in a comfortable but firm bed. A significant problem for some patients is simply inadequate time allowed for sleeping, either because it is considered a waste of time, or because of jobs with rotating shifts, for instance which interfere with sleep routines. Specific counselling can often result in significantly improved sleep, even without drugs.

Tricyclic antidepressant agents

Deep sleep-promoting medications, such as low-dose tricyclic antidepressant (TCA) agents, often help (Goldenberg, 1989b), especially in patients with recognized poor sleep, i.e. those who awaken physically more tired than when they went to bed. Amitriptyline hydrochloride or doxepin hydrochloride, taken two hours before bedtime in a dose of 10–25 mg (and sometimes less), may be quite effective. In a minority of patients somewhat higher doses are helpful, but should only be used after testing the lower doses initially.

Two short-term, double-blind therapy trials have shown significant improvement in sleep quality and significant overall benefits in fibromyalgia patients from amitryptyline given at bedtime in doses of 25 mg (Goldenberg et al, 1986) or 50 mg (Carette et al, 1986). In the latter study, the tender point count also showed significant improvement. Cyclobenzaprine hydrochloride 10 mg has also been found to be helpful (Bennett et al, 1988; Quimby et al, 1989). Sedative or hypnotic sleep aids such as benzodiazepines should not be used routinely, because of their habituating properties and their tendency to decrease stage 3 or 4 sleep (Harvey, 1985). However, such compounds may be useful in low dosage, combined with a tricyclic antidepressant, for promoting sleep, or may be used in low doses to help control overt daytime anxieties.

Mode of action of tricyclic antidepressant agents. The mechanisms of action of tricyclic antidepressant agents in relieving depression (Sethy and Harris, 1982; Pinder, 1985; Willner, 1985) or in improving sleep are not clearly understood. In vitro, these drugs block receptor reuptake of serotonin (5HT) and noradrenaline (norepinephrine) at the presynaptic nerve endings and also block α_2-adrenergic, histamine H_1 and histamine H_2 receptors. The various chemical compounds have different spectra of receptor affinities and pharmacological potencies, resulting in somewhat different clinical effects and particularly varied side-effects. Sedation is the most common side-effect of H_1 receptor antagonism, and may play a role in appetite stimulation. Doses used in the studies by Goldenberg et al (1986) and Carette et al (1986) were too small (25 mg and 50 mg respectively) and the effects occurred too soon to have been due to a clear-cut antidepressant effect (Goldenberg, 1989c). Tricyclics in low doses may improve sleep by blocking reuptake of brain serotonin (Russell, 1989). This sedative effect occurs early and with low doses, as opposed to an antidepressant effect. Another, more specific, serotonin receptor (5HT$_2$) antagonist, ritanserin, increases human slow wave sleep (Idzikowski et al, 1986), and may offer promise in FMS. Following improved sleep, patients often claim an improvement in mood and decreased fatigue. Depressed patients, however, require larger doses of tricyclics, suggesting that the poor sleep may be a secondary manifestation in them. Such patients may require phenothiazine drugs, on a short-term basis, and be followed concurrently by a psychiatric consultant.

Sleep problems, depression and the chronic pain connection

Interestingly, alterations in sleep physiology may precede clinical expression of psychiatric disorders such as depression (Reynolds and Kupfer, 1987). Also, the risk of developing new major depression was much higher in persons who had indicated sleep complaints at baseline and at follow-up one year later than in persons who had resolution of their sleep problems at the one-year evaluation (Ford and Kamerow, 1989). Also, patients having chronic pain, sleep disturbance or depression all showed objective polysomnographic findings, raising questions concerning interrelationships among these traits (Wittig et al, 1982). It seems reasonable to expect, therefore, that a subset of FMS patients with depression will have improvement in chronic pain from any medication that relieves the depression, not only the 'serotonergic' and more sedating TCAs, e.g. amitriptyline hydrochloride and doxepin hydrochloride. More recently approved selective serotonin reuptake inhibitors, such as fluoxitine hydrochloride (taken in low dosage, because of its tendency to promote anxiety and insomnia), may benefit carefully selected FMS patients. Presumably, patients with greater depressive and lesser anxiety or sleep-arousal problems would be considered. However, clinical trial data are not yet available to support such clinical impressions.

9. Anti-inflammatory and analgesic agents

Anti-inflammatory analgesics, e.g. salicylates or one of the non-steroidal anti-inflammatory drugs (NSAIDs), which might be tolerated, may be tried, but are usually of limited clinical benefit. This impression is supported by two controlled trials (Goldenberg et al, 1986; Yunus et al, 1989d). However, since some patients claim symptomatic relief from these drugs, and since decreased prostaglandins might theoretically modulate effects of bradykinin in nociception, empiric trials would seem to be reasonable, although possibly of placebo benefit. Medications should be taken on regular dosage schedules for greater efficacy, rather than as required.

An uncontrolled trial reported benefit of phenylbutazone and oxyphenbutazone in treatment of primary fibrositis (Klinefelter, 1972). Further study of these compounds in FMS might be useful. Paracetamol may be considered if side-effects preclude use of NSAIDs, but controlled data are not available. Systemic oral corticosteroids do not provide significant symptomatic relief in fibromyalgia (Clark et al, 1985b), which supports its non-inflammatory nature, and these compounds are not indicated. Narcotic analgesics are also not advised in this condition, because of the potential for addiction. The same may be said for chronic, high doses of muscle relaxant drugs.

The role of endorphins and brain serotonin in possibly modifying pain tolerance requires further study, as well as the possible effects of salicylates (or NSAIDs) and TCAs on these endogenous compounds.

10. Injection of disabling tender points or trigger points; osteopathic and other somatic treatments

Tender point or trigger point (TP) injections

Precisely localized injections can provide prompt, dramatic relief of incapacitating TPs (Masi, 1987; Sheon et al, 1987; Yunus, 1988). However, the disabling and most symptomatic TPs must be exactly localized with firm finger palpation (sufficient to cause the nailbed to blanch). TPs that do not respond to more conservative therapy, e.g. exercise, warmth and stretching, usually improve with injection. However, since an average fibromyalgia patient may have a dozen or more TPs, many unknown to the patient, random TP injections cannot be expected to be of much benefit. A small minority of FMS patients may need TP injections at any particular visit.

Hypersensitivity to a local anaesthetic agent should be excluded before attempting injection. The exact site of the intended injection should be marked on the overlying skin, using rotary pressure and the back end of the sterilizing swab. Sterile technique, but not necessarily gloves, should be used. Dilute local anaesthetic is first infiltrated intracutaneously with the narrowest available needle (e.g. 30 gauge). The localized, intramuscular TP is then radially ('fan' or 'spoke-wheel') infiltrated with a longer needle. The narrowest gauge needle consistent with tissue resistance and depth of the TP (under the fatty layer) should be used. A 27-gauge, 32-mm or 38-mm length may be used in a thin person or a 25-gauge, 89-mm length (spinal needle) in an obese patient. Local anaesthetic alone may be used or followed with a combination of a depot corticosteroid (recommended for soft tissue injections) mixed with a local anaesthetic (in a ratio of steroid to anaesthetic of 1:3 to 1:5). Precautions should be taken to avoid penetrating cavities, particularly the pleural space.

After the most acute TP has been anaesthetized, re-examination of the area may uncover another significant, adjacent TP, which could not be detected earlier because of generalized tenderness and reflex spasm. Further symptomatic relief in this area can be achieved after the second injection. Usually, not more than three or four TPs should be injected at one time.

Injection will often result in elimination of a disabling TP for a month or two or longer, especially if a regular stretching programme is maintained. Rarely, patients may have increased pain for one or two days at the injection site. Such postinjection flares can be minimized by application of cold compresses and rest of the local area for a day or two.

Patients, especially older ones, should lie down for a few minutes after injection of a local anaesthetic, since a few may experience transient dizziness. Rarely, panic reactions may occur, which may last up to half an hour. Rapid accumulation of local anaesthetic or inadvertent intravenous injection can cause serious side-effects, such as shock. For this reason, the plunger on the syringe should *always* be pulled back, to note any aspiration of blood, before each infiltration, to avoid direct intravascular injection.

Osteopathic manipulative treatment

Perhaps the oldest and most comforting physical treatment is the 'laying on of hands', be it a compassionate touch, gentle massage or muscle manipulation. Within the latter category, some therapists recommend anaesthetic spray and direct muscle stretch to relieve trigger points rather than injection (Travell and Simons, 1983; Simons, 1986). Such a manoeuvre is but one of many other osteopathic manipulative treatment techniques (Korr, 1978, 1986). Controlled studies are needed to determine the most effective approach to relieving TPs under various clinical circumstances.

Transcutaneous electrical nerve stimulation

In resistant cases, transcutaneous electrical nerve stimulation (TENS) may be of some benefit (McCain, 1989), but further study is required, especially in view of the absence of benefit to sufferers from chronic low back pain (Deyo et al, 1990).

Chiropractic treatment

No controlled study of chiropractic treatment in FMS has been reported and its possible benefits are unknown. Patients with chronic, severe low back pain of mechanical origin were reported to benefit more from chiropractic treatment than from hospital outpatient treatment in a randomized comparison study (Meade et al, 1990). These techniques and osteopathic manipulative treatment (Korr, 1978) deserve further investigation in FMS.

Acupuncture

Although acupuncture has been reported to be effective in an uncontrolled study of myofascial pain syndromes and fibrositis (Waylonis, 1977), scientific confirmation is lacking for this technique.

Oestrogen replacement therapy

In an uncontrolled, observational study, 65 of 100 fibromyalgia patients had onset of menopause (mean age 42 years) before diagnosis of fibromyalgia (mean age 46), suggesting that oestrogen deficit might be a promoting factor which should be treated in the management of fibromyalgia (Waxman and McSherry Zatzkis, 1986).

11. Psychological therapy and improvement of coping strategies

Patients typically require some degree of emotional support, but not usually formal psychological therapy (Table 5). Referral for psychological intervention, if necessary, should be done skilfully. Focus should be maintained on the reality of the physical problems in fibromyalgia and on continuing an established patient–physician relationship. Such consultations need not generally be obtained at an early phase of management.

Table 5. Psychological and coping strategies to help control fibromyalgia.

- Engage in pain-distracting activities and cultivate good spirits (develop behavioural habits that combat depression)
- Develop optimistic attitudes and try not to fear the worst (think positively and maintain faith)
- Strive to maintain calmness and control of anxiety (address problems or crises 'one step at a time')
- Practice self-assurance and self-confidence, but be realistic (avoid unwarranted panic and despair)
- Strengthen interactions with family and friends (basic interpersonal support relationships and human assets)
- Control unreasonable inhibitions or insecurities (promote outgoing traits in social support relationships)
- Cultivate a tolerance for emotional stresses and strains (try to 'toughen up', downplay self-incrimination and guilt)
- Be active, take action, but try not to 'settle' crises when unprepared (face each day's 'ups and downs' as smoothly as possible)

Psychological consultation and stress management programmes

Some patients do require consultation for significant psychological disturbance, including anxiety, stress or depression. Consultants, particularly those trained and interested in the management of chronic pain and other functional somatic disorders, may successfully use various measures such as biofeedback (Ferraccioli et al, 1987) and cognitive–behavioural therapy (Bradley, 1989). Although one study reported efficacy of biofeedback methods in PFS (Ferraccioli et al, 1987), this modality has not been tested adequately. Interestingly, hypnosis has been reported to be effective in treatment of a patient with myofibrositis and anxiety (Elkins, 1984).

Role conflicts

Professional mothers and wives, for example, can engender considerable psychological stresses and anxieties, which may be seen among fibromyalgia patients. In addition, such persons may display physical fatigue or 'burn-out' from actual or perceived excessive demands. The astute physician commonly encounters such problems in various functional disorders and must question whether or not the patient feels psychologically trapped within her or his life's circumstances. If so, the possibility that such circumstances may be contributing to FMS should be explored in a supportive manner.

Specialized pain centres

The resources of a specialized pain centre may be considered for difficult fibromyalgia patients. A multidisciplinary approach is used, employing a team of anaesthetists, psychiatrists, psychologists, physical therapists, occupational therapists and social workers, who are usually well-trained to give intensive care to chronic pain patients. However, specialized knowledge without caring, supportive attitudes and rehabilitative programmes may not necessarily achieve better results than the informed, compassionate primary physician.

12. Encourage the patient's commitment to assume management responsibility

Last but not least, successful management is highly dependent upon the patient making a commitment to assume positive attitudes in the process of self-rehabilitation. An attitude of 'pain behaviour' must be actively translated into 'well behaviour'. Passive dependence upon a care-giver is counterproductive! Care-givers who convey compassion and reasoned optimism are more likely to mobilize the patient's responsibility and initiatives in their management plan.

Restful sleep, improved posture, moderate physical activities, increased aerobic conditioning and emotional strengthening can all be important ingredients in the recipe for improvement. Although difficult, these examples are not impossible to achieve. However, patients must make the commitment to change their predisposing behaviour, in the hope of alleviating their painful condition. Loved ones can also help motivate patients. Specialist consultation of a rheumatologist, psychiatrist or pain clinic may be needed for difficult patients who do not respond to the primary physician's programme. However, one must avoid medicalization of social problems (Hadler, 1986) and be wary of symptoms generated for secondary gains, even if unintentionally, by the patient (Fordyce, 1976, 1988).

COURSE AND PROGNOSIS

Limited quantitative information is available on the prognosis, course and outcome of fibromyalgia (Felson and Goldenberg, 1986; Hawley et al, 1988). Yearly telephone interviews of 39 fibromyalgia patients over three years revealed that 60% had continued moderate or severe symptoms. Initially mild symptoms were indicators of a better prognosis (Felson and Goldenberg, 1986). Questionnaires mailed monthly to 75 fibromyalgia patients, for 12 months, revealed that individuals were generally stable over time, although variability was found among them. Global disease severity correlated with pain and psychologic status (anxiety and depression) scales and also with an indicator of functional status (Hawley et al, 1988). Further research in this area is important to patient management and health care planning.

One clinical opinion is that 'fibromyalgia is forever' (Smythe and Sheon, 1990). As fibromyalgia is usually chronic, care-givers and patients should understand that once the foundations of an effective management programme are established, continued intermittent monitoring and reinforcement are important for successful maintenance.

CONCLUSION

Chronic pain is a personal and emotional experience. Fibromyalgia may not be adequately explained (or understood) by abnormalities at any one level of the host's biology, such as the peripheral muscles or nerves, the intermediary neurohormones influencing pain transmission and sleep quality, or the ultimate cognitive perceptions and affective reactions. Personal imbalances may exist in some or all of these areas, as well as in the relationships of the individual to social and physical environments. This holistic view (Masi, 1978) suggests that primary fibromyalgia syndrome may be (at least in part) a 'maladaptive' phenomenon. It may result from aberrant patterns of general systems reactivity, rather than from specific tissue abnormalities or predispositions *per se*. Proper study and management of fibromyalgia may require a general systems theory approach (Von Bertalanffy, 1968) and a new medical model (Engel, 1977, 1980). For the present, critical research in each area of relevance to fibromyalgia is welcomed. Effective integration of such information can lead to meaningful concepts of this disorder and improved management, if not prevention, in the future.

The best treatment of fibromyalgia now available is a personalized, comprehensive, ambulatory management programme, in which the patient assumes the major responsibilities for self-rehabilitation. A detailed, personalized history of factors affecting manifestations is essential, more to help patients understand their pain dynamics and dysfunctions, and how these may be rationally managed, than simply to make a diagnosis. A complete examination is equally important, to detect the degree of physical contributors and support a firm diagnosis. The extent of the patient's tender points or disability may be documented, as well as any associated or underlying conditions. Laboratory testing should be guided by any abnormalities found on clinical evaluation, but is usually of limited value.

After arriving at a firm and convincing diagnosis, the next priority is to reassure the patient of its benign nature. Then the patient should be educated in simple terms as to how various physical and personal factors contribute to fibromyalgia manifestations. The patient should be offered emotional support and motivation to pursue behavioural changes necessary for self-rehabilitation. Somatic management often includes correction of postural abnormalities and other factors to reduce chronic stresses on the lower cervical and lower lumbar regions; alleviation of other perpetuating physical stresses; physical conditioning; maintaining body warmth (i.e. avoidance of chilling); and other measures, e.g. promoting deep sleep, as indicated and reviewed. These measures can all offer some benefits.

Importantly, some patients will require more emotional support than others. Care-givers should assess and provide personally or through consultation of colleagues, the necessary psychological support and behavioural guidance. Formal psychotherapy is seldom needed in this condition; rather, empathy, compassion, understanding and personal counselling are beneficial.

Patients must understand and be willing to assume the serious, continuing responsibility for maintaining their individualized management programmes. When presented in a personalized, supportive fashion, patient responsibilities are more likely to be accepted in this chronic disorder. Management of fibromyalgia patients is challenging and largely intuitive, depending upon the care-givers' perceptions of the major contributory factors. Often, this care is effective and assuring to patients, especially when offered with a measure of human kindness, clinical experience and judgment.

Acknowledgements

We wish to express our sincere appreciation of the Word Processing Center Staff of the University of Illinois College of Medicine at Peoria for their excellent cooperation in preparation of this manuscript, to Jo Dorsch and Bobbi Vanover for their generous help with literature searches and documentation, and to our secretary, Margaret Walsh, for general assistance. Also, we would like to thank Drs Brian Curtis, Anthony M. Masi, Christopher M. Masi and Walter L. Norton for their critical reviews of the manuscript and suggestions, as well as several FMS patients who have contributed essential insights into this perspective.

REFERENCES

Agnoli A, Canonico PL, Milhaud G & Scapagnini V (eds) (1985) *Spasmophilia: Calcium Metabolism and Cell Physiology*. Proceedings of the First International Symposium, Rome, 28–29 April 1984. London: John Libbey.

Ahles TA, Yunus MB, Riley SD, Bradley JM & Masi AT (1984) Psychological factors associated with primary fibromyalgia syndrome. *Arthritis and Rheumatism* 27: 1101–1106.

Ahles TA, Khan SA, Yunus MB, Spiegel DA & Masi AT (submitted for publication). Psychiatric status of primary fibromyalgia and rheumatoid arthritis patients and nonpain controls: comparison of data from the psychiatric diagnostic interview and the MMPI.

American Psychiatric Association (1987) Generalized anxiety disorder. In *Diagnostic and Statistical Manual of Mental Disorders*, 3rd edn, revised, pp 251–253. Washington, DC: American Psychiatric Association.

Beighton P, Grahame R & Bird H (1989) *Hypermobility of Joints*, 2nd edn. London: Springer-Verlag.

Bengtsson A & Henriksson KG (1989) The muscle in fibromyalgia—a review of Swedish studies. *Journal of Rheumatology* 16 (supplement 19): 144–149.

Bengtsson A, Henriksson KG & Larsson J (1986) Reduced high-energy phosphate levels in the painful muscles of patients with primary fibromyalgia. *Arthritis and Rheumatism* 29: 817–821.

Bennett RM (1981) Fibrositis: misnomer for a common rheumatic disorder. *Western Journal of Medicine* 134: 405–413.

Bennett RM (1989a) Fibrositis. In Kelley WN, Harris ED, Ruddy S & Sledge CB (eds) *Textbook of Rheumatology*, 3rd edn, pp 541–553. Philadelphia: W.B. Saunders.

Bennett RM (1989b) Beyond fibromyalgia: ideas on etiology and treatment. *Journal of Rheumatology* 16 (supplement 19): 185–191.

Bennett RM (1989c) Muscle physiology and cold reactivity in the fibromyalgia syndrome. *Rheumatic Disease Clinics of North America* 15: 135–147.

Bennett RM, Gatter RA, Campbell SM et al (1988) A comparison of cyclobenzaprine and placebo in the management of fibrositis. *Arthritis and Rheumatism* **31:** 1535–1542.

Bennett RM, Clark S, Goldberg L et al (1989) Aerobic fitness in patients with fibrositis: a controlled study of respiratory gas exchange and xenon[133] clearance from exercising muscle. *Arthritis and Rheumatism* **32:** 454–460.

Blumer D & Heilbronn M (1982) Chronic pain as a variant of depressive disease: the pain-prone disorder. *Journal of Nervous and Mental Diseases* **170:** 381–406.

Bradley LA (1989) Cognitive-behavioral therapy for primary fibromyalgia. *Journal of Rheumatology* **16** (supplement 19): 131–136.

Breier A, Albus M, Pickar D et al (1987) Controllable and uncontrollable stress in humans: alterations in mood and neuroendocrine and psychophysiological function. *American Journal of Psychiatry* **144:** 1419–1426.

Campbell SM (1989) Regional myofascial pain syndromes. *Rheumatic Disease Clinics of North America* **15:** 31–44.

Campbell SM, Clark S, Tindall EA, Forehand ME & Bennett RM (1983) Clinical characteristics of fibrositis: I. a 'blinded', controlled study of symptoms and tender points. *Arthritis and Rheumatism* **26:** 817–824.

Carette S, McCain GA, Bell DA & Fam AG (1986) Evaluation of amitriptyline in primary fibrositis: a double-blind, placebo-controlled study. *Arthritis and Rheumatism* **29:** 655–659.

Caro XJ (1989) Is there an immunologic component to the fibrositis syndrome? *Rheumatic Disease Clinics of North America* **15:** 169–186.

Clark S, Campbell SM, Forehand ME et al (1985a) Clinical characteristics of fibrositis: II. a 'blinded', controlled study using standard psychological tests. *Arthritis and Rheumatism* **28:** 132–137.

Clark S, Tindall E, Bennett RM (1985b) A double blind crossover trial of prednisone versus placebo in the treatment of fibrositis. *Journal of Rheumatology* **12:** 980–983.

Deyo RA, Walsh NE, Martin DC et al (1990) A controlled trial of transcutaneous electrical nerve stimulation (TENS) and exercise for chronic low back pain. *New England Journal of Medicine* **322:** 1627–1634.

Elkins GR (1984) Hypnosis in the treatment of myofibrositis and anxiety: a case report. *American Journal of Clinical Hypnosis* **27:** 26–30.

Emre M & Mathies H (eds) (1988) *Muscle Spasms and Pain*. Park Ridge, NJ: Parthenon.

Engel GL (1977) The need for a new medical model: a challenge for biomedicine. *Science* **196:** 129–136.

Engel GL (1980) The clinical application of the biopsychosocial model. *American Journal of Psychiatry* **137:** 535–544.

Felson DT & Goldenberg DL (1986) The natural history of fibromyalgia. *Arthritis and Rheumatism* **29:** 1522–1526.

Fletcher DJ (1986) Coping with insomnia: helping patients manage sleeplessness without drugs. *Postgraduate Medicine* **79:** 265–274.

Ford DE & Kamerow DB (1989) Epidemiologic study of sleep disturbances and psychiatric disorders: an opportunity for prevention? *Journal of the American Medical Association* **262:** 1479–1484.

Fordyce WE (1976) *Behavioral Methods for Chronic Pain and Illness*. St Louis: C.V. Mosby.

Fordyce WE (1988) Pain and suffering: a reappraisal. *American Psychologist* **43:** 276–283.

Ferraccioli G, Ghirelli L, Scita F et al (1987) EMG–biofeedback training in fibromyalgia syndrome. *Journal of Rheumatology* **14:** 820–825.

Garrett RA (1989) Chronic pain syndromes. In Kelley WN, Harris ED, Ruddy S & Sledge CB (eds) *Textbook of Rheumatology*, 3rd edn, pp 1860–1903. Philadelphia: W.B. Saunders.

Goldenberg DL (1987) Fibromyalgia syndrome: an emerging but controversial condition. *Journal of the American Medical Association* **257:** 2782–2787.

Goldenberg DL (1989a) Treatment of fibromyalgia syndrome. *Rheumatic Disease Clinics of North America* **15:** 61–71.

Goldenberg DL (1989b) A review of the role of tricyclic medications in the treatment of fibromyalgia syndrome. *Journal of Rheumatology* **16** (supplement 19): 137–139.

Goldenberg DL (1989c) Psychiatric and psychologic aspects of fibromyalgia syndrome. *Rheumatic Disease Clinics of North America* **15:** 105–114.

Goldenberg DL, Felson DT & Dinerman H (1986) A randomized controlled trial of amitriptyline and naproxen in the treatment of patients with fibromyalgia. *Arthritis and Rheumatism* **29:** 1371–1377.

Goldenberg DL, Simms RW, Geiger A & Komaroff AL (1990) High frequency of fibromyalgia in patients with chronic fatigue seen in a primary care practice. *Arthritis and Rheumatism* **33:** 381–387.

Gowers WR (1904) Lumbago: its lessons and analogues. *British Medical Journal* **1:** 117–121.

Grahame R (1990) The hypermobility syndrome. *Annals of the Rheumatic Diseases* **49:** 199–200.

Guyton AC (1986) *Textbook of Medical Physiology*, 7th edn. Philadelphia: W.B. Saunders.

Hadler NM (1986) A critical reappraisal of the fibrositis concept. *American Journal of Medicine* **81** (supplement 3A): 26–30.

Harvey SC (1985) Hypnotics and sedatives. In Gilman AG, Goodman LS, Rall TW & Murad F (eds) *Goodman and Gillman's The Pharmacological Basis of Therapeutics*, 7th edn, pp 340–371. New York: Macmillan.

Harvey JA, Schlosberg AJ & Yunger LM (1975) Behavioral correlates of serotonin depletion. *Federation Proceedings* **34:** 1796–1801.

Hawley DJ, Wolfe F & Cathey MA (1988) Pain, functional disability, and psychological status: a 12-month study of severity in fibromyalgia. *Journal of Rheumatology* **15:** 1551–1556.

Hench PK (1989) Evaluation and differential diagnosis of fibromyalgia: approach to diagnosis and management. *Rheumatic Disease Clinics of North America* **15:** 19–29.

Hench PK & Mitler MM (1986) Fibromyalgia. 2. Management guidelines and research findings. *Postgraduate Medicine* **80:** 57–69.

Hudson JI & Pope HG (1989) Fibromyalgia and psychopathology: is fibromyalgia a form of 'affective spectrum disorder?' *Journal of Rheumatology* **16** (supplement 19): 15–22.

Idzikowski C, Mills FJ & Glennard R (1986) 5-Hydroxytryptamine-2 antagonist increases human slow wave sleep. *Brain Research* **378:** 164–168.

International Association for the Study of Pain Subcommittee on Taxonomy (1986) Fibrositis or diffuse myofascial pain syndrome (I-9) (Non-articular rheumatism, fibromyalgia). *Pain* **25** (supplement 3): S33–36.

Jacobsen S & Danneskiold-Samsøe B (1987) Isometric and isokinetic muscle strength in patients with fibrositis syndrome. *Scandinavian Journal of Rheumatology* **16:** 61–65.

Jacobsen S & Danneskiold-Samsøe B (1989) Inter-relations between clinical parameters and muscle function in patients with fibromyalgia. *Clinical and Experimental Rheumatology* **7:** 493–498.

Kaplan PE & Tanner ED (1989) *Musculoskeletal Pain and Disability*. Norwalk: Appleton & Lange.

Kessler RM & Hertling D (1988) *Management of Common Musculoskeletal Disorders: Physical Therapy Principles and Methods*. Philadelphia: J.B. Lippincott.

Klinefelter HE (1972) Primary fibrositis and its treatment with the pyrazolone derivatives, butazolidin and tanderil. *Johns Hopkins Medical Journal* **130:** 300–307.

Klug GA, McAuley E & Clark S (1989) Factors influencing the development and maintenance of aerobic fitness: lessons applicable to the fibrositis syndrome. *Journal of Rheumatology* **16** (supplement 19): 30–39.

Korr IM (1978) *The Neurobiologic Mechanisms in Manipulative Therapy*. New York: Plenum Press.

Korr IM (1986) Somatic dysfunction, osteopathic manipulative treatment, and the nervous system: a few facts, some theories, many questions. *Journal of the American Osteopathic Association* **86:** 109–114.

Kushmerick MJ (1989) Muscle energy metabolism, nuclear magnetic resonance spectroscopy and their potential in the study of fibromyalgia. *Journal of Rheumatology* **16** (supplement 19): 40–46.

Lal H, LaBella F & Lane J (eds) (1985) *Endocoids*. New York: Alan R. Liss.

Littlejohn GO (1989) Fibrositis/fibromyalgia syndrome in the workplace. *Rheumatic Disease Clinics of North America* **15:** 45–60.

Lund N, Bengtsson A & Thorborg P (1986) Muscle tissue oxygen pressure in primary fibromyalgia. *Scandinavian Journal of Rheumatology* **15:** 165–173.

Manu P, Matthews DA & Lane TJ (1988a) The mental health of patients with a chief complaint of chronic fatigue: a prospective evaluation and follow-up. *Archives of Internal Medicine* **148:** 2213–2217.

Manu P, Lane TJ & Matthews DA (1988b) The frequency of the chronic fatigue syndrome in patients with symptoms of persistent fatigue. *Annals of Internal Medicine* 109: 554–556.

Masi AT (1978) An holistic concept of health and illness: a tricentennial goal for medicine and public health (editorial). *Journal of Chronic Diseases* 31: 563–572.

Masi AT & Yunus MB (1986) Concepts of illness in populations as applied to fibromyalgia syndromes. *American Journal of Medicine* 81 (supplement 3A): 19–25.

Masi AT (1987) Nonarticular rheumatism. In Berkow R & Fletcher AJ (eds) *The Merck Manual of Diagnosis and Therapy*, 15th edn, p 1268. Rahway NJ: Merck, Sharp & Dohme.

Mau W (1988) Primary functional causes of soft tissue pain (primary fibromyalgia). In Emre M & Mathies H (eds) *Muscle Spasms and Pain*, pp 33–42. Park Ridge, NJ: Parthenon.

Mayer TG, Gatchel RJ, Mayer H, Kishino ND, Keeley J & Mooney V (1987) A prospective two-year study of functional restoration in industrial low back injury. *Journal of the American Medical Association* 258: 1763–1767.

McCain GA (1989) Nonmedicinal treatments in primary fibromyalgia. *Rheumatic Disease Clinics of North America* 15: 73–90.

McCain GA, Bell DA, Mai FM & Holliday PD (1989) A controlled study of the effects of a supervised cardiovascular fitness training program on the manifestations of primary fibromyalgia. *Arthritis and Rheumatism* 31: 1135–1141.

Meade TW, Dyer S, Browne W, Townsend J & Frank AO (1990) Low back pain of mechanical origin: randomized comparison of chiropractic and hospital outpatient treatment. *British Medical Journal* 300: 1431–1437.

Melzack R (1981) Myofascial trigger points: relation to acupuncture and mechanism of pain. *Archives of Physical Medicine and Rehabilitation* 62: 114–117.

Melzack R, Stillwell DM & Fox EI (1977) Trigger points and acupuncture points for pain: correlations and implications. *Pain* 3: 2–23.

Miller DR & Seifert RD (1987) Management of fibromyalgia, a distinct rheumatologic syndrome. *Clinical Pharmacy* 6: 778–786.

Moldofsky H (1982) Rheumatic pain modulation syndrome: the inter-relationships between sleep, CNS serotonin and pain. In Critchley M, Friedman AP, Sicuteri F et al (eds) *Advances in Neurology*, vol. 33, *Headache: Physiopathological and Clinical Concepts*, pp 51–57. New York: Raven Press.

Moldofsky H (1989a) Sleep and fibrositis syndrome. *Rheumatic Disease Clinics of North America* 15: 91–103.

Moldofsky H (1989b) Sleep-wake mechanisms in fibrositis. *Journal of Rheumatology* 16 (supplement 19): 47–48.

Moldofsky H & Lue FA (1980) The relationship of alpha and delta EEG frequencies to pain and mood in 'fibrositis' patients treated with chlorpromazine and L-tryptophan. *Electroencephalography and Clinical Neurophysiology* 50: 71–80.

Moldofsky H, Scarisbrick P, England R & Smythe H (1975) Musculoskeletal symptoms and non-REM sleep disturbance in patients with 'fibrositis' syndrome and healthy subjects. *Psychosomatic Medicine* 37: 341–351.

Moldofsky H, Lue FA & Smythe HA (1983) Alpha EEG sleep and morning symptoms in rheumatoid arthritis. *Journal of Rheumatology* 10: 373–379.

Newham DJ (1988) The consequences of eccentric contractions and their relationship to delayed onset muscle pain. *European Journal of Applied Physiology* 57: 353–359.

Nixon PGF (1989) Hyperventilation and cardiac symptoms. *Internal Medicine for the Specialist* 10: 67–84.

Paul SM (1988) Anxiety and depression: a common neurobiological substrate? *Journal of Clinical Psychiatry* 49 (10 supplement): 13–16.

Pinder RM (1985) α_2-Adrenoceptor antagonists as antidepressants. *Drugs of the Future* 10: 841–857.

Quimby LG, Block SR & Gratwick GM (1988) Fibromyalgia: generalized pain intolerance and manifold symptom reporting. *Journal of Rheumatology* 15: 1264–1270.

Quimby LG, Gratwick GM, Whitney CD & Block SR (1989) A randomized trial of cyclobenzaprine for treatment of fibromyalgia. *Journal of Rheumatology* 16 (supplement 19): 140–143.

Reuler JB, Girard DE & Nardone DA (1980) The chronic pain syndrome: misconceptions and management. *Annals of Internal Medicine* 93: 588–596.

Reynolds MD (1983) The development of the concept of fibrositis. *Journal of History of Medicine and Allied Sciences* **38:** 5–35.

Reynolds CF & Kupfer DJ (1987) Sleep research in affective illness: state of the art circa 1987. *Sleep* **10:** 199–215.

Russell IJ (1989) Neurohormonal aspects of fibromyalgia syndrome. *Rheumatic Disease Clinics of North America* **15:** 149–168.

Schumacher HR (1988) Classification of the rheumatic diseases. In Schumacher HR, Klippel JH & Robinson DR (eds) *Primer on the Rheumatic Diseases*, 9th edn, pp 81–82. Atlanta: Arthritis Foundation.

Sethy VH & Harris DW (1982) Role of beta-adrenergic receptors in the mechanism of action of second-generation antidepressants. *Drug Development Research* **2:** 403–406.

Sheon RP, Moskowitz RW & Goldberg VM (1987) Intralesional soft tissue injection technique. In *Soft Tissue Rheumatic Pain: Recognition, Management, Prevention*, 2nd edn, pp 293–300. Philadelphia: Lea & Febiger.

Siegler EL & Beck LH (1989) Stiffness: a pathophysiologic approach to diagnosis and treatment. *Journal of General Internal Medicine* **4:** 533–540.

Sigal LH (1990) Summary of the first 100 patients seen at a Lyme disease referral center. *American Journal of Medicine* **88:** 577–581.

Simons DG (1986) Fibrositis/fibromyalgia: a form of myofascial trigger points? *American Journal of Medicine* **81** (supplement 3A): 93–98.

Smythe HA (1989a) Fibrositis syndrome: a historical perspective. *Journal of Rheumatology* **15** (supplement 19): 2–6.

Smythe HA (1989b) Nonarticular rheumatism and psychogenic musculoskeletal syndromes. In McCarty DJ (ed) *Arthritis and Allied Conditions: a Textbook of Rheumatology*, pp 1241–1254. Philadelphia: Lea & Febiger.

Smythe HA & Sheon RP (1990)0 Fibrositis/fibromyalgia: a difference of opinion. *Bulletin on the Rheumatic Diseases* **39:** 1–8.

Sola AE (1981) Myofascial trigger point therapy. *Resident and Staff Physician* **27:** 38–46.

Travell JG & Simons DG (1983) *Myofascial Pain and Dysfunction: The Trigger Point Manual.* Baltimore: Williams & Wilkins.

Turk DC & Flor H (1989) Primary fibromyalgia is greater than tender points: toward a multiaxial taxonomy. *Journal of Rheumatology* **16** (supplement 19): 80–86.

Vaerøy H, Sakurada T, Førre Ø, Kass E & Terenius L (1989) Modulation of pain in fibromyalgia (fibrositis syndrome): cerebrospinal fluid (CSF) investigation of pain related neuropeptides with special reference to calcitonin gene related peptide (CGRP). *Journal of Rheumatology* **16** (supplement 19): 94–97.

Vitali C, Tavoni A, Rossi B et al (1989) Evidence of neuromuscular hyperexcitability features in patients with primary fibromyalgia. *Clinical and Experimental Rheumatology* **7:** 385–390.

Von Bertalanffy L (1968) *General Systems Theory.* New York: Braziller.

Wall PD & Melzack R (eds) (1989) *Textbook of Pain*, 2nd edn. Edinburgh: Churchill Livingstone.

Waxman J & McSherry Zatzkis S (1986) Fibromyalgia and menopause: examination of the relationship. *Postgraduate Medicine* **80:** 165–171.

Waylonis GW (1977) Long-term follow-up on patients with fibrositis treated with acupuncture. *Ohio State Medical Journal* **73:** 299–302.

Willner P (1985) Antidepressants and serotonergic neurotransmission: an integrative review. *Psychopharmacology* **85:** 387–404.

Wittig RM, Zorick FJ, Blumer D, Heilbronn M & Roth T (1982) Disturbed sleep in patients complaining of chronic pain. *Journal of Nervous and Mental Disease* **170:** 429–431.

Wolf S (1990) Studying the person in the patient: a look back at developments. *Pharos* **53:** 38–40.

Wolfe F (1988) Fibromyalgia: whither treatment? (editorial). *Journal of Rheumatology* **15:** 1047–1049.

Wolfe F (1989) Fibromyalgia: the clinical syndrome. *Rheumatic Disease Clinics of North America* **15:** 1–18.

Wolfe F, Smythe HA, Yunus MB et al (1990) The American College of Rheumatology 1990 criteria for classification of fibromyalgia: report of the multicenter criteria committee. *Arthritis and Rheumatism* **33:** 160–172.

Yunus MB (1983) Fibromyalgia syndrome: a need for uniform classification. *Journal of Rheumatology* **10**: 841–844.

Yunus MB (1988) Diagnosis, etiology, and management of fibromyalgia syndrome: an update. *Comprehensive Therapy* **14**: 8–20.

Yunus MB & Kalyan-Raman U (1989) Muscle biopsy findings in primary fibromyalgia and other forms of nonarticular rheumatism. *Rheumatic Disease Clinics of North America* **15**: 115–134.

Yunus M, Masi AT, Calabro JJ, Miller KA & Feigenbaun SL (1981) Primary fibromyalgia (fibrositis): clinical study of 50 patients with matched normal controls. *Seminars in Arthritis and Rheumatism* **11**: 151–171.

Yunus MB, Holt GS, Masi AT & Aldag JC (1988) Fibromyalgia syndrome among the elderly: comparison with younger patients. *Journal of the American Geriatrics Society* **36**: 987–995.

Yunus MB, Masi AT & Aldag JC (1989a) A controlled study of primary fibromyalgia syndrome: clinical features and association with other functional syndromes. *Journal of Rheumatology* **16** (supplement 19): 62–71.

Yunus MB, Masi AT & Aldag JC (1989b) Preliminary criteria for primary fibromyalgia syndrome (PFS): multivariate analysis of a consecutive series of PFS, other pain patients, and normal subjects. *Clinical and Experimental Rheumatology* **7**: 63–69.

Yunus MB, Berg BC & Masi AT (1989c) Multiphase skeletal scintigraphy in primary fibromyalgia syndrome: a blinded study. *Journal of Rheumatology* **16**: 1466–1468.

Yunus MB, Masi AT & Aldag JC (1989d) Short-term effects of ibuprofen in primary fibromyalgia syndrome: a double blind, placebo controlled trial. *Journal of Rheumatology* **16**: 527–532.

Yunus MB, Ahles TA, Aldag JC & Masi AT (1990) Clinical features in primary fibromyalgia: relationship with psychologic status. *Arthritis and Rheumatism* (in press).

Zidar J, Bäckman E, Bengtsson A & Henriksson KG (1990) Quantitative EMG and muscle tension in painful muscles in fibromyalgia. *Pain* **40**: 249–254.

10

Non-steroidal anti-inflammatory drugs versus simple analgesics in the treatment of arthritis

PAUL A. SANDERS
DAVID M. GRENNAN

Twenty million non-steroidal anti-inflammatory drugs (NSAIDs) are prescribed annually in the UK National Health Service; these drugs represent 5% of all such prescriptions, but 25% of all voluntary yellow card reports on side-effects. Between 1964 and 1985 there were 3500 reports of upper gastrointestinal bleeding or perforation thought to be caused by NSAIDs, nearly 75% of these were in patients aged 60 years or older. Six hundred deaths were reported, 90% of which occurred in patients over 60 years old (Committee on Safety of Medicines, 1986). Eighty-five per cent of long-term NSAID treatment is initiated by general practitioners. Often NSAIDs are prescribed to elderly patients or patients with important medical conditions which may be adversely affected by the prescription, for example hypertension, heart failure, renal impairment and upper gastro-intestinal symptoms (Day et al, 1987). Steele et al (1987) reported that 46% of patients on long-term NSAID therapy suffered from one or more of these medical conditions and 38% were taking potentially interacting medicines. In view of these figures it is perhaps surprising that severe problems and deaths caused by NSAIDs are not reported more commonly. Prescription of NSAIDs is often inappropriate and NSAID-associated morbidity might be markedly reduced by an increased usage of other methods of treatment, such as local steroid injection therapy, physiotherapy and other physical treatments. NSAIDs are often prescribed for conditions that are conven-tionally considered non-inflammatory; as simple analgesics in therapeutic dosage are generally associated with fewer side-effects, the risks of NSAIDs might be reduced by more selective prescribing of NSAIDs and more frequent prescribing of simple analgesics.

Definitions

Pharmacological dogma tells us that *simple analgesics* are drugs that relieve pain, but do not affect the other clinical symptoms or signs of inflammation (i.e. erythema, warmth, loss of function); whereas *NSAIDs* have an analgesic action, but also in high dosage have an effect on the other cardinal features of inflammation by mechanisms that are thought to include interruption of the

Baillière's Clinical Rheumatology—
Vol. 4, No. 2, August 1990
ISBN 0–7020–1480–X

arachidonic acid pathway by prostaglandin synthetase or cyclo-oxygenase inhibition.

However, in low dosage even NSAIDs may have a purely analgesic effect. Furthermore, it is salutary to remember that the initial clinical studies (Boardman and Hart, 1967) which showed an anti-inflammatory effect for high-dose salicylates (5.3 g per day) did so by demonstrating a reduction in finger swelling (proximal interphalangeal joint circumference). The same authors (Hart and Boardman, 1963) showed similar effects with indomethacin. However, many more recent NSAIDs have not been shown to be truly anti-inflammatory by this strict criterion, and some may be merely acting as analgesics in the dosages commonly used.

Tables 1 and 2 respectively indicate simple non-narcotic analgesics and NSAIDs currently available on National Health Service prescription in Great Britain (*British National Formulary*, 1990). Narcotic analgesics are not indicated in the management of chronic musculoskeletal conditions, and compounds containing dextropropoxyphene or codeine should be used with caution.

Table 1. Analgesics currently available.

Drug	Proprietary name	Notes
Non-narcotic single preparations		
Paracetamol	Calpol	
	Disprol	
	Paldesic	
	Panadol	
	Panaleve	
	Salzone	
Nefopam	Acupan	
Combination preparations		
Co-codamol		paracetamol 500 mg, codeine phosphate 8 mg
Co-codaprin		aspirin 400 mg, codeine phosphate 8 mg
Co-dydramol		dihydrocodeine tartrate 10 mg, paracetamol 500 mg
Co-proxamol		dextropropoxyphene 32.5 mg, paracetamol 325 mg
Aspirin, paracetamol and codeine tablets		aspirin 250 mg, paracetamol 250 mg, codeine phosphate 6.8 mg
	Aspav	aspirin 500 mg, papaveretum 10 mg
	Fomulix	paracetamol 120 mg, codeine phosphate 12 mg
	Tylex	paracetamol 500 mg, codeine phosphate 30 mg

EFFICACY OF SIMPLE ANALGESICS IN INFLAMMATORY ARTHRITIS

The definitions of these categories of drugs imply preferential prescription of NSAIDs in inflammatory arthritis and of simple analgesics in non-inflammatory conditions. Evidence for the efficacy of simple analgesics used alone in inflammatory joint diseases is not good. Thus Fremont-Smith and Bayles (1965) investigated 11 patients with early, active rheumatoid arthritis

Table 2. NSAIDs currently available.

Drug	Proprietary name
Aspirin	Caprin
	Nu-seals Aspirin
Aloxiprin	Paraprin Forte
Benorylate*	Benoral
Choline magnesium trisalicylate	Trilisate
Salsalate	Disalcid
Sodium salicylate	
Azapropazone	Rheumox
Diclofenac sodium	Rhumalgan
	Voltarol
Diflunisal	Dolobid
Etodolac	Lodine
Fenbufen	Lederfen
Fenoprofen	Fenopron
Flurbiprofen	Froben
Ibuprofen	Apsifen
	Brufen
	Fenbid
	Ibular
	Lidifen
	Motrin
	Paxofen
Indomethacin	Flexin Continus
	Imbrilon
	Indocid
	Indocid-R
	Indolar SR
	Indomod
	Mobilan
	Rheumacin LA
	Slo-Indo
Ketoprofen	Alrheumat
	Orudis
	Oruvail
Mefenamic acid	Ponstan
Nabumetone	Relifex
Naproxen	Laraflex
	Naprosyn
	Synflex
Phenylbutazone†	Butacote
	Butazolidin
Piroxicam	Feldene
	Larapam
Sulindac	Clinoril
Tenoxicam	Mobiflex
Tiaprofenic acid	Surgam
	Surgam SA
Tolmetin	Tolectin

* Aspirin-paracetamol ester.
† Licensed only for ankylosing spondylitis (in hospital).

and one with systemic lupus erythematosus, and showed a flare of disease activity following salicylate withdrawal and its replacement by either dextropropoxyphene or narcotics (codeine or pethidine). Similarly, in a later study, Lee et al (1975) showed no significant improvement in terms of pain relief or patient satisfaction for paracetamol compared with placebo in patients with rheumatoid arthritis.

It should be added that there are difficulties in interpretation of study results where pain relief is used as the main method of clinical assessment, as pointed out by Huskisson (1974) who showed that the effectiveness of soluble placebo depended on its colour, and in some cases this could make placebo appear as effective as active analgesic drugs in rheumatoid arthritis.

In contrast, some evidence for the effectiveness of simple analgesics in rheumatoid arthritis was provided by Hardin and Kirk (1979) who found aspirin, paracetamol, codeine, pentazocine and dextropropoxyphene to be superior to placebo in providing pain relief in patients who had ceased background anti-inflammatory drugs 24–48 hours prior to the study.

There is more evidence that some—but not all—analgesic drugs may be useful as supplements to NSAIDs in inflammatory joint disease. Nuki et al (1973) performed a double-blind controlled crossover trial comparing pentazocine with placebo as a supplement to NSAID treatment in rheumatoid arthritis patients and found that the majority preferred the placebo (43% versus 20%), but this was probably due to the high incidence of side-effects on pentazocine (51% compared with 23% on placebo).

Huskisson (1974) showed using a pain relief score that effective supplementary analgesics in rheumatoid arthritis included low-dose aspirin (600 mg), Codis (aspirin and codeine) and co-proxamol (paracetamol and dextropropoxyphene). Paracetamol alone and pentazocine were of intermediate efficacy compared with placebo.

Nefopam also has a high incidence of side-effects but has been shown to be superior to placebo as a supplementary analgesic in rheumatoid arthritis in a double-blind crossover study (Emery and Gibson, 1986). Surprisingly, this drug was found to improve grip strength and duration of early morning stiffness as well as providing pain relief.

Dextropropoxyphene used as a supplement to an NSAID was found to be more effective than placebo in producing pain relief in a mixed group of patients with rheumatoid arthritis or osteoarthritis (Brooks et al, 1982).

A study of usage of analgesics as supplements to NSAIDs, in the form of a questionnaire completed by rheumatoid arthritis patients and their physicians (Gibson and Clark, 1985), showed that both groups considered simple analgesic prescription worth while. Indeed, 48% of those receiving analgesics as well as NSAIDs considered analgesics to be the more effective. Half the patients on analgesics were taking them without the knowledge of their rheumatologists. It appears therefore that patients perceive a clear need to take simple analgesics in addition to NSAIDs, a need that may be underestimated by their doctors.

Overall it appears that some analgesics may have a mild additive effect used in combination with NSAIDs in rheumatoid arthritis, although side-effects may limit their use. This problem should, however, be balanced by the possibility of reducing the NSAID dose, which may result in the lessening of potentially dangerous NSAID-related side-effects.

EFFICACY OF SIMPLE ANALGESICS IN NON-INFLAMMATORY ARTHRITIS

Simple analgesics are usually regarded as the first choice drugs in non-inflammatory rheumatic conditions, such as simple osteoarthritis (Nuki, 1983). Paracetamol used alone has been shown in a controlled study to have an analgesic effect in the treatment of osteoarthritis of the knee (Cummings and Amadio, 1983). Similarly, dextropropoxyphene has been shown to be superior to placebo in relieving osteoarthritis pain (Strumia and Babbini, 1973).

There are few controlled data on the relative efficacy of different simple analgesics in defined non-inflammatory articular disorders, although in the study by Brooks et al (1982) discussed above, dextropropoxyphene appeared to give better analgesia than placebo, aspirin alone, paracetamol alone, or combinations of dextropropoxyphene with paracetamol or aspirin, in a mixed group of 12 rheumatoid arthritis and 12 osteoarthritis patients.

EFFICACY OF NSAID IN INFLAMMATORY ARTHRITIS

Inflammation is a complex reaction to injury. Following cell damage, chemical mediators such as histamine, bradykinin, 5-hydroxytryptamine, slow-reacting substance of anaphylaxis (SRS-A), chemotactic factors and prostaglandins are released locally. Phagocytic cells migrate into the affected area and contribute to the reaction by releasing lytic enzymes. The ability of NSAIDs to inhibit the production of prostaglandins (by cyclo-oxygenase inhibition) has been thought to account for their anti-inflammatory effects, but various mechanisms have been proposed over the years including interference with cellular metabolism, with release of inflammatory mediators, with sodium and potassium ion transfer across cell membranes, inhibition of chemical mediators other than prostaglandins, and stabilization of lysosomes.

Current thinking suggests that NSAIDs provide symptomatic relief only, do not slow the progression of rheumatoid arthritis and have little effect on acute phase reactants (erythrocyte sedimentation rate, C-reactive protein). Numerous studies since the 1960s have demonstrated the efficacy of these drugs in clinical inflammatory joint disease (Fremont-Smith and Bayles, 1965; Mainland and Sutcliffe, 1965). NSAIDs are now regarded as the first choice in the treatment of the inflammatory features of rheumatoid arthritis, the seronegative arthritides and the juvenile inflammatory joint disorders (Huskisson, 1977; Levinson et al, 1977; Liebling et al, 1975).

Comparative studies of NSAIDs with each other and with aspirin almost ·always show them to be of equal effectiveness, but most of the newer preparations are less toxic than aspirin in full dosage. Despite the apparent similarities between the different NSAIDs available, it has been shown that there is marked interpatient variability in response to these drugs (Huskisson et al, 1976). Similar results have been reported by other authors, including a study of 10 NSAIDs in RA by Scott et al (1982) who concluded that ranking NSAIDs according to potency was not a clinically useful exercise. Often a patient preference for a particular NSAID will be sustained for a long time. This interpatient variability of response may be multifactorial. It may depend on the patients' own perceptions, the patients' and doctors' knowledge of alternative preparations, or perhaps on the severity or type of disease treated. Additionally there may be pharmaco-kinetic reasons for the variability. For example, the degree and reversibility of cyclo-oxygenase inhibition can differ, also the degree of interference with leukotriene production. It would be expected that NSAIDs should show a clear relationship between plasma concentration and effect, but this has been surprisingly hard to demonstrate with these drugs (Grennan et al, 1983). This could be due to difficulty in accurately measuring disease activity, the dosage ranges studied, or the short half-life of many of the drugs. Additionally, for some drugs such as ibuprofen there may be inter-patient variability in the relative proportions of the active and inactive optical isomers which may affect the drug's efficacy (Lee et al, 1985). A major difficulty is that tissue or synovial fluid levels may relate more closely to clinical effectiveness, and the time course of concentration in synovial fluid is very different from that in plasma. Clinical studies of synovial fluid pharmacokinetics are limited by ethical considerations.

EFFICACY OF NSAIDs IN NON-INFLAMMATORY ARTHRITIS

There is little doubt that NSAIDs are effective in providing pain relief in a proportion of patients with osteoarthritis (Wanka and Dixon, 1964; Famaey and Colinet, 1976; Hubault et al, 1976; Calabro et al, 1977; Gillgrass and Grahame, 1984; Blechman, 1987; Williams et al, 1989). The evidence that NSAIDs are more effective than simple analgesics is more limited. In one study Doyle et al (1981) showed that ketoprofen 150 mg daily was more effective than co-proxamol six tablets daily in osteoarthritis as measured by joint tenderness.

Some NSAIDs may have detrimental effects on articular cartilage in osteoarthritis. Rashad et al (1989) investigated patients on a waiting list for hip arthroplasty surgery. They were treated either with indomethacin (a potent prostaglandin synthetase inhibitor) or azapropazone (a weak inhibitor). Those treated with azapropazone deteriorated less rapidly than the group treated with indomethacin. It was concluded that strong prosta-glandin synthetase inhibitors may be inappropriate for treatment of hip joint osteoarthritis. This study may be criticized for its apparent failure to be performed in double-blind fashion and for its arbitrary end-point of 'time to need for urgent arthroplasty'.

Osteoarthritic pain may be caused by a number of factors, including microfractures in subchondral trabeculae, irritation of periosteal nerve endings, ligamentous or muscular stress, venous congestion caused by remodelling of subchondral bone, or associated soft-tissue rheumatism, as well as by low-grade and probably secondary synovitis. It might be argued that osteoarthritis subjects who respond better to NSAIDs are likely to be those with a significant secondary inflammatory element. In order to address this question we compared the relative efficacy of paracetamol 3 g daily and diclofenac 200 mg daily in patients with osteoarthritis of the knee, after dividing the patients into those with and those without an inflammatory component (an inflammatory component was defined as the presence of morning stiffness of 30 minutes or more and the presence of definite soft-tissue swelling or tenderness). Diclofenac was more effective than paracetamol overall but these differences were mainly in subjects in the group with inflammatory features (unpublished data).

Similarly, NSAIDs have been shown to have some effect on pain relief in subjects with acute 'mechanical' low back pain with sciatica (Jacobs and Grayson, 1968; Amlie et al, 1987) and localized soft-tissue rheumatic conditions (Schorn, 1986) but there is little information to our knowledge concerning the relative efficacy of analgesics and NSAIDs in these conditions.

TOXICITY ASSOCIATED WITH ANALGESICS

The attraction of using analgesics rather than NSAIDs for arthritis lies in the lesser risk of gastrointestinal side-effects with analgesics. Simple analgesics, however, can be toxic, particularly in overdosage. Paracetamol is commonly taken in deliberate overdosage with an estimated mortality of 3.5%. As little as 10 g ingested may produce hepatic necrosis (Sherlock, 1985). The combination of paracetamol with dextropropoxyphene is particularly liable to fatal abuse. Meredith and Vale (1984) reported a figure of fewer than 200 deaths per annum in England and Wales attributed to paracetamol alone, and 293 deaths due to paracetamol and dextropropoxyphene in combination. In contrast, in recent years there has been a decline in the number both of hospital admissions and of deaths from aspirin poisoning. In 1983 acute salicylate poisoning caused 137 adult deaths in England and Wales (Meredith and Vale, 1986).

Another problem is the addictive potential of narcotic components of analgesics. Dextropropoxyphene has been the subject of a lively debate in the medical press for several years because of its side-effects as well as its efficacy. As long ago as 1960 Chernish and Gruber investigated the physical dependence potential of dextropropoxyphene and declared it safe at therapeutic doses (Chernish and Gruber, 1960). However, case reports of small numbers of physically addicted patients followed (Elson and Domino, 1963; Whittington, 1979; Harris and Harper, 1979; Wall et al, 1980). The risks to rheumatoid arthritis patients may be overestimated from these reports. In 1980 Owen and Hills investigated 31 patients with rheumatoid arthritis treated with regular dextropropoxyphene 32.5 mg in combination with paracetamol 325 mg. Treatment was withdrawn and patients completed a questionnaire on withdrawal symptoms. No evidence of withdrawal reactions was found (Owen and Hills, 1980).

Because of the adverse publicity, the combination of dextropropoxyphene and paracetamol has been withdrawn from some district formularies or made available for consultant prescription only. There is already evidence that these measures may not be worthwhile: Tennant (1983) reported that removal of dextropropoxyphene from a formulary merely led to an increase in codeine-related deaths! Shenfield et al (1980) showed that consultants still wished to prescribe the drug, and also mentioned the risk of increased codeine use where dextropropoxyphene is restricted.

Renal toxicity of non-narcotic analgesics

Chronic use of non-narcotic analgesics is associated with renal papillary necrosis. Experimental studies have produced this lesion using a variety of drugs including phenacetin (no longer available because of this side-effect), aspirin, paracetamol and most NSAIDs (Nanra, 1983; Wiseman and Reinert, 1975). The prevalence of analgesic-associated renal papillary necrosis has been assessed in several countries by autopsy studies. The highest prevalence recorded is in Australia (3.7–21.4%) compared with 0.07–0.41% in different studies from England (reviewed by Kincaid-Smith, 1986). The varying figures for different countries broadly parallel the quantity of analgesics consumed. A large, multicentre case-control study in the USA (Sandler et al, 1989) of 554 adults with newly diagnosed kidney disease (serum creatinine 130 μmol/l or over) showed that daily users of analgesics had significantly more renal disease than infrequent users (odds ratio 2.8, 95% confidence interval 1.9 to 4.2). The risk of renal disease was highest for phenacetin (odds ratio 5.1) and was also increased with paracetamol (odds ratio 3.2). There was no significant risk attributable to aspirin in this study.

Overall analgesic nephropathy is a potentially serious long-term side-effect, but as renal papillary necrosis may also occur with NSAID therapy (Munn et al, 1982; Robertson et al, 1980) this problem is unlikely to influence the clinician's decision on which type of drug to prescribe. It is conceivable that there may be an added risk in co-prescription of NSAIDs with simple analgesics, particularly if combination analgesics are used.

TOXICITY OF NSAID

Over the last few years NSAIDs have acquired a reputation for causing serious toxic side-effects and deaths. In fact the individual risk to each patient is very small indeed, but because these drugs are so commonly prescribed, often to elderly or ill patients, the extent of iatrogenic disease is considerable. It has been estimated that in the UK and Australia around 20% of all cases of, and deaths from peptic ulcer are directly attributable to NSAIDs (Somerville et al, 1986; Henry et al, 1987). NSAIDs also have significant toxicity outside the gastrointestinal tract, and may cause renal, hepatic, haematological and cutaneous problems (Table 3).

ANALGESICS VERSUS ANTI-INFLAMMATORY DRUGS IN THE ELDERLY

The withdrawal of benoxaprofen from the market in 1982 after reports of hepatic and renal toxicity resulting in deaths in elderly patients has highlighted the dangers of giving NSAIDs to this age group. All NSAIDs should be used with caution in the elderly, particularly drugs with long half-lives, and in patients with pre-existing hepatic, renal or cardiac dysfunction. There are also important drug interactions which may result in destabilization of coexisting medical disease (for example inhibition of the action of diuretic drugs). Unfortunately a large number of NSAID prescriptions are still given to this age group.

NSAID therapy in the elderly

Pharmacokinetics

Protein binding of several NSAIDs has been shown to be reduced in elderly

Table 3. Toxicity of NSAIDs.

System	Side-effects
Gastrointestinal	Dyspepsia Gastric/duodenal ulceration (including perforation/haemorrhage) Small bowel perforation/haemorrhage Colonic perforation/haemorrhage Diarrhoea
Renal	Interstitial nephritis Acute renal failure Tubular damage Papillary necrosis Decreased renal blood flow
Biochemical	Salt and water retention Hyperkalaemia
Hepatic	Hepatocellular damage Cholestatic jaundice
Haematological	Inhibition of platelet aggregation Thrombocytopenia Aplastic anaemia Haemolytic anaemia
Allergic	Anaphylaxis
Nervous system	Headache (indomethacin) Tinnitus, deafness (salicylate)
Skin	Pruritus Macular erythematous rashes Urticaria Photosensitivity (rare) Rarely Stevens–Johnson syndrome, erythema multiforme, pemphigus
Cartilage	? acceleration of cartilage loss in OA

patients, which may lead to enhanced sensitivity to the drugs (Lesko et al, 1983; Verbeeck and DeSchepper, 1980; Upton et al, 1984). There have been several studies of the pharmacokinetics of NSAIDs in elderly populations. Plasma clearance of NSAIDs in the elderly may be slower and the concentration of unbound drug may be higher. It is therefore recommended that some NSAIDs, including naproxen (Upton et al, 1984) and azapropazone (Ritch et al, 1982), should be given in reduced dosage in the elderly. Other drugs appear to have approximately equal half-lives in old and young subjects; these include piroxicam (Woolf et al, 1983), indomethacin (Traeger et al, 1973) and diclofenac (Willis and Kendall, 1978).

Toxicity

The elderly have been over-represented in many studies of gastrointestinal NSAID toxicity. Caradoc-Davies (1984) investigated 33 cases of upper gastrointestinal bleeding presenting to an acute geriatric unit in England and found that 52% were taking NSAIDs at the time of diagnosis. In another study confined to the elderly, Booker (1983) reported an association of haematemesis or melaena with NSAID use in 17 out of 43 patients. These results suggest an increased risk to the elderly stomach from NSAIDs.

Hepatic toxicity also appears to be increased. Although a reversible rise in transaminases is relatively common, it may if ignored herald more serious damage including toxic hepatitis, cholestasis and irreversible liver damage.

As people in this age group are likely to have arteriosclerotic cardiovascular disease and many patients are taking diuretics, it is to be expected that there is a greater risk of renal toxicity, including renal failure. This has been confirmed in clinical practice (Blackshear et al, 1983). Older people also appear to be more prone to the development of interstitial nephritis (Blackshear et al, 1985).

It has also been shown that the elderly, particularly elderly women, are at increased risk of phenylbutazone-related agranulocytosis and aplastic anaemia (Fowler, 1976).

Central nervous system effects of indomethacin such as dizziness, confusion, depression, drowsiness and seizures may lead to falls and serious fractures in this age group, and for this reason indomethacin should rarely, if ever, be used in the elderly.

Analgesic therapy in the elderly

Age may be an important factor in determining responsiveness to potent analgesics. Bellville et al (1971) studied 712 patients given either morphine or pentazocine for postoperative pain relief and reported an increased response with increasing age. It has been suggested that the enhanced effect of analgesics in old age may be due to age-related differences in pain perception (Vestal, 1978).

Pharmacokinetics

Briant et al (1976) showed that the mean plasma half-life for paracetamol was increased in the elderly to a mean of 2.2 hours compared with 1.8 hours in the young. Whether this slight difference is of any clinical importance is unclear.

Toxicity

In the absence of either overdosage or coexisting chronic liver disease, paracetamol has not been shown to be more toxic in older patients (Schlegel and Paulus, 1986). Dextropropoxyphene and codeine, which act centrally as opioid receptor agonists, are likely to cause particular problems, however, with central nervous system toxicity, respiratory depression and constipation. They also have the potential to produce physical dependence and addiction, which may be particularly relevant to an elderly 'at risk' population.

In general the use of NSAIDs should be reduced in the elderly and alternatives to their prescription should be considered carefully. Simple analgesics such as paracetamol might be a suitable alternative.

ANALGESICS VERSUS ANTI-INFLAMMATORY DRUGS IN PREGNANCY

Analgesics and anti-inflammatory drugs have frequently been taken during pregnancy, although recently potentially serious problems have come to light with NSAIDs used in the third trimester.

Slone et al (1976) conducted a large study in the USA of aspirin use in pregnancy, in which over 50 000 pregnancies were observed. There was found to be no increase in congenital malformations in the 15 000 fetuses exposed to the drug. The same group (Shapiro et al, 1976) also found no evidence for an increase in stillbirths, neonatal deaths or reduced birth weight associated with aspirin. Presumably most mothers were taking aspirin intermittently in analgesic rather than anti-inflammatory doses, and it would appear from the above work that this is safe practice.

In 1979 Wilkinson and colleagues reported three infants with persistent pulmonary hypertension following NSAID treatment (naproxen) which had been given to delay labour (Wilkinson et al, 1979). At the time this was a recognized use for NSAIDs. An editorial in the *Lancet* the following year (Editorial, 1980) drew attention to the risk and reported that similar effects occurred with indomethacin. NSAIDs were also recognized to delay closure of the ductus arteriosus after birth. It was recommended therefore that NSAIDs be contraindicated in pregnancy. Fortunately rheumatoid arthritis often goes into remission at this time.

It has been suggested that the effects on the fetal ductus arteriosus may be unique to acidic NSAIDs. Momma and Takeuchi (1983) gave 24 different NSAIDs to full-term pregnant rats. All 16 acidic NSAIDs constricted the fetal ductus (which it is thought then predisposes to primary pulmonary hypertension), whereas 6 out of 8 experimental basic NSAIDs did not.

Paracetamol appears to be safe in pregnancy. A survey by the Royal

College of General Practitioners (Crombie et al, 1970) on pregnancy outcome showed no increase in congenital abnormalities or stillbirths.

CONCLUSION

Current therapeutic thinking inherent in the definitions of simple analgesics and NSAIDs implies preferential prescription of the latter group of drugs in subjects with inflammatory joint problems and of simple analgesics in those with non-inflammatory problems. Current evidence supports the continued use of NSAIDs as first-choice drugs in subjects with inflammatory joint disease. There is limited evidence that such drugs may be more efficacious in some subjects with osteoarthritis, although on logical grounds it seems more likely that this will be mainly true in subjects with an inflammatory component to their disease. By contrast, there is little evidence that simple analgesics alone have a significant role in the management of inflammatory joint disease, although their use in a supplementary role is popular and frequently practised by patients, often without the knowledge of their doctors. Paracetamol alone or in combination with dextropropoxyphene is a popular choice of supplementary analgesic. The latter combination may be preferred by patients, but there are worries about its addictive potential and excessive toxicity in overdosage. Particular cases for the use of analgesics rather than NSAIDs can be made in the elderly and during pregnancy.

REFERENCES

Amlie E, Weber H & Holme I (1987) Treatment of acute low back pain with piroxicam: results of a double-blind placebo controlled trial. *Spine* **12:** 473–476.

Bellville JW, Forrest WH, Miller E et al (1971) Influence of age on pain relief from analgesics. *Journal of the American Medical Association* **217:** 1835–1841.

Blackshear JL, Davidman M & Stillman MT (1983) Identification of risk factors for renal insufficiency from nonsteroidal antiinflammatory drugs. *Archives of Internal Medicine* **143:** 1130–1134.

Blackshear JL, Napier JS, Davidman M et al (1985) Renal complications of nonsteroidal antiinflammatory drugs: identification and monitoring of those at risk. *Seminars in Arthritis and Rheumatism* **14(3):** 163–175.

Blechman WJ (1987) Nabumetone therapy of osteoarthritis. *American Journal of Medicine* **83 (supplement 4B):** 70–73.

Boardman PL & Hart FD (1967) Clinical measurement of the anti-inflammatory effects of salicylates in rheumatoid arthritis. *British Medical Journal* **4:** 264–268.

Booker JA (1983) Haematemesis and melaena in the elderly. *Age and Ageing* **12:** 49–54.

Briant RH, Dorrington RE, Cleal J et al (1976) The rate of acetaminophen metabolism in the elderly and the young. *Journal of the American Geriatrics Society* **24:** 359–361.

British National Formulary (1990) London: No. 19 (March). British Medical Association and Royal Pharmaceutical Society of Great Britain.

Brooks PM, Dougan MA, Mugford S et al (1982) Comparative effectiveness of 5 analgesics in patients with rheumatoid arthritis and osteoarthritis. *Journal of Rheumatology* **9:** 723–726.

Calabro JJ, Andelman SY, Caldwell JR et al (1977) A multicenter trial of sulindac in osteoarthritis of the hip. *Clinical Pharmacology and Therapeutics* **22:** 358–363.

Caradoc-Davies TH (1984) Nonsteroidal antiinflammatory drugs: arthritis and gastrointestinal bleeding in elderly patients. *Age and Ageing* **13:** 295–298.

Chernish SM & Gruber CM (1960) Demonstration of absence of physical dependence to therapeutic doses of dextropropoxyphene hydrochloride (Darvon) using the 'allyl test'. *Antibiotic Medicine and Clinical Therapy* **7**: 190–192.

Committee on Safety of Medicines (1986) CSM update: non-steroidal anti-inflammatory drugs and serious gastrointestinal adverse reactions—1. *British Medical Journal* **292**: 614.

Crombie DL, Pinsent RJFH, Slater BC et al (1970) Teratogenic drugs—RCGP survey. *British Medical Journal* **4**: 178–179.

Cummings DM & Amadio P (1983) Evaluation of acetaminophen in the symptomatic management of osteoarthritis of the knees (abstract). *Clinical Pharmacology and Therapeutics* **33**: 266.

Day RO, Graham GG, Williams KM et al (1987) Clinical pharmacology of non-steroidal anti-inflammatory drugs. *Clinical Pharmacology and Therapeutics* **33**: 383–433.

Doyle DV, Dieppe PA, Scott J et al (1981) An articular index for the assessment of osteoarthritis. *Annals of the Rheumatic Diseases* **40**: 75–78.

Editorial (1980) PG-synthetase inhibitors in obstetrics and after. *Lancet* **ii**: 185–186.

Elson A & Domino EF (1963) Dextropropoxyphene addiction: observations of a case. *Journal of the American Medical Association* **183**: 482–485.

Emery P & Gibson T (1986) A double-blind study of the simple analgesic nefopam in rheumatoid arthritis. *British Journal of Rheumatology* **25**: 72–76.

Famaey JP & Colinet E (1976) A double-blind trial of ketoprofen in the treatment of osteoarthritis of the hip. *Rheumatology and Rehabilitation* (supplement) 45–49.

Fowler PD (1976) Marrow toxicity of the pyrazoles. *Annals of the Rheumatic Diseases* **26**: 344.

Fremont-Smith P & Bayles TB (1965) Salicylate therapy in rheumatoid arthritis. *Journal of the American Medical Association* **192**: 1133–1136.

Gibson T & Clark B (1985) Simple analgesic use in rheumatoid arthritis. *Annals of the Rheumatic Diseases* **44**: 27–29.

Gillgrass J & Grahame R (1984) Nabumetone: a double-blind study in osteoarthrosis. *Pharmotherapeutica* **3**: 592–594.

Grennan DM, Aarons L, Siddiqui et al (1983) Dose-response study with ibuprofen in rheumatoid arthritis: clinical and pharmacokinetic findings. *British Journal of Clinical Pharmacology* **15**: 311–316.

Hardin JG & Kirk KA (1979) Comparative effectiveness of five analgesics for the pain of rheumatoid arthritis. *Journal of Rheumatology* **6**: 405–412.

Harris B & Harper M (1979) Psychosis after dextropropoxyphene (letter). *Lancet* **ii**: 743.

Hart FD & Boardman PL (1963) Indomethacin: a new non-steroid anti-inflammatory agent. *British Medical Journal* **2**: 965–970.

Henry DA, Hall PR, Johnston A et al (1987) NSAIDs as a cause of morbidity and mortality from peptic ulcer complications in New South Wales. *Proceedings of the Third International Conference on Pharmacoepidemiology*, Minneapolis.

Hubault A, Caroit M, Forette B et al (1976) Double-blind trial of ketoprofen compared with placebo in osteoarthritis of the hip. *Rheumatology and Rehabilitation* (supplement) 52–55.

Huskisson EC, Woolf DL, Balme HW et al (1976) Four new anti-inflammatory drugs: responses and variations. *British Medical Journal* **1**: 1048–1049.

Huskisson EC (1974) Simple analgesics for arthritis. *British Medical Journal* **4**: 196–200.

Huskisson EC (1977) Anti-inflammatory drugs. *Seminars in Arthritis and Rheumatism* **7**: 1–20.

Jacobs JH & Grayson MF (1968) Trial of an anti-inflammatory agent (indomethacin) in low back pain with and without radicular involvement. *British Medical Journal* **3**: 158–160.

Kincaid-Smith P (1986) Effects of non-narcotic analgesics on the kidney. *Drugs* **32** (supplement 4): 109–128.

Lee EJD, Williams K, Day R et al (1985) Stereoselective disposition of ibuprofen enantiomers in man. *British Journal of Clinical Pharmacology* **19**: 669–674.

Lee P, Watson M, Webb J et al (1975) Therapeutic effectiveness of paracetamol in rheumatoid arthritis. *International Journal of Clinical Pharmacology* **11**: 68–75.

Lesko LJ, Yeager RL, Narang PK et al (1983) Salicylate protein binding in young and elderly serum as measured by diafiltration (abstract). *Clinical Pharmacology and Therapeutics* **33**: 257.

Levinson JE, Baum J, Brewer E et al (1977) Comparison of tolmetin sodium and aspirin in the treatment of juvenile rheumatoid arthritis. *Journal of Pediatrics* **91**: 799–804.

Liebling MR, Altman RD, Benedek TG et al (1975) A double blind multi-clinic trial of sulindac

(MG-213) in the treatment of ankylosing spondylitis (abstract). *Arthritis and Rheumatism* **18:** 411.

Mainland D & Sutcliffe MI (1965) Aspirin in rheumatoid arthritis, a seven-day double blind trial—preliminary report. *Bulletin on the Rheumatic Diseases* **16:** 388–391.

Meredith TJ & Vale JA (1984) Epidemiology of analgesic overdose in England and Wales. *Human Toxicology* **3:** 61S–74S.

Meredith TJ & Vale JA (1986) Non-narcotic analgesics. Problems of overdosage. *Drugs* **32 (supplement 4):** 177–205.

Momma K & Takeuchi H (1983) Constriction of fetal ductus arteriosus by non-steroidal anti-inflammatory drugs. *Prostaglandins* **26:** 631–643.

Munn E, Lynn KL & Bailey RR (1982) Renal papillary necrosis following regular consumption of non-steroidal anti-inflammatory drugs. *New Zealand Medical Journal* **95:** 213–214.

Nanra RS (1983) Renal effects of antipyretic analgesics. *American Journal of Medicine* **75(5A):** 70–81.

Nuki G (1983) Non-steroidal analgesic and anti-inflammatory agents. *British Medical Journal* **287:** 39–43.

Nuki G, Downie WW, Dick WC et al (1973) Clinical trial of pentazocine in rheumatoid arthritis. Observations on the value of potent analgesics and placebos. *Annals of the Rheumatic Diseases* **32:** 436–443.

Owen M & Hills LJ (1980) How safe is dextropropoxyphene? (letter). *Medical Journal of Australia* **i:** 617–618.

Rashad S, Revell P, Hemingway A et al (1989) Effect of non-steroidal anti-inflammatory drugs on the course of osteoarthritis. *Lancet* **ii:** 519–522.

Ritch AES, Perera WNR & Jones CJ (1982) Pharmacokinetics of azapropazone in the elderly. *British Journal of Clinical Pharmacology* **14:** 116–119.

Robertson CE, Van Someren V, Ford MJ et al (1980) Mefenamic acid and nephropathy. *Lancet* **ii:** 232–233.

Sandler DP, Smith JC, Weinberg CR et al (1989) Analgesic use and chronic renal disease. *New England Journal of Medicine* **320:** 1238–1243.

Schlegel SI & Paulus HE (1986) NSAID and analgesic treatment in the elderly. *Clinics in Rheumatic Diseases* **12:** 245–273.

Schorn D (1986) Tenoxicam in soft-tissue rheumatism. *South African Medical Journal* **69:** 301–303.

Scott DL, Roden S, Marshall T et al (1982) Variations in responses to non-steroidal anti-inflammatory drugs. *British Journal of Clinical Pharmacology* **14:** 691–694.

Shapiro S, Siskind V, Monson RR et al (1976) Perinatal mortality and birthweight in relation to aspirin taken during pregnancy. *Lancet* **i:** 1375–1376.

Shenfield GM, Jones AN & Paterson JW (1980) Effect of restrictions on prescribing patterns for dextropropoxyphene. *British Medical Journal* **281:** 651–653.

Sherlock S (1985) Drugs and the liver. In Diseases of the Liver and Biliary System, 7th edn, p. 311. Oxford: Blackwell.

Slone D, Siskind V, Heinonen OP et al (1976) Aspirin and congenital malformations. *Lancet* **i:** 1373–1375.

Somerville K, Faulkner G & Langman M (1986) Non-steroidal anti-inflammatory drugs and bleeding peptic ulcer. *Lancet* **i:** 462–464.

Steele K, Mills K & Gilliland A (1987) Repeat prescribing of non-steroidal anti-inflammatory drugs excluding aspirin: how careful are we? *British Medical Journal* **295:** 962–964.

Strumia E & Babbini M (1973) A comparative evaluation of mefenamic acid, propoxyphene, flufenisal and placebo in osteoarticular pain. *Journal of International Medical Research* **1:** 258–260.

Tennant FS (1983) Adverse effects on codeine prescriptions in California arising from governmental regulations (letter). *New England Journal of Medicine* **308:** 288.

Traeger A, Kunze M, Stein G et al (1973) Pharmacokinetics of indomethacin in the aged. *Zeitschrift für Alternsforschung* **27:** 151–155.

Upton RA, Williams RL, Kelly J et al (1984) Naproxen pharmacokinetics in the elderly. *British Journal of Clinical Pharmacology* **18:** 207–214.

Verbeeck RK & DeSchepper PJ (1980) Influence of chronic renal failure and haemodialysis on diflunisal plasma protein binding. *Clinical Pharmacology and Therapeutics* **27:** 628–634.

Vestal RE (1978) Drug use in the elderly: a review of problems and special considerations. *Drugs* **16**: 358–382.

Wall R, Linford SMJ & Akhter MI (1980) Addiction to Distalgesic (dextropropoxyphene). *British Medical Journal* **i**: 1213–1214.

Wanka J & Dixon ASJ (1964) Treatment of osteoarthritis of the hip with indomethacin: a controlled clinical trial. *Annals of the Rheumatic Diseases* **23**: 288–290.

Whittington RM (1979) Dextropropoxyphene addiction. *Lancet* **ii**: 743–744.

Wilkinson AR, Aynsley-Green A & Mitchell MD (1979) Persistent pulmonary hypertension and abnormal prostaglandin E levels in preterm infants after maternal treatment with naproxen. *Archives of Disease in Childhood* **54**: 942–945.

Williams PI, Hosie J & Scott DL (1989) Etodolac therapy for osteoarthritis: a double-blind placebo-controlled trial. *Current Medical Research and Opinion* **11**: 463–470.

Willis JV & Kendall MJ (1978) Pharmacokinetics studies on diclofenac sodium in young and old volunteers. *Scandinavian Journal of Rheumatology* **22**: (supplement) 36–41.

Wiseman EH & Reinert H (1975) Anti-inflammatory drugs and renal papillary necrosis. *Agents and Actions* **5**: 322–325.

Woolf AD, Rogers HJ, Bradook ID et al (1983) Pharmacokinetic observations on piroxicam in young adults, middle-aged and elderly patients. *British Journal of Clinical Pharmacology* **16**: 433–437.

11

Are there any antirheumatic drugs that modify the course of ankylosing spondylitis?

RODGER LAURENT

The most significant advances in the management of ankylosing spondylitis have been the introduction of non-steroidal anti-inflammatory drugs (NSAIDs) and the use of regular exercise programmes. The majority of patients can be successfully managed with these treatments, but there is a small group for whom they are inadequate. It is not known what percentage of patients with ankylosing spondylitis require disease-modifying drugs, but they are usually those who have a peripheral arthritis in addition to spinal disease. The first attempt at disease modification was with radiotherapy, which was probably the mainstay of treatment until the 1950s when an association with malignancy—particularly leukaemia—was recognized. Numerous medications, which are all disease-modifying drugs used in rheumatoid arthritis, have been used in ankylosing spondylitis. Most of the studies are case reports or uncontrolled and only sulphasalazine and D-penicillamine have been evaluated with adequate placebo-controlled studies.

Ankylosing spondylitis is a more difficult disorder in which to assess disease activity than rheumatoid arthritis. This has produced problems in the design and interpretation of ankylosing spondylitis clinical studies. There are several factors responsible for these difficulties, and because they influence the interpretation of studies they are discussed here before the studies on antirheumatic drugs are reviewed. These factors are the pathological heterogeneity of ankylosing spondylitis, disease duration of patients included in studies, definition of a peripheral joint and the appropriate clinical and laboratory assessments.

PROBLEMS ASSOCIATED WITH ANKYLOSING SPONDYLITIS CLINICAL STUDIES

Pathological heterogeneity

Ankylosing spondylitis consists of two distinct pathological processes: enthesitis and synovitis. The aetiology is the same even though the histology and clinical features are different, depending on the nature of the involved tissue. It is important, therefore, to assess each component separately.

Baillière's Clinical Rheumatology—
Vol. 4, No. 2, August 1990
ISBN 0–7020–1480–X

Peripheral joint symptoms often have not been separated into an enthesitis or synovitis so that the effect of the treatment on each component cannot be compared. Enthesitis is the major pathology in the spinal disease, but about 45% of patients have a peripheral enthesitis at some stage in their disease (Burgos-Vargas et al, 1989). An enthesis index has been recently described which could be a useful measurement for inclusion in clinical trials (Mander et al,1987).

Synovitis not only involves the peripheral joints, but can also occur in the zygapophyseal joints, although how this contributes to the back pain is unknown (Ball, 1980). If it parallels the peripheral arthritis, it is probably more important in the early stages of the disease and contributes little in a patient whose disease duration is greater than ten years.

All the drugs that have been used to try to modify the course of ankylosing spondylitis are effective in controlling synovitis in other arthritides, particularly rheumatoid arthritis. The major question being asked in ankylosing spondylitis is whether these drugs have an effect on the enthesitis rather than the synovitis. Therefore, any study of ankylosing spondylitis must clearly separate spinal from peripheral disease, and subdivide the latter into enthesitis and synovitis.

Duration of disease

Patients included in most studies have had their disease for at least ten years; only a few studies have included patients with shorter disease duration. There are two important consequences of this: the first is that patients will probably have irreversible loss of spinal movement, and measurement is unlikely to detect any change. In the studies reviewed, most measurements of spinal movement did not change significantly. The second is that patients with disease of more than ten years' duration are less likely to have a peripheral synovitis or enthesitis. A peripheral arthritis, which occurs in about 55% of patients at some stage of the disease, is usually present at disease onset in about 38%. Similarly, a peripheral enthesopathy, which occurs in 45% of patients, is present in about 28% of patients at disease onset (Burgos-Vargas et al, 1989). Synovitis occurs within the first ten years of the disease, and persists and becomes chronic in only a minority of patients (Wilkinson and Bywaters, 1958). Therefore, if a study is to assess the effect of treatment on synovitis and peripheral enthesitis, it should include patients with disease of shorter duration so that adequate information can be obtained. In the studies of antirheumatic drugs, most had insufficient patients with a peripheral arthritis or enthesitis for meaningful analysis.

The main reason for patients with established disease being included in most studies is that in order to fulfil the New York diagnostic criteria for ankylosing spondylitis patients must have at least grade 2 sacroiliitis. Because symptoms can precede grade 2 radiological changes by a mean duration of nine years (Mau et al, 1988), only patients with late disease are likely to meet these requirements.

There needs to be a radical change in the type of patient included in antirheumatic drug studies in ankylosing spondylitis, with the inclusion of more patients with early disease. Some will turn out not to have ankylosing spondylitis, and can be excluded before the studies are analysed. However, this group must be studied to establish whether antirheumatic drugs have any major effect on enthesitis or peripheral arthritis, or modify the long-term outcome of ankylosing spondylitis.

Peripheral arthritis

A source of confusion has been the definition of a peripheral joint, with the limb girdle or rhizomelic joints (the shoulders and hips) often being considered separately from other peripheral joints. The hip and shoulder joints are more commonly affected than other joints and are more likely to have cartilage loss and bone erosion (Hart, 1980). It is unclear why this distinction exists, and it would be more appropriate to include these joints with the other peripheral joints.

Clinical assessment

There is no universal agreement as to the most reliable and sensitive method for the assessment of ankylosing spondylitis. Numerous methods for measuring spinal movement have been described, although the reliability and validity of many of these methods have not been reported. Several commonly used measurements have been found to be unreliable (Pile et al, 1990). Measurements used in NSAID trials are poor at detecting differences and are not sensitive enough to be of value (Laurent et al, 1990). The appropriate measurements for the assessment of antirheumatic drugs and the lack of sensitivity of these measurements may also be a limiting factor in the assessment of antirheumatic drugs.

Laboratory assessment

Numerous acute phase proteins have been used in the assessment of ankylosing spondylitis without finding one that is an accurate measure of spinal disease activity. C-reactive protein and the erythrocyte sedimentation rate (ESR), the most common measurements used, correlate poorly with spinal disease and are more likely to be elevated in patients with a peripheral arthritis (Scott et al, 1981; Laurent and Panayi, 1983; Nashel et al, 1986; Sheehan et al, 1986; Will et al, 1989b). There is a correlation between different acute phase proteins even though they do not correlate with the clinical measurements of disease activity.

Serum immunoglobulin levels, particularly IgA and IgG, have been considered as a marker of disease activity. Immunoglobulin A levels do not correlate with the C-reactive protein or ESR which suggests that a different mechanism may be responsible for the hypergammaglobulinaemia and the elevated acute phase proteins (Franssen et al, 1985; Sanders et al, 1987). The stimulus for IgA production is probably in the gastrointestinal tract, and because IgA has a short half-life, its continuous presence suggests chronic stimulation. Elevated IgA levels may reflect antigen persistence rather than disease activity.

The poor correlation between acute phase proteins and clinical measurements is probably because the latter are not an assessment of disease activity but are a marker of spinal function. Whether it is the enthesitis or the synovitis of the zygapophyseal joints that produces the increase in acute phase proteins is unknown. Inflammation in the spine is a poor stimulus for an acute phase response, and measurement of acute phase proteins is of limited value.

ANTIRHEUMATIC TREATMENTS USED IN ANKYLOSING SPONDYLITIS

All the antirheumatic treatments (with the exception of radiotherapy) have been extensively used in rheumatoid arthritis. Most of the reports are of studies with small numbers of patients and only sulphasalazine and D-penicillamine have been evaluated with controlled clinical trials.

Radiotherapy

The first attempt at disease modification was with radiotherapy, which benefited ankylosing spondylitis but not osteoarthritis or rheumatoid arthritis (Sinclair, 1971). It was of value in relieving pain, with a quarter of patients having relief for three years, but did not improve spinal movement or prevent further exacerbations (Desmarais, 1953; Wilkinson and Bywaters, 1958). It was widely used until the 1950s, when the association with an increased risk of leukaemias and cancers was recognized. The peak incidence of leukaemias was three to five years after treatment, and for other cancers nine years after treatment (Darby et al, 1987). Radiotherapy has not been used in recent years, although it has occasionally been advocated for use in patients who have a localized area of severe back pain unresponsive to other treatments (Ward, 1963; Calman and Berry, 1980). A retrospective study of patients treated with radiotherapy, using an ankylosing spondylitis assessment questionnaire and an arthritis impairment measurement scale, showed a poorer outcome for those who received radiotherapy. This survey could not take into account whether patients who had radiotherapy had more severe disease and were therefore expected to have a worse outcome. However, the differences were small and the conclusion is that radiotherapy does not produce any significant long-term benefit (Calin and Elswood, 1989). Local radiotherapy may benefit recalcitrant enthesitis in the feet of patients with HLA-B27 related arthropathy (Grill et al, 1988). Radiotherapy appears to be effective in controlling enthesitis and may have a role in the treatment of localized inflammation unresponsive to other treatments.

Sulphasalazine

The current interest in the treatment of ankylosing spondylitis with sulphasalazine is another example of the unusual paths that treatment for the rheumatic diseases has followed. This therapy is based on the observation that 57% of patients with ankylosing spondylitis have inflammatory lesions in their terminal ileum, ileocaecal valve and caecum. In some, these lesions were similar to those seen in Crohn's disease, and were more common in patients with a peripheral arthritis (Mielants et al, 1988). It was concluded that these patients had a subclinical form of Crohn's disease, with ankylosing spondylitis being the only clinical expression. Treating the inflammatory lesions in the bowel with sulphasalazine might therefore help the peripheral arthritis and perhaps the spondylitis. An uncontrolled study suggested that the peripheral arthritis improved with sulphasalazine (Mielants et al, 1986). The most important studies are the five placebo-controlled studies and one interventional study discussed below.

The first report of sulphasalazine in ankylosing spondylitis was an open study in 8 patients treated for 16 weeks. There were reductions in early morning stiffness, NSAID dosage and ESR. The improvement occurred after 4 to 8 weeks of treatment, and the two patients with a peripheral arthritis had a reduction in the number of painful joints (Amor et al, 1984). As a result of this open study, the authors then carried out a double-blind, placebo-controlled study for 6 months in 60 patients, which demonstrated the importance of a placebo control group. The patients had only spinal disease with a median disease duration of 10 years. The NSAID dosage was reduced to a minimum prior to the study although there were no other disease activity criteria used for inclusion. The sulphasalazine group showed significant improvement in pain, joint index, an indicator of tender areas, daily dose of NSAIDs, a functional index and hand-to-ground distance. When compared with the placebo group, however, the only significant differences were minor changes in the functional index and in serum IgG concentration. The ESR fell significantly in both groups but the fall was only 2 mm/h from an original value of 11 mm/h or 13 mm/h, which is clinically insignificant. Improvement in the sulphasalazine group was not noted until the third month (Dougados et al, 1986). The conclusion from this study is that sulphasalazine administration gave marginal benefit in spinal disease as measured by the functional index without any significant improvement in pain or spinal movement.

The second study involved 37 patients, mean disease duration 11.3 years, who were treated for 3 months. Only patients with active disease were included, active disease being morning stiffness of more than 30 minutes duration or disturbance of sleep due to pain, an ESR greater than 30 mm/h or an increase in serum orosomucoid or haptoglobin levels. The sulpha-salazine group showed a reduction in pain, morning stiffness, chest expansion and sleep disturbance, but there were no significant changes in any variable in the placebo group. The only significant differences between the placebo and sulphasalazine groups were a small reduction in sleep disturbance, and a fall in haptoglobin and orosomucoid levels. The effect of sulphasalazine on peripheral synovitis could not be determined because there was only one patient with this in each treatment group. Sulphasalazine may produce haemolysis so that it is not possible to determine whether the improvement in haptoglobin levels is due to a reduction in the acute phase response or secondary to haemolysis. The greatest improvement in the sulphasalazine group was in patients with an ESR greater than 20 mm/h or haptoglobin greater than 3.8 g/l. The study also showed only minimal benefit for spinal disease (Feltelius and Hallgren, 1986).

A multicentre, multiassessor study of 85 patients treated for 26 weeks included patients with a short disease duration, the mean being 4.6 years. They included 55 patients who had peripheral joint symptoms, which were subdivided into swollen joints and painful joints, although the distribution of the involved joints was not indicated. The study also had similar inclusion criteria, which were an elevated ESR greater than 30 mm/h, C-reactive protein greater than 20 mg/l or morning stiffness for more than 30 minutes. Patients with fused sacroiliac joints of more than three fused syndesmophytes in the lumbar spine were excluded, thus eliminating patients who could not improve spinal function. The only significant differences between sulphasalazine and placebo were a reduction in morning stiffness (which was small, with a mean improvement of 15 minutes), a mean increase in chest expansion of 12 mm, and reductions in ESR and immunoglobins.

This study demonstrates the importance of including a placebo control group. There were improvements in duration and severity of morning stiffness, severity of spinal pain, chest expansion, Schober test, fingertips-to-floor distance and the number of swollen joints in the sulphasalazine group. However, in the placebo group, there were improvements in Schober's test, fingertips-to-floor and the number of swollen joints.

Clinical and laboratory measurements showed improvement more commonly in patients with peripheral arthritis than in those with only spinal involvement, but the differences were not significant. Even though sulphasalazine produced significant changes compared to the placebo group, the changes were only minimal. There was a tendency for it to be more helpful in those with a peripheral arthritis but it gave little benefit to those with spinal disease (Nissila et al, 1988).

A further open study of sulphasalazine administration for 6 months to patients with a wide range of disease duration (1 to 24 years) demonstrated significant improvement in several measurements including those of spinal movement and ESR. Patients with a peripheral arthritis were included although they were not evaluated separately (Coelho-Andrade et al, 1989). However, the lack of a placebo control group makes these results of little significance.

The next double-blind, placebo-controlled study had fewer patients (28), and criteria similar to those in previous studies were used for including patients with active disease. Patients were treated for 3 months and the mean disease duration was 8.5 years. Seven patients had peripheral joint involvement, but there was no comment as to whether this group derived any significant improvement from the sulphasalazine. An improvement was noted in inactivity stiffness, severity of pain, occiput-to-wall distance and sleep disturbance. There was no change in the placebo group, and unfortunately no comparison was made between the two treatment groups. In the sulphasalazine group there was an improvement in ESR, C-reactive protein and serum IgA and IgA α-antitrypsin complex levels (Davis et al, 1989).

The study was expanded to 40 patients, treated for 1 year, with similar improvements to those in the short-term study. There were no radiological changes, but the duration of treatment was too short for these to have occurred. Unfortunately, the two treatment groups were not compared and this makes it impossible to interpret the results adequately (Taylor et al, 1989).

The most recent placebo-controlled study involved 62 patients treated for a duration of 48 weeks (Corkhill et al, 1990). They had a long disease duration, the mean being 14.1 years. Peripheral arthritis was present in 4 of the active group and 7 of the placebo group, the numbers being too small for analysis. At 48 weeks, there was no significant improvement in either group or significant difference between the groups. Analysis of patients with an ESR over 20 mm/h—5 in the active group and 7 in the placebo group—did not show any significant change. There was a small reduction in the ESR but immunoglobulin levels did not change. The conclusion from this study is that sulphasalazine does not help spinal disease in patients with long disease duration.

The latest study was an interventional study in 20 patients, whose median disease duration was 9 years (Fraser and Sturrock, 1990). They were treated for 24 weeks with sulphasalazine which was then discontinued and assessments made at 30 and 36 weeks, which is up to 12 weeks after treatment. The inclusion criteria for active disease were similar to those in other studies. At 24 weeks, there were improvements in the number of active joints (from four to two), chest expansion, ESR, C-reactive protein and serum IgA levels. After sulphasalazine was discontinued, the ESR, C-reactive protein and platelet levels returned to pre-treatment values. There were no changes in clinical parameters; in particular, there was no increase in the number of peripheral joints involved. Peripheral joint involvement was regarded as being due to synovitis or restricted movement, and the shoulder, hip and sternoclavicular joint were regarded as peripheral joints. This does not distinguish between a synovitis or an enthesitis of the surrounding structures as the cause of the joint involvement, and the improvement could have been due to control of either the enthesitis or the synovitis. The effect on spinal disease was minimal, benefiting only chest expansion. The value of this study is that it included patients with peripheral joint involvement, which may be the subgroup most likely to derive benefit from sulphasalazine.

The dosages of sulphasalazine used in the studies were 2–3 g a day. Side-effects were not a major problem, the most common being gastrointestinal, headaches or a skin rash.

Several studies noted a fall in the serum level of at least one immunoglobulin class with sulphasalazine treatment (Dougados et al, 1986; Nissila et al, 1988; Davis et al, 1989; Fraser and Sturrock, 1990). *In vitro* studies have shown that sulphasalazine inhibits spontaneous IgG secretion, pokeweed mitogen-induced B-cell proliferation and immunoglobulin G, A and M production. (Comer and Jasin, 1988; MacDermott et al, 1989). The levels of sulphasalazine required to produce a significant reduction in immunoglobulin secretion were higher than those normally found in blood or synovial fluid, although they may equate with levels in the synovium or lymph nodes. The reduction in serum immunoglobulin levels associated with sulphasalazine treatment could be due to a reduction in disease activity or as a result of a direct effect on B-cells which is unrelated to disease activity.

The conclusions from these studies are that sulphasalazine does not benefit spinal disease but may be useful for treating a peripheral arthritis. Only one or two measurements of spinal function improved in each study, and in each case the improvement was minimal. The course of the spondylitis associated with Crohn's disease is not influenced by treatment of the bowel disease (Moll, 1985), and the same relationship may apply in ankylosing spondylitis associated with ileocaecal inflammation.

D-Penicillamine

Therapy with D-penicillamine has been used predominantly in rheumatoid arthritis, and only occasionally in the seronegative spondarthritides. Its documented use in ankylosing spondylitis is limited to case reports and only one placebo-controlled study. Case reports have shown an improvement in pain and morning stiffness without altering spinal movement in two patients (Golding, 1974), improvement in the peripheral arthritis in one patient (Scharf and Nahir, 1976), or no benefit for either spinal disease or peripheral arthritis in five patients (Bird and Dixon, 1977).

The only double-blind, placebo-controlled study was of six months' duration in 17 patients with ankylosing spondylitis whose median disease duration was 15 years. Thirteen patients had peripheral joint involvement as determined by peripheral joint pain and tenderness, with the shoulder and hip not being regarded as peripheral joints. D-penicillamine did not benefit either the spinal disease or the peripheral arthritis (Steven et al, 1985). Forty-nine patients with a mean disease duration of 10.9 years were treated in an open study for nine months. There was improvement in spinal movement at one month as measured by the Schober test and the finger-to-floor distance. The patients received physiotherapy during the first month which is probably the reason for the improvement in spinal movement. There was no comment on pain or morning stiffness (Tytman et al, 1989). In the latter two studies, side-effects were similar to those experienced by patients with rheumatoid arthritis. The conclusions from these studies are that D-pencillamine does not benefit either the axial disease or the peripheral arthritis of ankylosing spondylitis.

Methotrexate

Methotrexate has been used in the treatment of Reiter's syndrome but rarely in ankylosing spondylitis. A report of three cases with psoriatic spondylitis, ankylosing spondylitis or possible ankylosing spondylitis, demonstrated improvement in all three. A placebo-controlled study is required to determine the value of methotrexate in ankylosing spondylitis (Handler, 1989).

Cyclophosphamide

Intravenous cyclophosphamide has been considered useful in systemic lupus erythematosus and vasculitis and is associated with fewer side-effects compared with oral treatment. An interesting open study used intravenous cyclophosphamide in 12 patients with severe ankylosing spondylitis and peripheral arthritis. The regimen consisted of 200 mg intravenously on alternate days for 20 days and then 100 mg intravenously once a week for three months to a total dose of 3.3 g. There were reductions in spinal pain, the number of swollen peripheral joints (from 12.9 to 2.7) and the mean ESR (from 90 mm/h to 50 mm/h), without any changes in the parameters of spinal movement. Three patients with secondary amyloid disease did not respond to treatment (Sadowska-Wroblewska et al, 1986).

Even though there was no control group, significant changes particularly in the peripheral arthritis and ESR suggest that cyclophosphamide may be useful in active disease. Intravenous cyclophosphamide may be useful for the occasional patient with severe disease in whom all other medications have failed. It is unlikely that the appropriate controlled trial will be done to assess the efficacy of cyclophosphamide in ankylosing spondylitis.

Levamisole

Levamisole is an anthelmintic drug that is an immunostimulant, particularly of cell-mediated immunity, used in the treatment of rheumatoid arthritis. An open study showed marginal clinical improvement in 4 of 13 patients with ankylosing spondylitis (Rosenthal et al, 1976).

A double-blind, placebo-controlled study of 12 weeks' duration in patients with spondyloarthropathy, which included psoriatic arthritis and reactive arthritis as well as ankylosing spondylitis, demonstrated an improvement in morning stiffness, low back movement and peripheral arthritis, when compared to placebo. As each subgroup was not analysed separately, it is uncertain as to how useful it was in ankylosing spondylitis (Goebel et al, 1977). Levamisole probably has little to offer in the management of ankylosing spondylitis.

Corticosteroids

Oral corticosteroids

Oral corticosteroids may be beneficial in ankylosing spondylitis (Ward, 1963) although it is considered that they should be used only in patients with uveitis or vasculitis (Calabro and Mody, 1966). Short courses of corticotrophin have also been used to control acute exacerbations of the disease (Hill, 1980). Spinal osteoporosis occurs in ankylosing spondylitis and this can be secondary to the systemic disease as well as inactivity. It could be made worse by long-term treatment with corticosteroids (Will et al, 1989a; Ralston et al, 1990). However, control of the systemic features of the disease by low-dose corticosteroids may alleviate rather than potentiate osteo-porosis. Oral corticosteroids probably have a role in the treatment of acute flares in the disease that do not respond to NSAIDs (Ward, 1963). A trial of low-dose corticosteroids in patients unresponsive to NSAIDs may be useful. The relative merits of oral corticosteroids or pulse methylprednisolone for the treatment of acute flares has not been evaluated.

Pulse methylprednisolone

Large, intermittent doses of intravenous methylprednisolone have been used in the treatment of several immunologically mediated diseases. This regimen has both an anti-inflammatory and an immunosuppressant effect, and has the advantage over oral corticosteroids in that it does not have the side-effects associated with chronic dosage.

There have been three open studies using methylprednisolone in anky-losing spondylitis (Mintz et al, 1981; Richter et al, 1983; Ejstrup and Peters, 1985). These studies had only small numbers of patients (5, 7 and 8 respectively) with disease duration of 13 years in two studies and 3.8 years in the third. In two studies 1 g was given on three consecutive days, and in the third, 1 g was given on consecutive days up to a total dose of 4 g. The latter study noted that dosages of 1 or 2 g gave benefit that lasted for only two weeks; at least 3 g was required for the benefit to last more than two weeks. There was a dramatic initial improvement—usually maximal at one week—in pain, morning stiffness and measurements of spinal mobility. Even though all studies showed a dramatic early improvement, there were differences between them in the measurements in which the improvement was maintained. Pain was the measurement most likely to maintain the improvement, this lasting from 3 to 21 months (Mintz et al, 1981; Richter et al, 1983). Improvement in morning stiffness and spinal mobility lasted for 10 months to 21 months after treatment (Mintz et al, 1981). Richter et al (1983) noted that it took 4 weeks before overall spinal movement significantly improved, with all movements returning to pre-treatment values at 3 months. Ejstrup and Peters (1985) noted an initial improvement in pain, chest expansion and Schober test, which all returned to pre-treatment values by 2 months. Cervical spine flexion and finger-to-floor distance remained significantly improved at 6 months.

The conclusion from these studies is that there is a dramatic improvement in all measurements at one week, but the improvement in pain relief is the one most likely to be maintained. It is interesting that a powerful anti-inflammatory agent can produce some improvement in spinal mobility in patients with established disease. Whether or not it is possible to maintain this improvement by commencing an intensive course of exercises at this time is unknown. Pulse methylprednisolone may have a role in controlling pain when other treatments have failed, allowing the commencement of an intensive exercise regimen. It may then facilitate subsequent management with exercise and NSAIDs. Pulse methylprednisolone in lower doses is just as effective as the 1 g dose in the treatment of rheumatoid arthritis and this could also be sufficient for ankylosing spondylitis (Iglehart et al, 1990).

OTHER TREATMENTS

Gold salts and the antimalarials chloroquine and hydroxychloroquine do not provide any benefit in ankylosing spondylitis. However, they have not been evaluated by appropriate studies (Ward, 1963; Calabro and Mody, 1966; Smythe, 1979).

CONCLUSION

There is no convincing evidence that antirheumatic drugs, in particular sulphasalazine, benefit spinal disease in ankylosing spondylitis. Those studies reporting significant changes found them in only one or two measurements, and even though they were statistically significant, the changes were very small and of little clinical relevance.

The outcome for the peripheral arthritis is slightly better, with some evidence suggesting that patients may benefit from antirheumatic drugs. However, the major problems with these studies were the small number of patients, and the failure to distinguish between an arthritis and other causes of joint pain, including enthesitis of the surrounding tissues. Further placebo-controlled studies with larger numbers are required to determine clearly the effect of antirheumatic drugs on peripheral arthritis.

The major question as to whether antirheumatic drugs modify the long-term outcome of the disease, in particular radiological changes, has not been answered.

The reports so far clearly demonstrate the importance of placebo-controlled studies. The active treatment showed changes compared with baseline assessments, but when compared with the placebo group most of these improvements were not significant. It is doubtful whether open studies are of any value in the assessment of these drugs.

Several problems associated with studies of medication in ankylosing spondylitis need to be considered. These include clearly determining whether peripheral joint pain is due to an arthritis or an enthesitis, and the inclusion of patients with a shorter disease duration because they are more likely to have a peripheral arthritis as well as potentially reversible spinal disease. The problem as to the appropriate clinical and laboratory assessments has yet to be solved, as evidenced by the large number of measurements that are used, and this is an area that needs to be addressed in the future.

The number of patients with ankylosing spondylitis who require a disease-modifying drug is small, but at present there is no satisfactory treatment for those with severe spinal disease. Drugs that have been shown to suppress inflammation other than that due to synovitis, for example methotrexate or low-dose corticosteroids, need to be evaluated with the appropriate trials.

REFERENCES

Amor B, Kahan A, Dougados M & Delrieu F (1984) Sulfasalazine and ankylosing spondylitis. *Annals of Internal Medicine* **101:** 878.

398   R. LAURENT

Ball J (1980) Pathology and pathogenesis. In Moll JMH (ed.) *Ankylosing Spondylitis*, pp 96–112. Edinburgh: Churchill Livingstone.

Bird HA & Dixon AStJ (1977) Failure of D-penicillamine to affect peripheral joint involvement in ankylosing spondylitis or HLA-B27 associated arthropathy (letter). *Annals of the Rheumatic Diseases* 36: 289.

Burgos-Vargas R, Naranjo A, Castillo J & Katona G (1989) Ankylosing spondylitis in the Mexican mestizo: patterns of disease onset according to age of onset. *Journals of Rheumatology* 16: 186–191.

Calabro JJ & Mody RE (1966) Management of ankylosing spondylitis. *Bulletin on the Rheumatic Diseases* 16: 408–411.

Calman FMB & Berry H (1980) The present position of radiotherapy. In Moll JMH (ed.) *Ankylosing Spondylitis*, pp 243–248. Edinburgh: Churchill Livingstone.

Calin A & Elswood J (1989) Retrospective analysis of 376 irradiated patients with ankylosing spondylitis and nonirradiated controls. *Journal of Rheumatology* 16: 1443–1445.

Coelho-Andrade LE, Atra E & Bosi Ferraz M (1989) Sulphasalazine and ankylosing spondylitis: an open pilot study. *Clinical and Experimental Rheumatology* 7: 661–662.

Comer SS & Jasin HE (1988) *In vitro* immuno-modulatory effects of sulphasalazine and its metabolites. *Journal of Rheumatology* 15: 580–586.

Corkill MM, Jobanputra P, Gibson T & MacFarlane DG (1990) A controlled trial of sulphasalazine treatment of chronic ankylosing spondylitis: failure to demonstrate a clinical effect. *British Journal of Rheumatology* 29: 41–45.

Darby SC, Doll R, Gill SK & Smith PG (1987) Long term mortality after a single treatment course with x-rays in patients treated for ankylosing spondylitis. *British Journal of Cancer* 55: 179–190.

Davis MJ, Danes PT, Beswick E, Lewin IV & Stanworth DR (1989) Sulphasalazine therapy in ankylosing spondylitis: its effect on disease activity, immunoglobulin A and the complex immunoglobulin A-alpha-1-antitrypsin. *British Journal of Rheumatology* 28: 410–413.

Desmarais MHL (1953) Radiotherapy in arthritis. *Annals of the Rheumatic Diseases* 12: 25–28.

Docker WP (1989) Low dose prednisone therapy. *Rheumatic Disease Clinics of North America* 15: 569–576.

Dougados M, Bomier P & Amor B (1986) Sulphasalazine in ankylosing spondylitis: a double blind controlled study in sixty patients. *British Medical Journal* 293: 911–914.

Ejstrup L & Peters ND (1985) Intravenous methylprednisolone pulse therapy in ankylosing spondylitis. *Danish Medical Bulletin* 32: 231–233.

Feltelius W & Hallgren R (1986) Sulphasalazine in ankylosing spondylitis. *Annals of the Rheumatic Diseases* 45: 396–399.

Franssen MJAM, Van de Puffe LBA & Gribnau FWJ (1985) IgA serum levels and disease activity in ankylosing spondylitis: a prospective study. *Annals of the Rheumatic Diseases* 44: 766–721.

Fraser SM & Sturrock RD (1990) Evaluation of sulphasalazine in ankylosing spondylitis—an interventional study. *British Journal of Rheumatology* 29: 37–39.

Goebel KM, Goebel FD, Schubotz R, Hahn G & Neurath F (1977) Levamisole-induced immunostimulation in spondyloarthropathies. *Lancet* ii: 214–217.

Golding DN (1974) D-penicillamine in ankylosing spondylitis and polymyositis. *Postgraduate Medical Journal* (supplement 2) 50: 62–64.

Grill V, Smith M, Ahern M & Littlejohn G (1988) Local radiotherapy for pedal manifestation of HLA-B27 related arthropathy. *British Journal of Rheumatology* 27: 390–392.

Handler RP (1989) Favourable results using methotrexate in the treatment of patients with ankylosing spondylitis (letter). *Arthritis and Rheumatism* 32: 234.

Hart FD (1980) Clinical features and complications. In Moll JMH (ed.) *Ankylosing Spondylitis*. Edinburgh: Churchill Livingstone.

Hill AGS (1980) Drug therapy. In Moll JMH (ed.) *Ankylosing Spondylitis*, pp 163–175. Edinburgh: Churchill Livingstone.

Iglehart IW, Sutton ID, Bender JC et al (1990) Intravenous pulsed steroids in rheumatoid arthritis: a comparative dose study. *Journal of Rheumatology* 17: 159–162.

Laurent MR & Panayi GS (1983) Acute phase proteins and serum immunoglobulins in ankylosing spondylitis. *Annals of the Rheumatic Diseases* 42: 524–528.

Laurent MR, Buchanan WW & Bellamy N (1990) Methods of assessment used in ankylosing spondylitis clinical trials: a review. *British Journal of Rheumatology* (in press).

MacDermott RP, Schloemann SR, Bertovich MJ, Nash GS, Peters M & Stenson WF (1989) Inhibition of antibody secretion by 5-aminosalicylic acid. *Gastroenterology* **96**: 442–448.

Mander M, Simpson JM, McLellan A, Walker D, Goodacre JA & Dick WC (1987) Studies with an enthesis index as a method of clinical assessment in ankylosing spondylitis. *Annals of the Rheumatic Diseases* **46**: 197–202.

Mau W, Zeidler H, Mau R et al (1988) Clinical features and prognosis of patients with possible ankylosing spondylitis. Results of a 10 year follow-up. *Journal of Rheumatology* **15**: 1109–1114.

Mielants H, Veys EM & Joos R (1986) Sulphasalazine in the treatment of enterogenic reactive synovitis and ankylosing spondylitis with peripheral arthritis. *Clinical Rheumatology* **5**: 80–83.

Mielants H, Veys EM, Corvelier C & DeVos M (1988) Ileocolonoscopic findings in sero-negative spondyloarthropathies. *British Journal of Rheumatology* **27** (supplement II): 95–105.

Mintz G, Enriquez RD, Mercado U, Robles EJ, Jimenez FJ & Gutievrez G (1981) Intravenous methylprednisolone pulse therapy in severe ankylosing spondylitis. *Arthritis and Rheumatism* **24**: 734–736.

Moll JMH (1985) Inflammatory bowel disease. *Clinics in Rheumatic Diseases* **11**: 87–111.

Nashel DJ, Petrone DZ, Ulmer CC & Sliwinski AJ (1986) C-Reactive protein: a marker for disease activity in ankylosing spondylitis and Reiter's syndrome. *Journal of Rheumatology* **13**: 364–367.

Nissila M, Lehtinen K, Leivisalo-Repo M, Laukkainen R, Mutru O & Yli-Kerttula U (1988) Sulphasalazine in the treatment of ankylosing spondylitis. *Arthritis and Rheumatism* **31**: 1111–1116.

Pile KD, Laurent MR, Salmond CE, Best MJ, Pyle EA & Moloney RO (1990) Clinical assessment of ankylosing spondylitis. A study of observer variation in spinal assessments. *British Journal of Rheumatology* (in press).

Ralston SH, Urquhart GDK, Brzeski M & Sturrock RD (1990) Prevalence of vertebral compression fractures due to osteoporosis in ankylosing spondylitis. *British Medical Journal* **300**: 563–565.

Richter MB, Woo P, Panayi GS, Trull A, Unger A & Shepherd P (1983) The effects of intravenous pulse methylprednisolone on immunological and inflammatory processes in ankylosing spondylitis. *Clinical and Experimental Immunology* **53**: 51–59.

Rosenthal M, Trabert U & Muller W (1976) Immunotherapy with levamisole in rheumatic diseases. *Scandinavian Journal of Rheumatology* **5**: 216–220.

Sadowska-Wroblewska M, Garwolinska H & Maczynska-Rusiniak B (1986) A trial of cyclo-phosphamide in ankylosing spondylitis with involvement of peripheral joints and high disease activity. *Scandinavian Journal of Rheumatology* **15**: 259–264.

Sanders KK, Hertzman A, Escobar MR & Littman BA (1987) Correlation of immunoglobulin and C-reactive protein levels in ankylosing spondylitis and rheumatoid arthritis. *Annals of the Rheumatic Diseases* **46**: 273–276.

Scharf Y & Nahir M (1976) Penicillamine in ankylosing spondylitis (letter). *Arthritis and Rheumatism* **19**: 122.

Scott DGI, Ring EFJ & Bacon PA (1981) Problems in the assessment of disease activity in ankylosing spondylitis. *Rheumatology and Rehabilitation* **20**: 74–80.

Sheehan NJ, Slarin BM, Donovan MP, Mount JN & Matthews JA (1986) Lack of correlation between clinical disease activity and erythrocyte sedimentation rate, acute phase protein or protease inhibitors in ankylosing spondylitis. *British Journal of Rheumatology* **25**: 171–172.

Sinclair RJG (1971) Treatment of rheumatic disorders with special reference to ankylosing spondylitis. *Proceedings of the Royal Society of Medicine* **64**: 1031–1038.

Smythe H (1979) Therapy of the spondyloarthropathies. *Clinical Orthopaedics and Related Research* **143**: 84–89.

Steven MM, Morrison M & Sturrock RD (1985) Penicillamine in ankylosing spondylitis: a double blind placebo controlled trial. *Journal of Rheumatology* **12**: 735–737.

Taylor HG, Beswick EJ, Davis MJ & Dawes PT (1989) Sulphasalazine in ankylosing spondylitis—effective in early disease? *British Journal of Rheumatology* **28** (supplement 1): 6 (Abstract).

Tytman K, Bernacka K & Sierakowski S (1989) D-penicillamine in the therapy of ankylosing spondylitis. *Clinical Rheumatology* **8:** 419–420.

Ward LE (1963) Rheumatoid spondylitis. *Arthritis and Rheumatism* **6:** 650–657.

Wilkinson M & Bywaters EGL (1958) Clinical features and course of ankylosing spondylitis. *Annals of the Rheumatic Diseases* **17:** 209–228.

Will R, Palmer R, Ring F & Calin A (1989a) Ankylosing spondylitis is associated with masked osteopeania of the lumbar spine and femoral neck in patient with mobile spines and normal hips (abstract). *British Journal of Rheumatology* **28 (supplement 1):** 19.

Will R, Magaro L, Elswood J & Calin A (1989b) Ankylosing spondylitis and acute phase reactant: a measure of peripheral joint inflammation—not axial disease (abstract). *British Journal of Rheumatology* **28 (supplement 2):** 11.

Index

Note: Page numbers of article titles are in **bold** type.